Mechanisms and Machine Science

Volume 20

Series editor

Marco Ceccarelli, Rome, Italy

For further volumes:
http://www.springer.com/series/8779

Aleksandar Rodić · Doina Pisla
Hannes Bleuler
Editors

New Trends in Medical and Service Robots

Challenges and Solutions

Springer

Editors
Aleksandar Rodić
Robotics Laboratory
Mihailo Pupin Institute
Belgrade
Serbia

Hannes Bleuler
LSRO—Robotic Systems Laboratory
École Polytechnique Fédérale de Lausanne
Lausanne
Switzerland

Doina Pisla
Research Center for Industrial Robots Simulation and Testing
Technical University of Cluj-Napoca
Cluj-Napoca
Romania

ISSN 2211-0984 ISSN 2211-0992 (electronic)
ISBN 978-3-319-37582-3 ISBN 978-3-319-05431-5 (eBook)
DOI 10.1007/978-3-319-05431-5
Springer Cham Heidelberg New York Dordrecht London

Softcover reprint of the hardcover 1st edition 2014

Printed on acid-free paper

Springer is part of Springer Science+Business Media (www.springer.com)

This book is dedicated to the memory of Prof. Miomir Vukobratović, one of the most famous world-recognized pioneers of humanoid robotics, founder of the "Belgrade school of robotics" in the early 1970s and author of one of the first research Monograph Series in robotics "Scientific Fundamentals of Robotics" published by Springer from 1982 to 1990.

Preface

With progress in microprocessor, sensor and actuator technology, production of new composite materials, as well as with permanent progress of scientific knowledge in the field of Robotics, new trends in development of service and medical robots appear and push things strongly forward.

The increasing complexity of our society and economy places greater emphasis on artificial systems such as intelligent robotic systems, which can deal autonomously with our needs and with the peculiarities of the environments we inhabit and construct. This challenge is to extend systems engineering methods to deal with open-ended and frequently changing real-world environments. In order to meet this challenge, a mix of innovative scientific theory and technology is needed, based on natural and artificial cognition, in conjunction with new engineering principles and implementations for robots that are robust and versatile enough to deal with the real world. Artificial cognitive systems and intelligent robots can extend the capabilities of people to perform routine, dangerous or tiring tasks, especially in previously inaccessible, uncharted or remote indoor or outdoor environments.

The need to substitute humans working on delicate, tiresome and monotonous tasks, or working with potentially health-damaging toxic materials, requires intelligent, high-performance service robots with the ability to cooperate, advanced communication and sophisticated perception and cognitive capabilities. In particular, broad class of service robotic systems are expected to be involved in everyday life within the public domain, in applications as diverse as: security, flexible manufacturing, market, entertainment, delivery, nursing, home keeping or elderly assisted tasks accomplishing, etc. All of these demanding applications mean that the research community should consider robotic systems in a quite different way, in the sense of their integration and networking to bring them together into the so called multi-agent collaborative teams capable of performing a variety of complex tasks as required together or without humans.

The book also concerns with new trends in medical robotics in light of involving new technologies and use of scientific innovations to gain advanced, non-invasive medical practice. In particular, the book regards to innovations and improvements in design, development and implementation of sophisticated surgical, rehabilitation and bio robots. Surgical robots allow surgeons greater access to areas under operation using more precise and less-invasive methods. Rehabilitation robots facilitate and support the lives of infirm, elderly people, or those with dysfunction of body parts effecting movement. These robots are also used for rehabilitation and related procedures, such as training and therapy. Bio robots are designed to imitate the cognition of humans and animals. Nowadays, medical robotic devices are used to replace missing limbs, perform delicate surgical procedures, deliver neurorehabilitation therapy to stroke patients, teach children with learning disabilities and perform a growing number of other health-related tasks.

This book represents the second one published in the Series of MeSRoB workshop proceedings to be printed annually beginning from 2013. The first workshop MeSRoB 2012 was organised by the TU Cluj-Napoca, Romania, in June 2012. The second MeSRoB 2013 was organised by Institute "Mihailo Pupin" in Belgrade, Serbia in July, 2013. The third MeSRoB 2014 is planned to be held in July, 2014, in Lausanne, Switzerland to be organised by EPFL. The chapters in this book represent the best selected papers from the workshop program "New Trends in Medical and Service Robotics (MeSRoB 2013)". The book is published by support of the Swiss National Scientific Foundation, grant no. IZ74Z0_137361/1 and partially by support of the Ministry of Education, Science and Technology Development of Republic Serbia as official sponsors of the MeSRoB 2013.

The editors express their kind appreciation to Prof. Dr. Duško Katić (Mihailo Pupin Institute, Belgrade, Serbia) for the professional help in book preparation as well as to Prof. Dr. Marco Ceccarelli (University of Casino and South Latium, Italy), Editor in Chief of the book series "Mechanisms and Machine Science" for advisory and valuable suggestions. Editors believe that this interesting book series will be extended in the next few years to the satisfaction of its readers.

Aleksandar Rodić
Doina Pisla
Hannes Bleuler

Contents

Robotic Assistance for Senior People for Safe Mobility and Work Support

Daniel Eck, Florian Leutert and Klaus Schilling

Abstract Worldwide demographic trends of aging societies raise the demand for assistive technologies for senior people, including in particular robotic aids. Here, specifically the fields of robotic assistance for support of mobility and for workers in industrial assembly tasks are emphasized. In mobility assistance a vehicle provides navigation functionalities for route planning and for safe driving. In case of the industrial workplace, a manipulator cooperates with the worker to take the major load in lifting heavy objects, while the human provides the guidance in placing the objects. Performance tests have been performed with a user group of more than 100 seniors.

Keywords Aging technology · Mobility scooter · Manipulator-based assistance · Human-robot-interaction · Human-robot-cooperation

1 Introduction

Aging societies worldwide (Germany's population by 2050: Results of the 11th coordinated population projection 2006; Forlizzi et al. 2004; Muramatsu and Akiyama 2011) raise challenging requirements for extending the working life and to enable self-sustained living at the own home. Robotic assistive systems are seen as one possible future contribution to support senior people in specific tasks, as

D. Eck (✉) · F. Leutert · K. Schilling
University of Wuerzburg, Wuerzburg, Germany
e-mail: eck@informatik.uni-wuerzburg.de

F. Leutert
e-mail: leutert@informatik.uni-wuerzburg.de

K. Schilling
e-mail: schi@informatik.uni-wuerzburg.de

A. Rodić et al. (eds.), *New Trends in Medical and Service Robots*,
Mechanisms and Machine Science 20, DOI: 10.1007/978-3-319-05431-5_1,

evidenced by the growing number of international research projects that address related technologies. The topics covered in this field range from sustaining the mobility of elderly people indoors and outdoors, supporting them in their daily household life, providing means to assist or relieve them at their workplaces or even as therapeutic means for patients with dementia (Wada and Shibata 2007). In the topics related to this chapter—mobility and work support—research was done on different robotic walking aid systems (SmartCane/SmartWalker) (Spenko et al. 2006), independent mobile home care robots (Care-O-bot) Graf et al. (2009) (autonomous) wheelchairs (Ding and Cooper 2005) or similar vehicles. Robotic support systems for cooperative work environments were for example considered in form of mobile (Khatib 1999; Hägele et al. 2002) or stationary manipulators (Thiemermann 2005).

In a joint effort of Bavarian industry and academia, the project Fit4Age also focused on technologies to support senior people in a self-determined, independent daily life. In this context, robotic assistance systems supported—among other aspects—elders in mobility and industrial work places. Demonstrators were developed and tested by senior users in typical environments.

Safe mobility is a key requirement to participate in social life. For this demand, a robotic vehicle for robust short range mobility in an urban environment was realized. Navigation equipment was adapted for pedestrian environments with focus on safety aspects. Preferences for route planning emphasize the inclusion of park areas, pedestrian zones and safe street crossings at traffic lights or cross-walks, but also avoid difficult routes that include stairs or other barriers. The navigation system and ranging sensors for collision avoidance and path tracking are addressed in the first part of this chapter.

Industrial production is confronted with an increasing average age of its personnel, too. While the experience of senior workers is appreciated, robotic assistance systems are needed to relieve personnel from arduous physical burdens like carrying heavy loads, but—due to their size and mass—require sensor systems to allow appropriate reactions in safety critical situations. Robotic arms should act as a "third hand" to the worker, meeting the high safety requirements with sensor and control approaches. In order to make the involved complex robotic data quickly and easily understandable, an intuitive interface using Augmented Reality was realized.

Robotic assistant systems for these two crucial areas—mobility and industrial work environment—will be addressed in detail in the following.

2 The Fit4Age Project

Due to increasing lifetime, the average age of most European populations increases. Especially the amount of senior people will rise dramatically in the next years. In Germany, the percentage of people older than 65 years will increase from 16 % in 2000 to about 25 % in 2030 (Germany's population by 2050: Results of the 11th coordinated population projection 2006). The cognitive and physical deprivation often associated with normal aging processes constitute a number of challenges to support senior people, to enable them to stay active in their normal working routine and allow for a self-determined and independent way of life. Furthermore, the amount of senior people in need of home care will also increase in the future, leading to rising costs in social spending. For all these reasons, the Fit4Age project (Fit4Age: Zukunftsorientierte Produkte und Dienstleistungen für die demographischen Herausforderungen 2007) was initiated in 2007, focusing on the development of technical aids for senior people. To increase the acceptance of these aids, a senior committee consisting of more than 100 senior people was integrated in the project. This senior committee supported the development phase by means of discussion of particular functions and evaluation of the resulting demonstrators. Altogether, 12 university institutes and more than 30 companies in Bavaria cooperated to drive the development of assistive technologies for elderly people. The two main aims of this project were: 1. design, implementation and evaluation of technical aids to enable a self-determined and independent life, and 2. advancements of the acceptance of products for the support of senior people. The project was subdivided into three main aspects: Fit4Life, Fit4Mobility and Fit4Work. In the following, two parts of those are introduced in detail, the mobility scooter, which was part of the Fit4Mobility scope and the collaboration of workers and manipulators in industrial production, which was part of the Fit4Work scope.

3 The Mobility Scooter

This section introduces a vehicle extended with assistance functions to relieve the operator from challenging control issues, to support and preserve the mobility of senior people. Mobility is one of the biggest issues and prerequisite for social participation and normal daily living, like shopping or visiting a doctor. Normal aging processes are associated with changing cognitive and physical abilities that might impair older adults' mobility and independence (Spirduso et al. 2005). Powered wheelchairs were already used to support mobility; however, these kinds of devices are mainly used by people with movement disorders or otherwise handicapped people. Accordingly, these devices are often associated with degenerative illness; hence healthy people will not use such devices, worrying about stigmatization. Thus, in the Fit4Mobility project a mobility scooter was used, which is described in the next subsection. Afterward, drive assistance and autonomous functions are explained, including the evaluation of the individual functions.

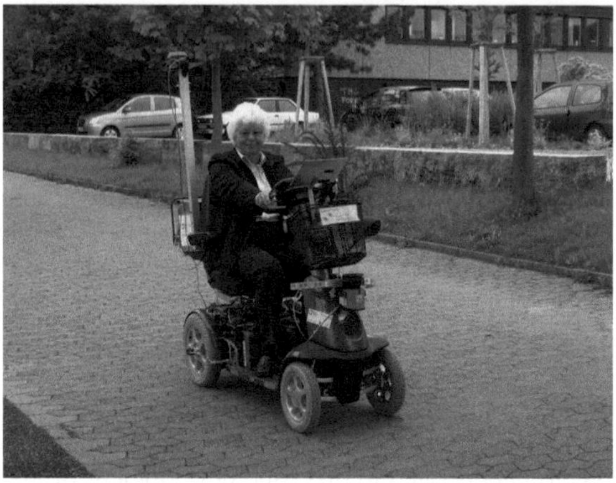

Fig. 1 The mobility scooter Trophy 4W with all hardware extensions during a test run with a member of the senior committee

3.1 Hardware

The Trophy 4W, manufactured by Handicare GmbH, was used as the base vehicle. This car-like vehicle drives up to 15 km/h and can cover a distance of 60 km on one battery charge. The vehicle is actuated at the rear axis with a set of differential gear between the wheels. Figure 1 illustrates the vehicle with all mounted sensors (Laser Range Finder (LRF), GPS, gyroscope, incremental sensors and hall sensor).

Furthermore, a portable GPS navigator manufactured by Navigon AG was mounted on the vehicle for autonomous navigation purposes. For further information about the hardware please refer to Eck and Schilling (2010), Eck et al. (2011, 2012).

3.2 Drive Assistance Functions

Next to basic assistance functions like steering control and velocity control several further functions were developed and implemented on the vehicle. One of these assistance functions is a new regulation of the hand throttle. The hand throttle is mounted on the steering wheel and controls the velocity of the vehicle. This assistance function changes the relation between the hand throttle position and the corresponding velocity. Originally, the relation was linear, so the displacement of the hand throttle between 0 and 2 km/h is the same as between 12 and 14 km/h. This makes a proper control of the vehicle at low velocities very challenging (Nitz 2008). For that reason, a new regulation of the hand throttle was implemented to relieve the operator of speed control in that range.

The new regulation of the hand throttle was distributed in three intervals. During the first 30 % of the movement of the hand throttle, the velocity is limited to a maximum of 2 km/h, compared to more than 5 km/h in the original version. The next interval of the new regulation is again much slower compared to original: the first 80 % of the hand throttle movement is limited to 8 km/h, compared to 13.5 km/h originally. In the last interval, the slope of ID1 is higher resulting in velocities up to 15 km/h. Due to the new regulation of the hand throttle it is easier to control the mobility scooter at low velocities. Fine grain control at high velocities is not required, since it is only possible to drive high velocities if there is enough free space. In such cases, it makes no difference whether the velocity is 13 or 14 km/h compared to a narrow environment, where a difference of 0.5 km/h can cause a collision.

This new regulation was evaluated with the senior committee. Several members of the committee (mean age 71.1 years) were invited to drive the vehicle in three different scenarios, once with the original speed regulation and once with the new one. The order of the regulations was counterbalanced to avoid influences of learning processes on the results. The scenarios consisting of a 180° turn, a narrow passage and a slalom and were built up using Styrofoam walls. Before starting the testing phase, each participant had to complete a training phase to get used to the vehicle. Still, the training phase was aimed to minimize the learning effects in the experiments. Three different aspects were recorded for the evaluation: run time, amount of collisions and the length of Styrofoam contacts. Regarding the amount of collisions and length of Styrofoam contacts, all participants performed better with the new speed regulation, resulting in a lesser amount of collisions and shorter contact length. Using the student t-test it can be shown that the new regulation is more safe with a probability of at least 99.5 % ($t = 2.84$, $\alpha < 0.01$). The run time was nearly equal with the new and the original regulation of the hand throttle. For more information please refer to Eck et al. (2012).

A further assistance function is a collision avoidance function. At the beginning of the Fit4Age project, it was planned to develop some collision avoidance algorithm which autonomously bypasses the obstacle. However, an interview with the senior committee revealed that the senior people want to control the vehicle by themselves continuously. They further want no impact of any assistance system on the handling of the vehicle during normal driving behaviors. Accordingly, a new collision avoidance algorithm was developed and implemented. The new approach determines the prospective path of the vehicle by means of the steering angle. If an obstacle on this prospective path is detected with the LRF, the vehicle will be slowed down according to the distance to this vehicle. In normal driving situations, such as on sidewalks without any obstacle, the assistance function will not influence the driving behaviors of the vehicle even if there is a wall next to the sidewalk. Obstacles next to the prospective path are ignored by the collision avoidance, which satisfied the senior committee.

However, in case the operator wants to drive through a narrow, it is possible that the obstacle avoidance slows down the vehicle because one border of the narrow is detected as an obstacle. This behavior influences the handling of the vehicle and is undesired by the target group. For this reason, the approach was extended with narrow passage detection. This detection is looking for passages

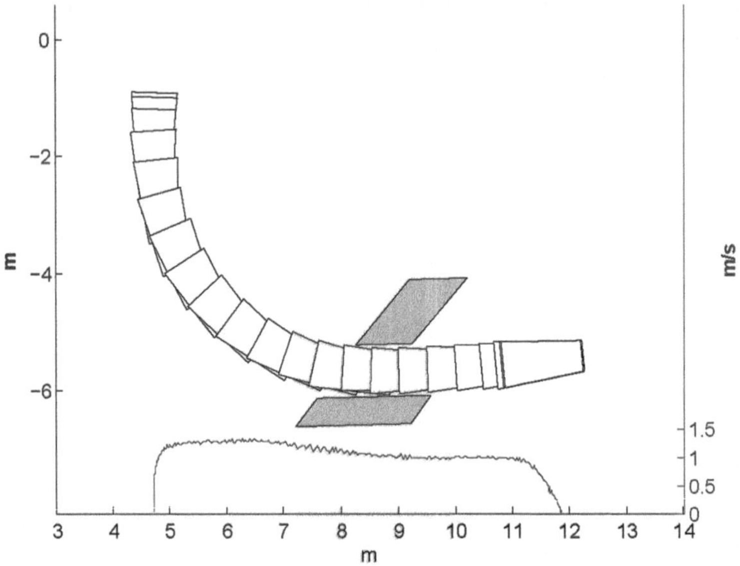

Fig. 2 Result of a single test run passing the narrow

close to the prospective path which are broad enough to drive through. If a traversable narrow is detected close to the prospective path, the collision avoidance is deactivated to enable an easy drive through. Although this deactivation does increase the risk of accidents to a certain degree, the senior committee wants no restrictions while they control the vehicle except in emergency situations. Therefore, this approach presumes that the operator will not cause an accident consciously.

The collision avoidance as well as the narrow passage detection was evaluated in several test runs. The result of a single run is depicted in Fig. 2. The maximum velocity was limited to 0.6 m/s, which enables the operator to control the vehicle with full throttle all the time. The green curve displays the velocity which did not change until the narrow was passed. For more information about the algorithm and the evaluation please refer to Eck et al. (2012).

3.3 Autonomous Functions

Besides drive assistance functions also some autonomous functions were implemented and integrated on the mobility scooter. Aim of the project was not to drive a senior person all the way from a start to a destination. As written at the beginning, the purpose of the vehicle is to support and maintain the available mobility of people. For this reason, one aim of the project was to enable the operator to walk in front of the vehicle, while the vehicle is following the operator autonomously. However, if the vehicle is driving behind some senior person, this person will continuously turn to monitor the vehicle. This continuous turning of the senior goes along with an increasing fall risk; after some discussion with the senior committee, this function was changed so that the vehicle will drive in front of the operator and the operator can walk behind the vehicle. In the changed scenario, the operator can always monitor the vehicle in front of him. To realize this function, the destination of the trip must be known beforehand.

To realize this function, a GPS navigator was integrated on the mobility scooter together with the project partner Navigon AG. The GPS navigator used a special map containing pedestrian specific information, such as pedestrian lights, sidewalks, cross-walks, paths in parks and steps. By the means of this information a pedestrian navigator was developed. The new navigator determines safe routes to a given destination, mainly using sidewalks and safe crossings of streets (crosswalks, pedestrian lights, …). Accordingly, the percentage of unsafe crossings was reduced from over 40 % in conventional GPS navigators to less than 3 %. For the usage on the mobility scooter, this pedestrian GPS navigator was extended in a way that steps were avoided completely. Furthermore, a new user interface of the GPS navigator was implemented, especially adapted to the demands of senior people. Only two big buttons are used, one for entering a destination and one back to home button, which directly navigates the operator home.

As soon as the route is traversing a park, the navigator is forwarding this information to the vehicle and an algorithm is looking for the path using the LRF. If a path can be detected, the operator is able to activate autonomous driving and can walk behind the vehicle. A project partner developed a device to determine the position of the person relative to the vehicle. In the autonomous mode, the mobility scooter is controlled according to the measured position and the velocity of the person. For more information about this autonomous function please refer to Eck et al. (2011).

4 Robotic Assistance in Industrial Production

With the increasing average age of the population also the age of working personnel will rise in companies. This is an especially critical point in sectors which impose a high physical workload on its personnel, e.g. in industrial assembling. Systems that reduce the physical burden on workers are needed to avoid age-related and chronic injuries, and also to allow elderly or already impaired staff to continue to perform tasks in working areas that are usually reserved for younger personnel. One approach here could be to employ a manipulator robot to assist a human coworker in order to support and relieve him in physically challenging tasks.

Systems that take over the weight of objects are already commonly used in industrial assembly; so called balancer systems mounted on rails or the ceiling stabilize heavy objects in a weightless state (compensation of the gravitational forces). Manipulators can provide that kind of gravitational balancing as well, with the additional benefit of the machine being able to also take over acceleration forces for sideways movement. Furthermore, robots—while in general being more expensive—have several additional advantages over simple load-balancing systems: for once, it is their ability for controlled and autonomous movement. Where applicable, simple parts of the assembling process can be executed by the robot autonomously so the worker can concentrate on other tasks in the meantime, effectively speeding up the assembly process or relieving the worker in terms of working cycle time. In more complex assembly steps, a human worker can manually guide the manipulator holding the workpiece: because of the robot's ability to precisely control its movement several helpful assistance functions can be realized here, to help the worker in his task. Some examples of how manipulators can be used to collaborate with a human coworker in industrial assembly are given later in this chapter.

It should not be neglected to mention that using a manipulator as a coworker also leads to additional challenges that need to be considered: the speed and mass of an industrial robot requires that sophisticated safety functions are in place, if a human is to be allowed to be sharing the same workspace and even working directly in contact with the robot. Besides making sure that the worker is safe in this collaboration it is also necessary to make sure that he does not see the robot or its safety functions as detrimental or laborious to use—otherwise the assistance systems might not be used at all, or safety devices might be avoided or overridden by the personnel (Sarodnick et al. 2005). The robotic assistance system should provide a benefit to the working task (Melenhorst et al. 2006) and needs to be as easy to use and comprehensible as possible.

However, when successfully realizing such a human-robot-interaction (HRI) system, one can combine the strength and accuracy of a robot with the understanding and perception of a human, and as such create a very effective and flexible working system, that is scant dependent on the physical capabilities of the human worker and thus enables elderly workers to stay productive longer in their working field.

4.1 The Fit4Work Assistance System

Central point of the developed assistance system (Fig. 3) is the manipulator robot, which can be adapted according to the assembly task; during the project, a RV60 Vertical articulated arm robot from Reis Robotics with a maximum admissible load of 60 kg was used. Attached to the end-effector of the robot was a two-hand guiding bar with enabling switches for manually guiding the manipulator (see subsection below), together with a 6D-force torque sensor for measuring the input forces. A laser range finder was used for person tracking in the work area, and an Augmented Reality-based user interface for more complex control inputs to the

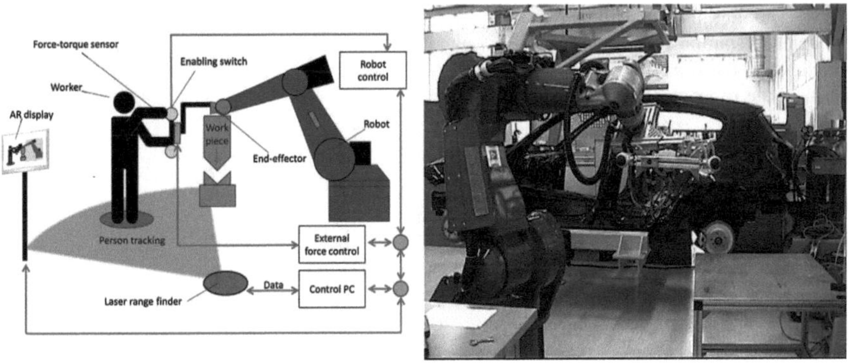

Fig. 3 Schematic (*left*) and actual (*right*) image of the manipulator-based assistance system developed in Fit4Work

assistance robot. Everything was connected to one another via a control PC. A more detailed description of individual system parts is given below.

4.2 Modes of Use

Central purpose of the robotic assistant in Fit4Work is to relieve a worker physically in industrial assembly by taking over the weight and inertness of the workpiece to be assembled. To achieve this, it can be used in three different control modes: autonomous, manually guided and hybrid movement mode.

Autonomous movement: One of the biggest advantages of a manipulator over a simple load balancing system is its ability for active, controlled movement. The robot can move autonomously without user input, e.g. picking up a work piece from a well-defined material storage, and deliver it to the assembly place independently. The human worker can concentrate on other process steps in the meantime, e.g. preparing the mounting frame, and can than take over the actual assembly step together with the robot once it has delivered the necessary part. After assembly is complete, the robot can leave the workspace independently to move to a standby position, or restart the working cycle. Autonomous movement can be programmed into the working cycle triggered by specific events, or as a reaction to given approval from the user (like pushing the robot outside the immediate assembly place to send it into standby position). Besides relieving the worker from the physical weight during this independent moving of the work piece, this means also alleviating the working cycle time in a production line.

While the robot is moving autonomously collisions are avoided using a person tracking system. No input or control from a human operator is necessary in this mode, though it can be included if desired.

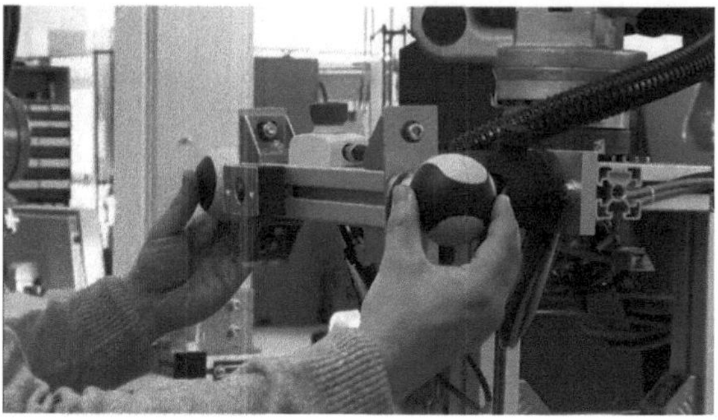

Fig. 4 The guiding bar with the attached enabling switches and the force-torque sensor at the robot flange

Manually guided movement: Some assembly steps are too complicated or change too often in order to perform them with predefined movement of the robot alone. In this case, the human worker has to manually guide the robot holding the component to the assembly spot. To achieve this, no complex commands in a graphical user interface should be necessary: the user should just be able to grasp the robot holding the work piece and push or pull it (with minimal force) in the direction he wants. This is achieved with a system developed by a project partner, consisting of a two-handed guiding bar with an attached force-torque sensor (FTS), mounted on the end-effector of the robot (Fig. 4). The forces the user applies to the guiding bar are measured with the FTS, filtered and amplified/dampened accordingly and then sent to the robot control in the form of directional speed vectors, i.e. the robot then drives in the direction it senses. The system also senses the amount of force employed by the user and accordingly allows for fast, rough positioned movements as well as sensitive small changes in the positioning. This enables an intuitive way of manually guiding the robot—and thus the workpiece—to the desired mounting position.

The two enabling switches also mounted on the guiding bar will block the robot's movement unless pressed. This on the one hand helps to avoid accidental pushing, while on the other hand ensuring that the hands of the user are in a safe spot and cannot be crushed during assembly steps.

While in manual mode the user is responsible for the robot's movement and thus for avoiding collisions; however, there are still some safety functions active to avoid injury or damage (see below).

Hybrid movement mode: The third mode of operation combines the advantages of the other two: the flexibility of manual guidance with the fast and precise automatic movements of the robot. One option here is that the robot—while being manually guided—keeps the work piece in a certain orientation (e.g. parallel to the ground) so that it aligns perfectly with the mounting frame—the user then just has to take care of the position of the component and need not care about its orientation. Another mode of use are complex assembly steps that cannot be done collision free or fast enough manually (e.g. the insertion of a car seat into a chassis, see Fig. 7). In this case the user can move the robot to a certain starting position and then start a predefined assembly motion executed by the robot. This predefined

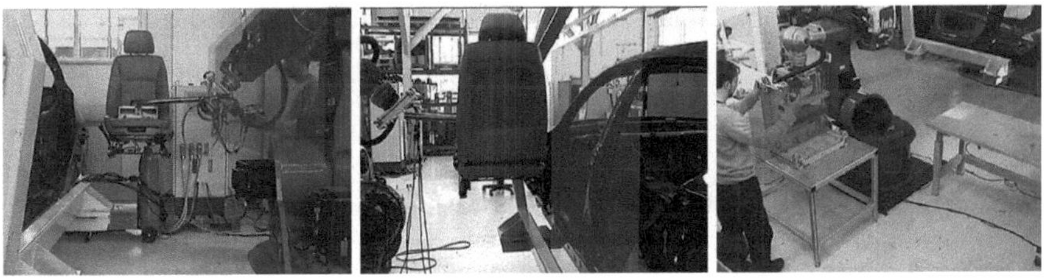

Fig. 5 Virtual barriers visualized using augmented reality, acting as safety boundaries during transport or as assistance stops during assembly

path of the manipulator can be controlled by the user (i.e. he can progress, stop or revert the insertion movement) while he does not have to control the precise path the robot takes. This allows for a controlled assembly with the user supervising the working area, which is at the same time fast and collision free.

4.3 Safety and Assistance Functions in Fit4Work

Current regulations (DIN EN ISO 10218) state that when working in close collaboration with a robot, certain safety aspects have to be followed to avoid or minimize damage in case of an accident. The latter, passive safety measures realized in Fit4Work include limiting (and monitoring) the movement speed of the manipulator to a certain margin to minimize injury potential as well as a dead-man system that shuts down movement when the connection to the control PC is lost.

An active safety measure that tries to avoid any collision during autonomous robot movement is realized with a person tracking system using a laser range finder: when a worker is detected in the trajectory of the autonomously moving manipulator it slows down in several steps up to a standstill. If the person clears the path again, movement is resumed. Automatic evasion movements could also be considered, however, in industrial environments there often is limited space to evade to, and movement is therefore restricted to predictable paths.

Another safety measure realized is the concept of virtual barriers/walls in the work environment: convex cartesian areas can be defined in the surroundings as needed. If the robot hits such a defined boundary all movement of its axes that would lead out of the defined area is locked, while movement back inside is still possible. As such, the robot can glide along such a wall or be moved back inside. This can be used in two ways: for once, objects can be secured against collisions because of careless guidance in manual mode (Fig. 5). Another option is using these barriers as a helping/guiding function during manual movement, marking a stop point above the mounting frame: the user can guide the robot with minimal attention towards the assembly until he hits the barrier; knowing he is directly above the correct mounting spot, he can then guide the work piece down along the wall onto the mounting. Another option would be a funnel shaped barrier to help with precise insertion.

4.4 User Interface with Augmented Reality

Although it is not necessary during normal working operation, sometimes adaptions to the working program of the assistance robot need to be made. For example, the position the robot autonomously delivers the work piece to needs to be changed, or safety barriers need to be adapted to a new mount. This should be possible without a reprogramming, feasible for a user even without in-depth knowledge of robotic systems. A graphical user interface can be used to guide the user through the adaptions; however, he also needs to be able to easily understand the often complex robotic data. One possibility to make this complex information easily understandable to the user is using Augmented Reality to simply visualize the data directly in the work environment (see also Sauer et al. 2010b).

Augmented Reality (AR) is a technology that enhances a user's perception of the environment, adding helpful virtual information into it to help the user in his tasks. It can be seen as a mixed form of a completely virtual environment (Virtual Reality/VR) and the standard, natural view of the surroundings; a commonly used definition by Azuma states that these additions to the environment should by dynamic in real-time and need to be correctly registered (aligned) to the environment (Azuma 1997). Different technologies exist that allow this enhanced view of the environment, like Headup-displays, projectors or enhanced camera images (Leutert et al. 2013; Sauer et al. 2010a). The latter were used in Fit4Work on a display in the work cell of the assistance robot.

Using AR, complex robotic data can simply be visualized directly in the work environment; the user then simply sees this information—there is no need to interpret this data or transfer it from some representation to the actual environment (as in VR). One application example is the pre-visualization of the robot's movement after the trajectory has been changed (e.g. after changing the delivery position): instead of having to interpret the position readings of the path in some unknown coordinate system, the user can simply see how the robot is going to move by superimposing a virtual model of the manipulator on top of the real one in the camera image and letting this virtual model perform the computed adapted motion (Fig. 6). The motion can be checked before actual execution to be collision-free. Another example is the visualization of virtual barriers in the work environment, so their location and dimension immediately becomes clear (Fig. 5) and needs not be construed from a set of plane-and vector data.

AR visualizations can be adapted to different data and for specific work purposes. With it, user operations involving complex robotic data can be made with higher efficiency and more intuitively than with traditional displays, especially for personnel untrained in robotics.

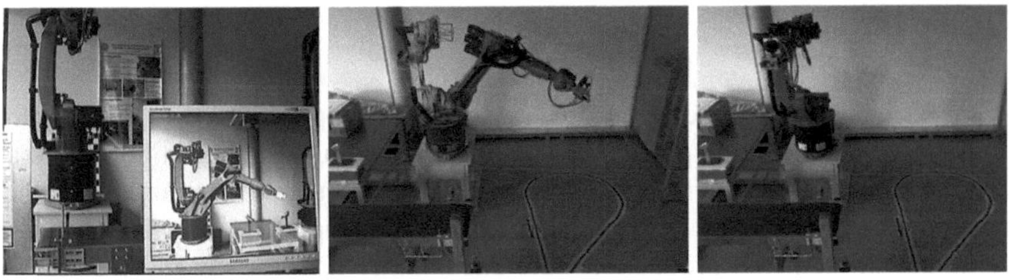

Fig. 6 Pre-visualization of robot movement with AR, using a virtual robot model superimposed onto the real robot

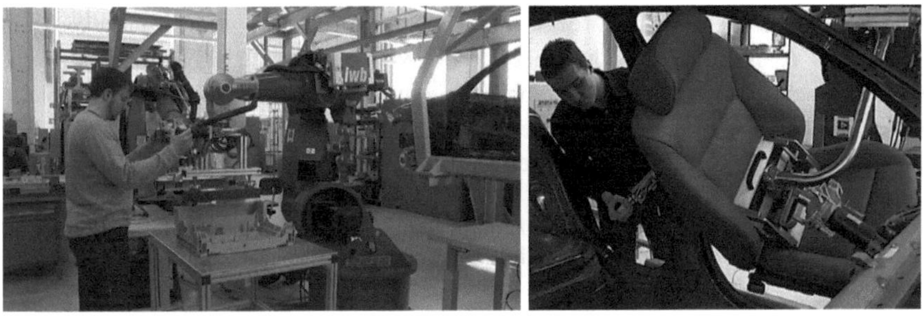

Fig. 7 The Fit4Work assistance system used in industrial use cases for assembly of dishwasher counter-weights and a car seat

4.5 Application Examples

The assistance system in Fit4Work that has been described here has been successfully tested in two application scenarios provided from industrial partners (Fig. 7). The first involved placing a counter-weight for a dishwasher into the corresponding mounting frame; the second scenario required the operator to place a heavy car seat ($\sim$32 kg) into a car chassis. The safety and assistance functions described earlier were adapted to both scenarios; afterwards, the assistant system was evaluated, and was successful in performing the industrial assembly with minimal physical strain in both cases.

The developed hybrid solution has several advantages over pure manual or completely automatic assembly operations: physical strain is a lot less compared to manual assembly while several assistance functions provide a lot of support during the individual assembly steps. Fully automatic assembly systems are almost always faster but often require pre-processing steps, need to be screened from human access which delays post-processing steps, and are difficult to adapt, while the hybrid system is very flexible and allows a human operator to work directly besides and with the robot.

5 Conclusions

Aging societies raise the demand for assistance to support daily life. In an integrated research effort, the project Fit4Age addressed crucial fields at home and at work to improve the environment for living by adequate technologies. In this contribution, two specific areas related to robotic support in mobility and at a workplace in industrial production were exemplarily discussed in more detail. A transport vehicle provides safe mobility on basis of advanced navigation and control technics. In particular, path and collision detection functions as well as path planning capabilities are integrated. At the workplace in industrial production a manipulator robot assists in lifting heavy parts. Next to safety functions to allow operation in the near vicinity of workers, an intuitive user interface on basis of augmented reality methods has been realized to visualize robotic data to the worker. These examples of robotic assistance have been tested by senior people to place emphasis on the development directions. Thus, appropriate technology should contribute to meet the challenges of a continuously aging society.

Acknowledgments The authors would like to thank their project partners in FitForAge for the fruitful and inspiring cooperation, as well as the Bavarian Research Foundation for their contribution to project funding.

References

R. T. Azuma. A Survey of Augmented Reality. In: Presence: Teleoperators and Virtual Environments, Jg. 6(4), pp. 355–385, 1997.

D. Ding, R. A. Cooper. A review of the current state of electric powered wheel-chairs. IEEE Control Systems Magazine (25), pp. 22–34, 2005.

D. Eck, K. Schilling, A. Abdul-Majeed, J. Thielecke, P. Richter, J. Gutierrez Boronat, I. Schens, B. Thomas, B. Williger, and F. Lang. Mobility assistance for elderly people. Journal of Applied Bionics and Biomechanics, 2011.

D. Eck, K. Schilling. Robotic and Telematic Assistant Technologies to Support Aging People. Journal of eHealth, Technology and Applications (8), pp. 152–155, 2010.

D. Eck, T. Heim, R. Hess and K. Schilling. A Narrow Passage Assistance Function on a Mobility Scooter for Elderly People. Robotik, 2012.

D. Eck, K. Schilling, B. Williger and F. R. Lang. Evaluation of a Drive Assistance Function for older Adults. CESCIT, 2012.

Fit4Age: Zukunftsorientierte Produkte und Dienstleistungen für die demographischen Herausforderungen. www.fit4Age.org. Accessed Jan 2007.

J. Forlizzi, C. DiSalvo, F. Gemperle. Assistive robotics and an ecology of elders living independently in their homes. Human-Computer Interaction 19 (1), pp. 25–59, 2004.

Germany's population by 2050: Results of the 11th coordinated population projection, 2006.

B. Graf, U. Reiser, M. Hägele, K. Mauz, P. Klein. Robotic Home Assistant Care-O-bot 3—Product Vision and Innovation Platform. IEEE Workshop on Advanced Ro-botics and its Social Impacts (ARSO), 2009.

M. Hägele, W. Schaaf, E. Helms. Robot assistants at manual workplaces: Effective co-operation and safety aspects. International Symposium on Robotics ISR, 2002.

O. Khatib. Mobile Manipulation: The Robotic Assistant. Journal of Robotics and Autonomous Systems, vol. 26, pp. 175–183, 1999.

F. Leutert, C. Herrmann, K. Schilling. A Spatial Augmented Reality system for intuitive display of robotic data. 8th ACM/IEEE International Conference on Human-Robot Interaction (HRI), 2013.

A.-S. Melenhorst, D. G. Bouwhuis, W. A. Rogers. Older Adults' Motivated Choice for Technological Innovation: Evidence for Benefit-Driven Selectivity. Psychology and Aging 21(1), pp. 190–195, 2006.

N. Muramatsu, H. Akiyama. Japan: Super-aging society preparing for the future. The Gerontologist (51), pp. 425–432, 2011.

J. C. Nitz. Evidence from a cohort of able bodied adults to support the need for driver training for motorized scooters before community participation. Patient Education and Counseling (70), pp. 276–280, 2008.

F. Sarodnick, P. Kohler, T. Lum, H. Schulze, R. Giessler. Sicherheit in der Mensch-Roboter-Kooperation. Zeitschrift für Arbeitswissenschaft 59(4), pp. 441–450, 2005.

M. Sauer, F. Leutert, K. Schilling. Occlusion Handling in Augmented Reality User Interfaces for Robotic Systems. Proceedings of the 41st International Symposium on Robotics (ISR 2010) and 6th German Conference on Robotics, pp. 177–183, 2010.

M. Sauer, F. Leutert, K. Schilling. An Augmented Reality Supported Con-trol System for Remote Operation and Monitoring of an Industrial Work Cell. Proceedings 2nd IFAC Symposium on Telematics Applications, pp. 63–68, 2010.

M. Spenko, H. Yu, S. Dubowsky. Robotic Personal Aids for Mobility and Monitoring for the Elderly. Neural Systems & Rehabilitation Engineering (14), pp. 344–351, 2006.

W. W. Spirduso, K. L. Francis, and P. G. MacRae. Physical Dimensions of Aging. Human Kinetics, 2005.

S. Thiemermann. Direkte Mensch-Roboter-Kooperation in der Kleinteilemontage mit einem SCARA-Roboter. PhD thesis, Univ. of Stuttgart, 2005.

K. Wada, T. Shibata. Living with Seal Robots-Its sociopsychological and physiological influences on the elderly at a care house. Robotics, vol. 23(5), pp. 972–980, 2007.

The Robot that Learns from the Therapist How to Assist Stroke Patients

M. D. Kostić, M. D. Popović and D. B. Popović

Abstract Results from clinical studies suggest that assisted training is beneficial for the recovery of functioning in patients with stroke and other central nervous system injuries. The training consists of the repetition of movements, which change the excitability of the brain, and due to cortical plasticity have carry-over effects. We are developing a 3D arm assistant that interfaces the patient at the hand/wrist. The development addresses three major issues: (1) the selection of the tasks that are appropriate for the training based on the level of motor abilities (2) the design of the visual feedback that enhances the motivation to train, and (3) the assessment of the performance. Therefore, our design integrates the new 3D robot assistant, various gaming based visual feedback, and software that acquires data on-line from sensors (position of the hand and force between the robot and the hand). The major novelties that the 3D arm assistant brings are the following: an automatic method of capturing movements presented by the therapist (expert), the use of the probabilistic movement representation for control of the robot, the incorporation of simple gaming with adjustable levels of difficulty, and finally, the assessment of differences between the achieved and target movements (kinematics) and interface force measured by a special handle with multiple sensors. The components of the new arm assistant in 2D have been tested and proved to work effectively in the clinical trials with stroke patients.

Keywords Stroke · Upper extremities · Rehabilitation · Robot assistance · Motivation · Gaming · Assessment

M. D. Kostić · D. B. Popović (✉)
Faculty of Electrical Engineering, University of Belgrade, Belgrade, Serbia
e-mail: dbp@etf.bg.ac.rs

M. D. Kostić
e-mail: thekostic@etf.bg.ac.rs

M. D. Popović
Faculty of Philosophy, Laboratory for Experimental Psychology, University of Belgrade, Belgrade, Serbia
e-mail: beumas@yahoo.com

A. Rodić et al. (eds.), *New Trends in Medical and Service Robots*,
Mechanisms and Machine Science 20, DOI: 10.1007/978-3-319-05431-5_2,

1 Introduction

The rising number of stroke patients with upper limb impairment and the development of new technologies influence the efforts to improve the recovery process of patients. There is evidence suggesting that the damaged motor system can be reorganized as a consequence of motor practice. Even though optimal training methodology is unclear, there is firm evidence suggesting that quantity of training is positively correlated with recovery (Kwakkel 2009). Personal robots have been identified as a possible way to automate and assist therapists in long training sessions. Hogan at MIT (1992) was among the first to exploit the idea of assisting stroke neurorehabilitation using dedicated robotic systems. This idea and the results obtained, influenced the development of several robot assistants [e.g., Bracio di Ferro (Casadio et al. 2006), ARMin (Nef and Riener 2005), Haptic-Master (Van der Linde et al. 2002)].

One of the challenges for the robot-assisted therapy is the selection of the appropriate tasks and translation of therapist skills into the control of a robot. Several control strategies have been proposed: assistance-based, challenge-based, haptic simulation, etc. The clinical evidence regarding the relative effectiveness of a specific control method is still limited (Marchal-Crespo and Reinkensmeyer 2009). It also became known that there are mechanisms by which some robotic control approaches might actually slow down the recovery when compared with conventional forms of training (Kahn et al. 2006; Kostić et al. 2011).

We need to emphasize that robot assistants aim to be an additional tool available to the physiotherapist and not their replacement. In this context, the physiotherapist would be making all the clinical decisions and when suitable, consider the use of the robot assistant (Loureiro et al. 2011).

The basics of our research can be formulated as follows: The robot assistant should be used to facilitate and speed up the acquisition of novel motor skills of patients with diminished motor control of upper limbs. We combined behavioral studies on motor learning with the design and implementation of robot assistants that behave as "therapists", capable of efficiently exploiting the adaptive properties of the human sensorimotor system and its structures. Regarding the behavioral studies, we focused on the cognitive and neural mechanisms underlying the acquisition of a variety of motor skills that involves the upper limb. In particular, we investigated the physical interaction strategies a human uses to assist the physical training of another human. To maximize the efficiency of the learning process in terms of its specified target outcome, the robot trainer needs to be capable of continuously regulating assistance in terms of the observed performance and of the neural and cognitive correlates of adaptation.

Several ideas that influenced this research follow the findings of the HUMOUR and MIMICS project where the use of robot assistant (Bracio di Ferro and Haptic Master, respectively) was combined with the challenging feedback presented in virtual reality (http://www.mimics.ethz.ch/index.php?page_id=10) (Kostić et al. 2011; Luttgen and Heuer 2012). In the MIMICS project, the three scenarios

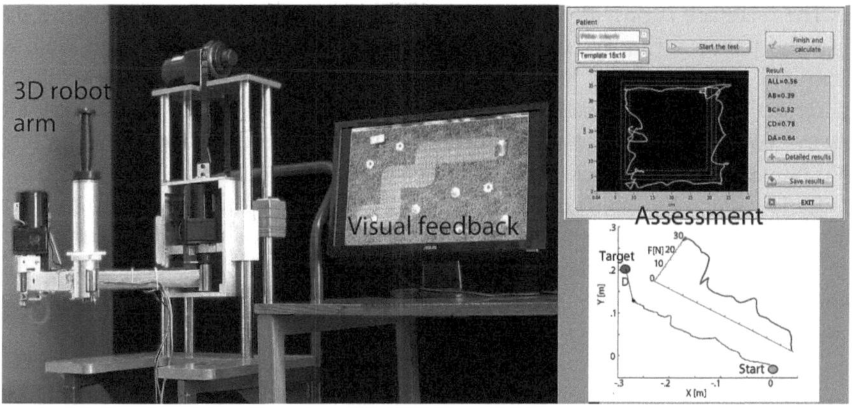

Fig. 1 The new 3D robot assistant (*left* panel) that mimics therapist assistance, visual feedback provided to the patient during the exercise allowing the adjusting of the level of difficulty of the task (*middle*), and two (out of several) measures of the quality of performance

combining motor and cognitive tasks of increasing complexity were compared (http://www.mimics.ethz.ch/index.php?page_id=10). The results indicate that the task during the exercise needs to be graded and to match the abilities of the patient. In short, the key for the success of learning from repetitions can be summarized: the task must be demanding but achievable, and the learning strategy should be from simple to complex. In the HUMOUR project, the question of defining the desired task was addressed from the perspective of motor knowledge transfer. Using research of robot aided motor learning (Došen et al. 2010; Luttgen and Heuer 2012) and human robot interaction (Zenzeri et al. 2011), a novel method for arm movement representation was defined (Kostić et al. 2013).

2 The 3D Robot: Training, Gaming and Assessment Tool

The robot that we are developing integrates a two-segment planar arm mounted on a vertical slider (Fig. 1). The joints of the planar arm were named shoulder (S) and elbow (E). The joints are instrumented with Hall-effect transducers and powered by 25 W asynchronous motors with the planetary gears (1:120 ratio). The motors can be decoupled and then the system operates in passive mode with low friction and inertia (Kostić et al. 2011). The handle (Fig. 1) comprises an in-house designed multi sensor system that measures the direction and amount of interaction force between the patient and the robot. All sensors data are acquired by NI USB-6009 DAQ. The software is developed using LabVIEW 2011. The sampling frequency for acquisition and control is 50 per second. The software integrates signal processing, control and communication in real time.

The feedback is provided by a PC based video game. The feedback shows the task and the actual movement, and shows the quality of movement measured by time and precision. The level of difficulty of the task is being automatically increased if the performance is good enough. The task and level of difficulty are always controlled by the therapist. The gaming that we developed includes also Wii Nintendo games described in detail elsewhere (Prodanović et al. 2012).

Right panels show two out of several screens relevant for the assessment, which are presented to the therapist and patient. The top one is a result of the modified drawing test (Kostić and Popović 2013) in which the ability to track sides of the square is estimated, while the bottom right panel shows the path of the hand and interface force with respect to the target trajectory.

2.1 Setup of the Training Scenario

The training scenario for the robot assistance is a replica of a conventional training provided by the therapist. This approach starts from the assumption that the experience and heuristics of an experienced physical/occupational therapist in managing the training of patients is near optimal. In a conventional training session, the therapist selects the appropriate movement based on the complete neurological status, clinical scores [Fugl-Meyer et al. (1974); ARAT (Van der Lee et al. 2001); Ashworth score (Pandyan et al. 1999)] of the patient, and experience. The therapist instructs the patient by guiding her/his paretic extremity along the target trajectory. Afterwards, the patient exercises this movement through numerous repetitions, while the therapist provides the assistance, again by leading the hand along the target trajectory. The robot assistant is anticipated as a replacement of the therapist from the tedious work. The use of the robot trainer should disturb neither the training protocol, nor the relationship between the patient and the therapist (Riener et al. 2005).

Therefore, the method that we developed follows the same training setup, and maintains the therapist as the dominant figure. It comprises the initial phase in which the therapist demonstrates the movement, and the training phase, where the patient receives assistance, but here the manual work is performed by the robot, leaving the therapist free to concentrate on patients.

During the "teaching the robot" phase, a therapist holds the top part of the handle mounted at the end point of the robot assistant, while the patient is holding (the hand could be attached to the handle if she/he is unable to grasp) the bottom part of the same handle (Fig. 2, left panel), which is instrumented with the force sensor. The therapist repeats the point-to-point movement in the horizontal plane (or in space—3D), while the patient is asked to contribute to the motion (or at least not to oppose it). The number of these repetitions is set to 15, which is sufficient for action representation used here, as we have shown in our earlier studies (Kostić and Popović 2011). The therapist selects the directions and distances in which the patient is provided assistance, based on the visual feedback on the screen.

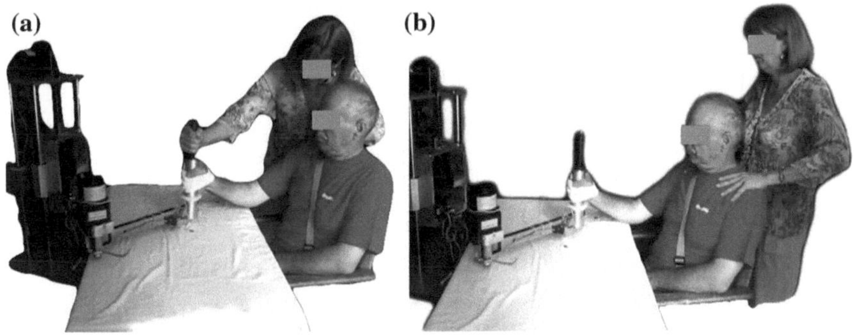

Fig. 2 *Phase A* the "teaching the robot" phase (therapist leads the movement of the robot). The selection of the target trajectory is based on feedback from the patient who holds the same handle. *Phase B* the "training the patient" phase in which robot provides assistance to the patient. The task given to the patient is to follow the trajectory shown on the screen (created during "teaching the robot" phase), while the robot assists only if the patient is unable to perform the task. The maximum assisting force is predefined to assure safety and comfort to the patient

The software allows that even short movements result with the ability to play the game. The trajectories are estimated from the Hall-effect sensors in the joints of the robot (sampling rate 100 per second, resolution of 0.01 rad). This data is filtered with no phase leg in real time and used for the synthesis of the target trajectory (Probability Tube action representation) used for closed-loop control (Kostić et al. 2013).

During the "training the patient" phase (Fig. 2, right panel), the patient is asked to move the hand in a manner to follow the trajectory shown on the feedback screen. The feedback is presented as a video game, which implements movements from the previous phase, and has positive impact on patient motivation, as shown in Popović et al. (2013). The robot is assisting this movement if the patient is not able to do so in a desired manner. The maximum assistance force is preset and limited for safety and comfort reasons (Kostić et al. 2013). The assistance force is acquired and presented on a separate screen to provide the quantified measure of the patient's contribution to the movement. If the interface force is low, then the patient is capable of executing the movement without assistance. This is the cue for the therapist to set a more demanding task. The therapist can readjust setup online without interrupting the training session. The detailed description of the methods to acquire data and generate the target points, trajectory and probability tube, are described elsewhere (Kostić et al. 2013; Kostić and Popović 2011).

2.2 Setup of the Games

The research results that indicate patient motivation as highly important for therapeutic outcome were the reason for integrating gaming into the robot-training scenario (Maclean and Pound 2000). Motivation is a multifaceted concept linked

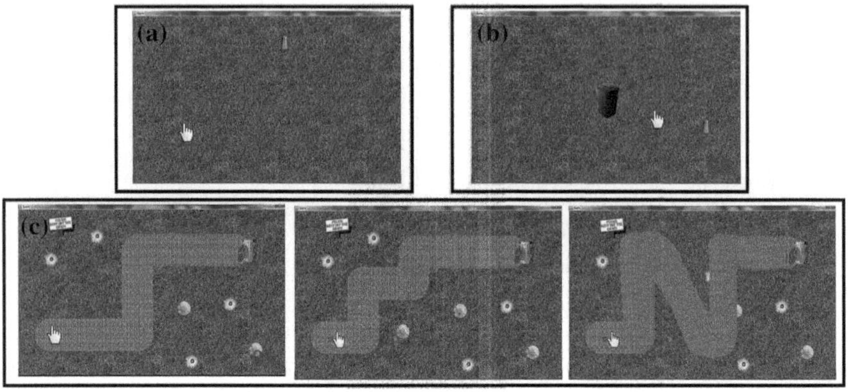

Fig. 3 The screens shown to the subject as tasks to be achieved. The complexity rises from **a** to **c**. The measure of success is the precision of the point-to-point movement/tracking and time to execute the task. The movement is continuously monitored in order to provide quantitative and qualitative measures to the clinician about the outcome of the training and for the introduction of changes of the level of difficulty to be appropriate to motor output

to several factors, including features inherent to the prescribed regimen, as well as personality traits of the patient, physician and therapist, and characteristics of the broader social environment (Maclean et al. 2002). Patients, who are highly motivated, in contrast to those who believe the outcomes of therapy depend on fate and the health system, restore their functioning to a larger extent (Campbell et al. 2001). Video games have long been known to be engaging to play; hence, developing rehabilitation games that can create a similar degree of interest can be highly beneficial for therapeutic outcome.

We are developing a feedback-mediated treatment, which uses gaming scenarios and allows on-line and off-line monitoring of both temporal and spatial characteristics of planar movements (Kostić et al. 2012). This treatment is a movement exercise, with visual feedback coming from the screen, showing targets and pathways to be followed. The targets and pathways are interactively set, as described earlier, to correspond to the abilities of the patient at any time during the treatment. The software and the user interface allow the setting of the level of difficulty of the task to be progressively increased, based on the success achieved in the game.

The gaming that we are describing here includes three types of exercises (Fig. 3) that required the activity of the proximal joints (shoulder and elbow) of the affected arm. Patients hold the handle as shown in Fig. 2 and move it in order to perform the task. Each game exercise lasts for about five minutes. This interval was heuristically found to correspond to the periods of increased motivation of the patents. However, patients can decide to stop after a shorter interval for any reason. Resting must be integrated into the training, and resting periods should be approximately as long as the actual training.

The coordinates of the end point of the robotic arm (handle) control the game. The position of the cursor on the screen shown to the patient corresponds to the position of the handle. The software allows amplification of the range of movement to allow patients with major disability to also participate in the training. The gain of amplification is decreased in parallel to the gain in functioning of the patient.

The first game (exercise) requires moving the cursor to reach targets, which are appearing in pseudo random positions on the screen (Fig. 3a). When the cursor would meet the target, it would disappear from the screen and trigger the "cash register" sound. This is followed by appearance of the next target in a pseudo random position on the screen. The minimal distance between two subsequent targets is defined to match the patient's workspace. The distance between targets gradually increases during the course of the game.

The second game (Fig. 3b) requires from patients to move the cursor to a given target, and then return to the initial position in order to trigger the next target appearance). The initial position is in the center of the workspace, and the targets are appearing in the same manner as in the first game.

In the third game, patients are presented with a target trajectory (path) which they had to follow with the cursor (Fig. 3c). Upon completion of one path, a new, more difficult path would appear. The shape and complexity of paths (varying from wide and straight paths, to narrow and complex paths) was designed by experienced therapists to match the abilities of patients.

The score (achieved speed and precision) is displayed during the game to allow patients to follow their performance. A high-score list, where patients could compare their performance to previous days and to performance of other patients, was shown after each session.

In the procedure of the development, the gaming was tested in 20 stroke patients with the 2D passive robot (Popović et al. 2013). The outcome measures were assessed from: (1) the modified drawing test—mDT; (2) received therapy time—RTT; and (3) Intrinsic Motivation Inventory—IMI. The overall conclusion is that gaming is beneficial, but that it must be tuned to match patient abilities; otherwise, it could be counterproductive.

2.3 Control of the Robot Trainer

We applied two single-input single-output Modified Internal Model Control (MIMC) liner digital controllers (Mataušek et al. 2002) to control the proximal (shoulder) and the distal (elbow) joint of the system robotic arm. Simple models G_{mpE}(s) of the elbow position p_E(t) [rad] and G_{mpS}(s) of the shoulder position p_S(t)

[rad] are developed from open-loop step response tests. Model G_{mpE}(s) is defined by the following transfer function:

$$G_{mpE}(s) = \frac{K_E e^{-L_e s}}{s(T_E^2 s^2 + 2\zeta_E T_E s + 1)},\\ K_E = 2.4 \times 10^{-4},\ L_E = 0.07,\ T_E = 0.04,\ \zeta_E = 0.7. \tag{1}$$

Model G_{mpS}(s) is defined by

$$G_{mpS}(s) = \frac{K_S e^{-L_S s}}{s(T_S^2 s^2 + 2\zeta_S T_S s + 1)},\\ K_S = 2.3 \times 10^{-4},\ L_S = 0.1,\ T_S = 0.08,\ \zeta_S = 0.7. \tag{2}$$

The controlled variables consist of the velocity of the elbow and the velocity of the shoulder. However, the measured variables on the patient are in the elbow and shoulder positions. Therefore, velocity of elbow v_E(t) [rad/s] and velocity of shoulder v_S(t) [rad/s] are obtained as first derivative of measured variables. Their dynamic characteristics are defined by the elbow velocity model G_{mvE}(s) and the shoulder velocity model G_{mvS}(s), which are obtained from (1) and (2). Model G_{mvE}(s) is defined by

$$G_{mvE}(s) = \frac{K_E e^{-L_E s}}{T_E^2 s^2 + 2\zeta_E T_E s + 1}. \tag{3}$$

Whereas model G_{mvS}(s) is defined by

$$G_{mvS}(s) = \frac{K_S e^{-L_S s}}{T_S^2 s^2 + 2\zeta_S T_S s + 1}. \tag{4}$$

The applied MIMC controller for elbow C_E and shoulder C_S can be derived from (1)–(4), as

$$C_E(s) = \frac{G_{mvE}^{-1}(s) F(s)}{1 - F(s) e^{-L_E s}}, \tag{5}$$

$$C_S(s) = \frac{G_{mvS}^{-1}(s) F(s)}{1 - F(s) e^{-L_S s}}, \tag{6}$$

where F(s) is a second order filter applied on error measurement. Detailed description of the control can be found in Kostić et al. (2013).

2.4 Assessment Provided by the Robot

The International Classification of Functioning, Disability and Health (ICF) relates to two domains: a list of body functions and structures, and a list of activities in daily life and social participation. The efforts of the European Experts group within the COST project TD 1006 (http://www.rehabilitationrobotics.eu/), created the lists with three categories: (1) capability measures, (2) pathophysiological measures, and (3) task performance measures.

The capability measures characterize the capacities such as range of motion (active/passive), overall workspace, maximum strength under isometric conditions, maximum joint power (non-isometric), and proprioception. The system that we developed allows the assessment of the range of motion and maximum strength under isometric conditions.

The pathophysiological measures quantify different impairments seen in neurological disorders such as abnormal synergies, spasticity, rigidity, ataxia, movement and postural asymmetries, and pain occurring or induced by the movement. The system that we developed allows the assessment of the abnormal synergies and spasticity.

The task performance measures quantify how well a task has been executed, including measures such as: execution time to complete a specific task, success rate of accomplishing the task, disturbance recovery, quality of movement for a specific task (smoothness, speed-accuracy curve, number and kind of unwanted collisions with objects, repeatability), and several measures related to grasping. The system that we developed allows the assessment of the execution time, smoothness, number of collisions, and speed-accuracy curve.

We present here one of the assessments that is facilitated with the 3D robot that we developed (Kostić and Popović 2013). The testing procedure comprised drawing a square based on the presented template, a 2-cm wide rectangular path. The path is formed by two concentric squares, with the side difference of 4 cm. The task is to complete the rectangular path (all four sides) as fast and precise as possible. The size of the template is determined by the initial measurement of subject's ROM.

The outcome measure of this test comprises three objective measures: movement speed, movement precision error, and movement smoothness. The average speed was calculated as the ratio of length of a single side of the square and the time used to complete that side. The precision error was calculated as the area of transgressions outside the path. Areas enclosed by the drawing and template lines outside the path were detected, counted, and measured automatically, using the image processing methods. Precision error was defined as the total area of transgressions multiplied by their number, normalized with respect to the area of the template square. Smoothness measure was defined as a function of four smoothness parameters proposed in Rohrer et al. (2002).

The entire testing procedure is supported by custom-made software with user-friendly interface (Fig. 4), which enables simple testing, and instant access to

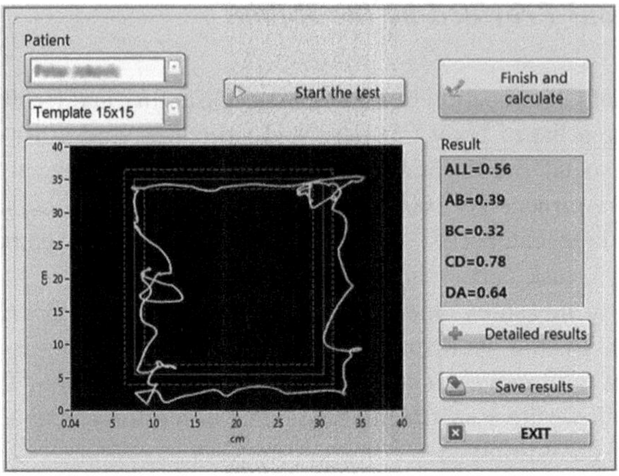

Fig. 4 User-friendly software for on-line assessment of performance. The window provides intuitive commands for the testing procedure and the score

results. In order to expedite the testing procedure, only basic commands and the score are provided in the main window, shown in Fig. 4, while detailed analysis of data can be performed by entering the advanced data analysis window. The results presented in Kostić and Popović (2013) indicate the applicability of this method in clinical assessment of patient performance.

Finally, we show here the assessment of the interface force and the "error" in reaching the target during the exercises. Figure 5 shows the setup and the processed output from the sensors. The position of the hand is being calculated from the measured joint angles, while the force is estimated based on the developed force sensor.

In the example shown in Fig. 5, it is clear that the patient was not able to follow the task and could not reach the target point (spastic patient, Ashworth grade 4). Though the robot was programmed to assist the movement in reaching the target point, for safety reasons the robot-generated force was limited to 30 N, hence the movement stopped before actually reaching the target. In the case of contralateral movement, the distance between the movement endpoint and the target was $D = 9.6$ cm, while in the ipsilateral direction the error was only $D = 2.9$ cm.

The interface force (Fig. 3, right panels) indicates that the robot was pulling the handle along the trajectory. Thus, the robot assisted the movement with strong force during the last 25 % of the actual movement ($F \approx 30$ N), whereas the force was approximately 10 N during the first 75 % of the movement. These two measures indicate the patient's ability to perform the target movement, as well as the generated force. They can be used for patient assessment, but also as feedback used by the therapist when selecting the level of difficulty for the robot-assisted rehabilitation.

The most important measure fed back to the patient is the game performance. This information is given by the time and number of repetitions within the preselected interval. This has been shown to influence patients in a highly competitive

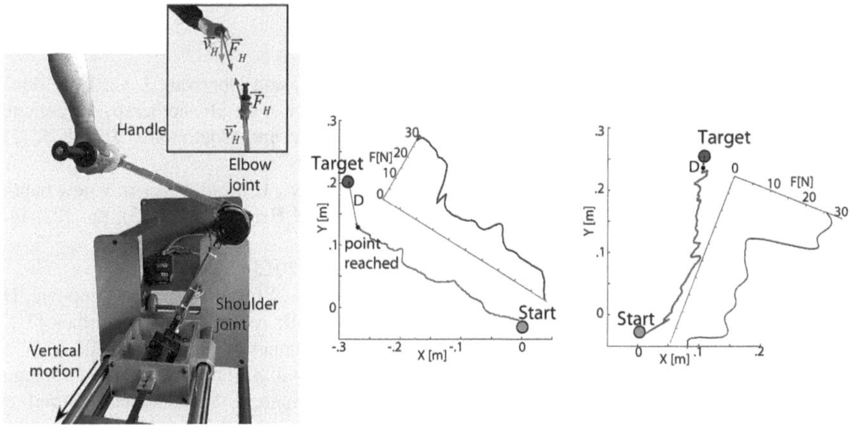

Fig. 5 The assessment of performance with the new robot assistant. The two *right* panels show the force estimated from the sensors in the handle, and the error (*D*) in reaching the target from the sensors in the robot joints. The recordings are from a patient that suffered stroke and is spastic (Ashworth grade 4). It is noticeable that the force generated by the robot (limited by controller to 30 N) is not adequate to move the spastic elbow, especially if the task was the movement from the point in front of the shoulder in the contralateral direction

manner (Popović et al. 2013). It allows patients to follow their own progress, but even more importantly, calls for competition with their peers.

3 Conclusions

We presented here the design and the methodology of use of the system in the clinical condition that could improve the rehabilitation of patients with upper extremity disability. The system that we are developing has an open architecture and allows simple integration with functional electrical stimulation systems that would control the grasping functions and possibly the hand orientation (Popović-Maneski et al. 2013). We developed earlier systems with array electrodes that allow selective activation of forearm and hand muscles, as well as the sensors system that can integrate easily into the 3D robot presented (Malešević et al. 2012).

We present the development of the 3D robot, which controls the position of the hand/arm. This could be seen as the replica of other robot assistants that control the end point trajectory. The novelties in the system presented are in control that integrates the selection of the trajectory, adaptation of the trajectory during the exercise, selection of the complexity of gaming by the therapist, and over all, the assessment features that are instrumental in judging if the training is appropriate or not. The reason why we decided to build our own robot is the necessity to have full control of all elements, having in mind that the robot assistant is to be used by clinicians without interference with the therapeutic session.

References

Campbell, R., Evans, M., Tucker, M., Quilty, B., Dieppe, P., and Donovan, J. L.: Why don't patients do their exercises? Understanding non-compliance with physiotherapy in patients with osteoarthritis of the knee. Journal of Epidemiology and Community Health 55(2), pp. 132–138 (2001)

Casadio, M., Sanguineti, V., Morasso, P. G., and Arrichiello, V.: Braccio di Ferro: a new haptic workstation for neuromotor rehabilitation. Technology and Health Care 14(3), pp. 123–142 (2006)

COST Action TD1006. http://www.rehabilitationrobotics.eu/ (2013)

Došen, S., Andersen, A., Kannik, K., Klausen, C., Nielesen, L., Wojtowicz, J., and Popović, D. B.: "Assistive" Forces for the Acquisition of a Motor Skill: Assistance or Disturbance? 1st International Conference on Applied Bionics and Biomechanics. Venice, Italy (2010)

Fugl-Meyer, A. R., Jaasko L., Leyman I., Olsson, S., and Steglind, S.: The post-stroke hemiplegic patient. 1. a method for evaluation of physical performance. Scandinavian journal of rehabilitation medicine 7(1), pp. 13–31 (1974)

Hogan, N., Krebs, H. I., Charnnarong, J., Srikrishna, P., and Sharon, A.: MIT-MANUS: a workstation for manual therapy and training. I. IEEE, pp. 161–165 (1992)

Kahn, L. E., Lum, P. S., Rymer, W. Z., and Reinkensmeyer, D. J.: Robot-assisted movement training for the stroke-impaired arm: Does it matter what the robot does? Journal of rehabilitation research and development 43(5), p. 619 (2006)

Kostić, M. D., Kovačević, P. S. and Popović, D. B.: Is the Haptic Tunnel Effective Tool for Motor Learning? In: Proc. of IFMBE2012 37, pp. 761–765 Budapest, Hungary (2011)

Kostić, M. D., Kovačević, P. S. and Popović, M. D.: Playing games in Virtual Reality: Motivation of patients during neurorehabilitation. In: Proc. of Infoteh 2012 Vol: 11, pp. 692–696 Jahorina, Bosnia & Herzegovina (2012)

Kostić, M. D., Mataušek, M. R., and Popović, D. B.: Therapeutic robot assistant for the arm: Modified internal model control. IEEE Trans Neur Syst and Rehab Eng (under review) (2013)

Kostić, M. D., Popović, D. B., and Popović, M. B.: Influence of planar manipulandum to the hand trajectory during point to point movement. In: Proc. of 12th International Conference on Rehabilitation Robotics, pp. 1–4. Zurich, Switzerland (2011)

Kostić, M. D. and Popović, D. B.: Action representation of point to point movements: Classification with probability tube. In: Proc. of IEEE 19th Telecomunacations Forum TELFOR, pp. 43–46. Belgrade, Serbia, (2011)

Kostić, M. D., Popović, M. B., and Popović, D. B.: A method for assessing the arm movement performance: probability tube. Medical & Biological Engineering & Computing DOI: 10.1007/s11517-013-1104-z (2013)

Kostić, M. D. and Popović, M. D.: The Modified Drawing Test for Assessment of Arm Movement Quality. Journal of Automatic Control 21(1), pp. 49–53 (2013)

Kwakkel, G.: Intensity of practice after stroke: More is better. Schweizer Archiv für Neurologie und Psychiatrie 160(7), pp. 295–298 (2009)

Loureiro, R. C., Harwin, W. S., Nagai, K., and Johnson, M.: Advances in upper limb stroke rehabilitation: a technology push. Medical & Biological Engineering & Computing 49(10), pp. 1103–1118 (2011)

Luttgen, J. and Heuer, H.: The influence of haptic guidance on the production of spatio-temporal patterns. Human movement science 31(3), pp. 519–528 (2012)

Maclean, N., Pound, P., Wolfe, C., and Rudd, A.: The concept of patient motivation a qualitative analysis of stroke professionals' attitudes. Stroke 33(2), pp. 444–448 (2002)

Maclean, N. and Pound, P.: A critical review of the concept of patient motivation in the literature on physical rehabilitation. Social Science and Medicine 50, pp. 495–506 (2000)

Malešević, N. M., Popović Maneski, L. Z., Ilić, V., Jorgovanović, N., Bijelić, G., Keller, T., Popović, D. B.: A Multi-Pad Electrode based Functional Electrical Stimulation System for Restoration of Grasp. J Neuro Eng Rehab 9–66, 10.1186/1743-0003-9-66 (2012)

Marchal-Crespo, L. and Reinkensmeyer, D. J.: Review of control strategies for robotic movement training after neurologic injury. Journal of NeuroEngineering and Rehabilitation 6(1), p. 20 (2009)

Mataušek, M. R., Micić, A. D., and Dačić, D. B.: Modified internal model control approach to the design and tuning of linear digital controllers. International Journal of Systems Science 33(1), pp. 67–79 (2002)

MIMICS project. http://www.mimics.ethz.ch/index.php?page_id=10 (2013)

Nef, T. and Riener, R.: ARMin-design of a novel arm rehabilitation robot. IEEE 9th International Conference on Rehabilitation Robotics, pp. 57–60 (2005)

Pandyan, A. D., Johnson, G. R., Price, C. I. M., Curless, R. H., Barnes, M. P., and Rodgers, H.: A review of the properties and limitations of the Ashworth and modified Ashworth Scales as measures of spasticity. Clinical rehabilitation 13(5), pp. 373–383 (1999).

Popović, M. D., Kostić, M. D., Mitrović, S. Z., and Konstantinović, L. M.: Feedback-mediated upper extremities exercise: Increasing patient motivation in post-stroke rehabilitation. BioMed Research International (under review) (2013)

Popović-Maneski, L., Kostić, M., Bijelić, G., Keller, T., Mitrović, S., Konstantinović, Lj., Popović, D. B.: Multi-pad electrode for effective grasping: Design. IEEE Trans Neur Sys Reh Eng 21(4), pp. 648–654 (2013)

Prodanović, M., Kostić, M. D., and Popović, D. B.: WiiMote control: gaming feedback for motivational training of the arm movements. IEEE Symposium on Neural Network Applications in Electrical Engineering (NEUREL), pp. 133–136 (2012)

Riener, R., Nef, T., and Colombo, G.: Robot-aided neurorehabilitation of the upper extremities. Medical and biological engineering and computing 43(1), pp. 2–10 (2005)

Rohrer, B., Fasoli, S., Krebs, H. I., Hughes, R., Volpe, B., Frontera, W. R., Stein, J., and Hogan, N.: Movement smoothness changes during stroke recovery. The journal of Neuroscience 22(18), pp. 8297–8304 (2002)

Van der Lee, J. H., De Groot, V., Beckerman, H., Wagenaar, R. C., Lankhorst, G. J., and Bouter, L. M.: The intra-and interrater reliability of the action research arm test: a practical test of upper extremity function in patients with stroke. Archives of physical medicine and rehabilitation 82(1), pp. 14–19 (2001)

Van der Linde, R. Q., Lammertse, P., Frederiksen, E., and Ruiter, B.: The HapticMaster, a new high-performance haptic interface. Proc. Eurohaptics., pp. 1–5 (2002)

Zenzeri, J., Basteris, A., Kostić, M. D., Popović, D. B., Sanguineti, V., Mohan, V., and Morasso, P.: Transferring complex motor skills from an expert to a novice through robotics platforms: A new methodology to approach neuromotor rehabilitation. Gait and posture 33, pp. s51–s52 (2011)

Lower Limbs Robotic Rehabilitation Case Study with Clinical Trials

M. Bouri, E. Abdi, H. Bleuler, F. Reynard and O. Deriaz

Abstract Robotic based lower limbs rehabilitation is addressed in this chapter. Different existing devices are presented to point out the context of mobilization of the limbs. The mechanical constructions of the systems "Lambda" and the "MotionMaker" developed at the Laboratoire de Systèmes Robotiques (LSRO-EPFL) are reviewed. The MotionMaker allows the mobilization of both legs with a twice 3 degrees of freedom orthosis (hip, knee and ankle of each leg). It has been developed for paraplegics and is the main concern in this chapter. The therapy, combining the mobilization of the legs through flexion/extension and the closed loop muscle electrostimulation is explained and clearly detailed. The results of three clinical studies are presented. In the first one, a simple knee orthosis is used to prove the possibility to follow an isotonic torque during an isokinetic knee extension by closed loop electrical stimulation. In the second clinical study, the academic MotionMaker has been used with 5 paraplegic subjects to evaluate the voluntary force progress and the reduction of the spastic behavior. Finally, the last clinical study describes the use of the commercial MotionMaker provided by the Swiss company Swortec during the last 5 years. More than 24 subjects have been considered and the increase of the voluntary force is clearly observed.

M. Bouri (✉) · E. Abdi · H. Bleuler
Laboratoire de Systèmes Robotique, Ecole Polytechnique Fédérale de Lausanne (EPFL), Station 9, 1015 Lausanne, Switzerland
e-mail: Mohamed.Bouri@epfl.ch

E. Abdi
e-mail: Elahe.Abdi@epfl.ch

H. Bleuler
e-mail: Hannes.Bleuler@epfl.ch

F. Reynard · O. Deriaz
Clinique Romande de Réadaptation (CRR), Ave. Grand-Champsec 90, CP 352, CH 1951 Sion, Switzerland
e-mail: Fabienne.Reynard@crr-suva.ch

O. Deriaz
e-mail: Olivier.Deriaz@crr-suva.ch

A. Rodić et al. (eds.), *New Trends in Medical and Service Robots*, Mechanisms and Machine Science 20, DOI: 10.1007/978-3-319-05431-5_3,

Keywords Robotics · Rehabilitation · Clinical results · Lower limbs · Closed loop · Electrical stimulation · Paraplegics

1 Introduction

Treating patients with mobility disabilities often consists of active, highly repetitive gestures, which require one-to-one manual interaction with the therapist.

Current technologies (e.g. robotics, electrical stimulation, video games) open new perspectives in the rehabilitation strategies by bringing the opportunity to create and implement intensive training in an efficient and safe manner, without increasing the therapists' workload.

Robotic technologies are becoming more prevalent in the clinics, assisting the therapy in tasks for motor re-learning, neurological recovery and muscle reinforcement for both upper and lower limbs.

Robotics has become an important tool for rehabilitation and assistance for the walking process. Indeed, robots execute known trajectories well and may actively move the legs along predefined locomotion trajectories: It is also possible to only provide an assistance that can automatically adapt to the patient's degree of impairment.

There are principally two types of leg mobilization devices for rehabilitation: (1) Sitting position devices and (2) Verticalized mobilization devices that can provide walking trajectories through motorized leg orthosis.

Verticalized leg mobilization devices let the patients carry out the exercises while in the verticalized posture. They are very attractive because they can provide real walking patterns and good feeling for the patients. We might highlight the Lokomat®[1] commercialized by Hokoma (Colombo and Dietz 2000) and the WalkTrainer®[2] initially developed in EPFL-LSRO and later commercialized by Swortec (Bouri et al. 2006; Stauffer 2009; Stauffer et al. 2007, 2008, 2009). These two devices provide a very complete rehabilitation with many degrees of freedom and weight support. Patients like this kind of devices because of the multi-degree of freedom mobilization and assistance (Pelvis, Legs, Body weight). Nevertheless, they are quite expensive because of the number of their components and the control complexity (Fig. 1).

In the sitting position rehabilitation devices, the subject is sitting or lying and the leg mobilization is carried out. Two simple examples of commercial sitting rehabilitation devices are the THERAvital machine (from Medica Medizinetechnik), which is a cycling motorized system and the Yaskawa TEM LX2 robot.

[1] Lokomat is a registered name of the HOKOMA Company.

[2] WalkTrainer and MotionMaker are registered names of the FSC (Swiss Foundation of Cyberthosis).

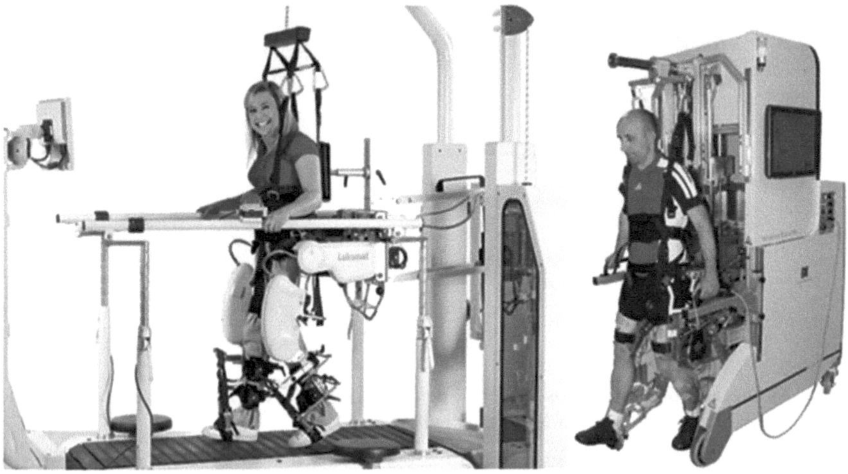

Fig. 1 Two examples of verticalized assistive devices: the Lokomat® (Hokoma) and the commercial version of the WalkTrainer® (Swortec)

These two devices have a relatively low price when compared with the above-verticalized solutions (Fig. 2).

Even though these devices are much more cost-efficient and portable, their rehabilitation strategies are intrinsically limited. The THERAlive (www.thera-trainer.de) device has only one degree of freedom (purely cycling devices) and the TEM LX2 (www.yaskawa.co.jp) can train only one leg at a time.

Continuing with sitting devices another noteworthy academic development is the robot called **"Lambda"**. This development consists of a lightweight parallel mobilization robot of the lower extremities of the patient during the rehabilitation session. The prototype is entirely instrumented with position and force sensors at each motorized articulation. This allows controlling all the movements and the corresponding generated force (Bouri and Clavel 2009) (Fig. 3).

The Lambda is promising because of its simplicity and the lack of anthropometric length adjustment for each subject. The generated motion trajectories are adjusted with respect to the segment lengths of the subject. In counterpart, this increases the safety analysis and risks because the joint space of the subject is totally dissociated with the joint space of the robot. Furthermore, the accessible workspace of the robot gets outside of the authorized feet workspace.

In this chapter, we will present the device **MotionMaker®**[3] and the associated therapy. This device provides the mobilization of the hip, knee and ankle joints of each leg. Both position and force control are taken into consideration. Muscles are electrostimulated in closed loop to reach the desired forces at the feet. The recruited muscles are presented and the clinical trials are discussed.

[3] The MotionMaker is a product commercialized by Swortec SA.

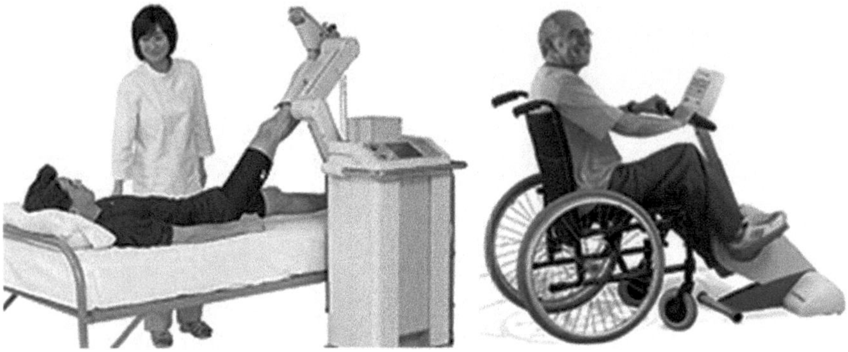

Fig. 2 Sitting and on-the-bed cost-effective devices: (*left*) the TEM LX2 from Yaskawa and (*right*) THERAvital from Medica Medizintechnik

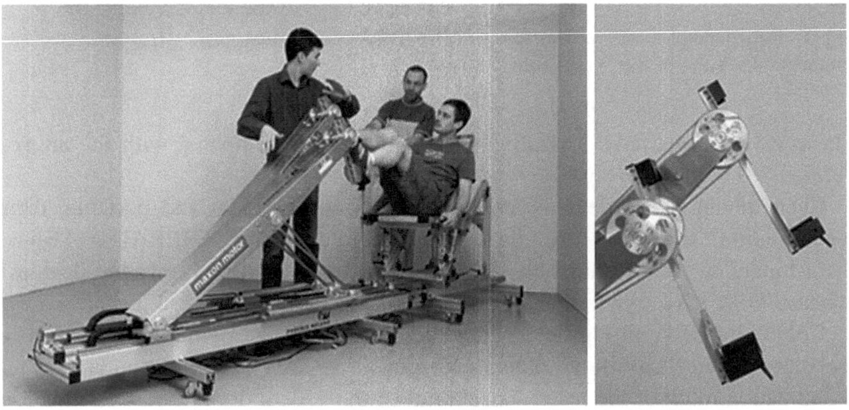

Fig. 3 The Lambda parallel robot for lower limb mobilization developed by LSRO

2 Presentation of the MotionMaker

The MotionMaker is a mobilization robotic device for lower limbs. This section introduces the MotionMaker device, its components and explains how the therapy combining motion and electrostimulation works.

2.1 The Mechanical Device

The MotionMaker is based on two leg orthosis (Fig. 4). Thanks to screw based transmission and a crank mechanism, each leg orthosis allows the mobilization of the hip, the knee and the ankle joints. Each joint is instrumented with a force sensor at the extremity of the screw for safety and control purposes.

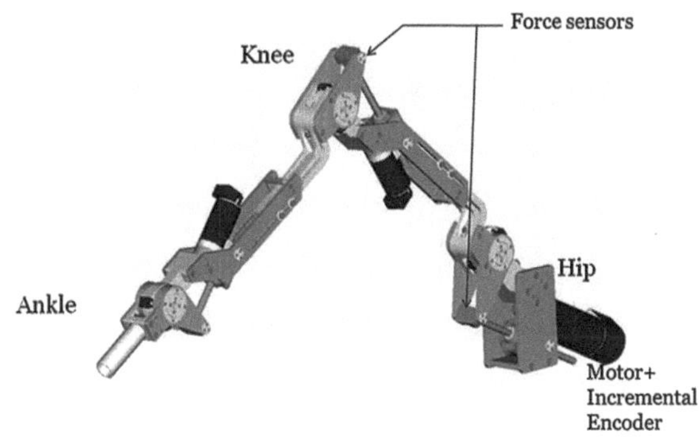

Fig. 4 The leg orthosis of the MotionMaker

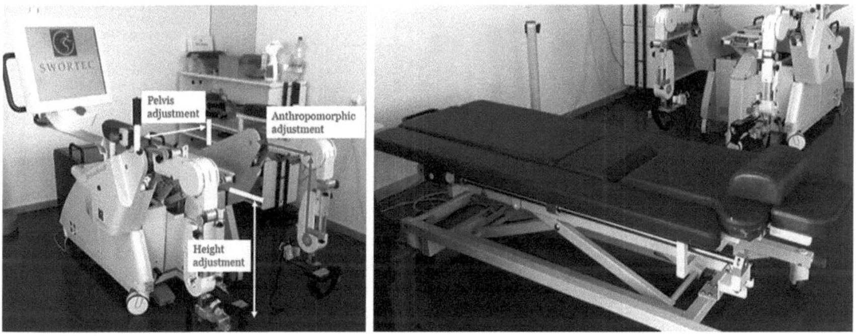

Fig. 5 The industrial MotionMaker and the transfer table

The subject is first transferred to the device by using a transfer table (Fig. 5) and is then adjusted in a sitting position thanks to different motors (vertical adjustment, pelvic adjustment and inclination of the back). The anthropomorphic lengths are also adjusted with respect to the subject. The MotionMaker carries out the mobilization of the legs through flexion/extension or cycling movements.

Figure 6 shows the academic and the industrial variants of the MotionMaker. The industrial device is commercialized by the company Swortec SA (www.swortec.ch).

2.2 Presentation of the Therapy

Conventional therapies are based on pure mobilization. Robotic based therapies often provide a mobilization that reproduces pre-programmed patterns. The Lokomat combines the movements with an adaptive compliance/stiffness,

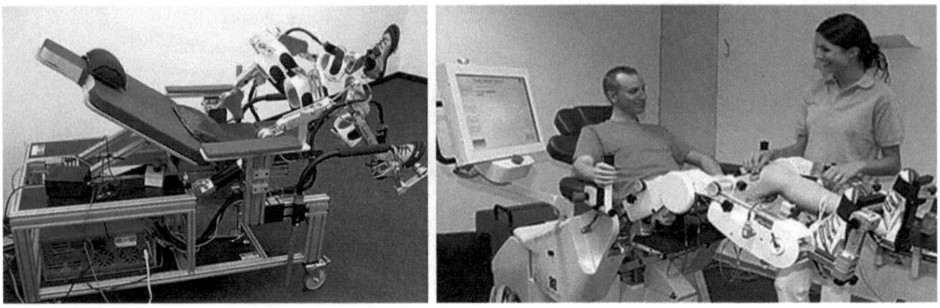

Fig. 6 (*left*) The academic prototype of MotionMaker developed at EPFL (*right*) The commercial version

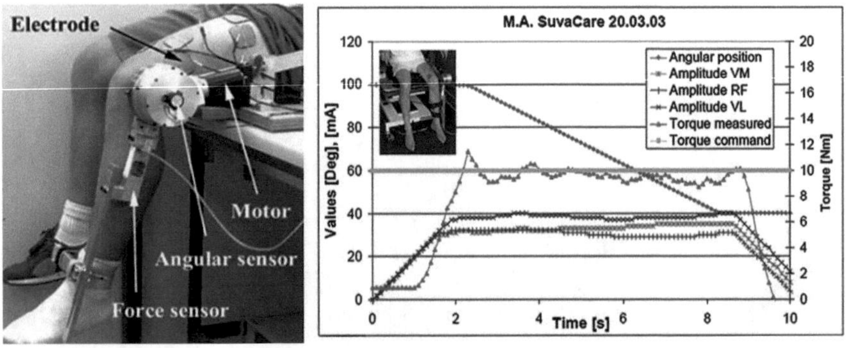

Fig. 7 The Knee orthosis (*left*) the mechanical device—(*right*) results of the CT—[Schmitt et al. 2004]

changing with the contribution of the subject during the walking assistance (Koenig et al. 2011; Riener et al. 2004; Bernhardt et al. 2005).

In our case, at the Laboratoire de Systèmes Robotiques (LSRO), we have adopted the combination between the leg mobilization and muscle electrostimulation to ensure both the contribution of the subject and that the muscles are active according to the movement phases (dynamic phases and when stopped). The muscles are electrostimulated in closed loop through the measurement of the force applied at each foot: the more the force exerted by the subject gets close to the targeted force, the less we electrostimulate the muscles (Schmitt et al. 2004; Metrailler et al. 2006; Metrailler 2005). This concept of bi-therapy approach, combining mobilization and closed loop electrostimulation has been patented (Brodard and Clavel 2002, 2004). The human is in the loop because the subject has to participate in the force application to reduce the electrostimulation current.

To understand the approach, Fig. 7 shows the knee motorized orthosis developed to implement the control strategy (Schmitt et al. 2004). Eight subjects with incomplete spinal cord lesion participated in this study. The desired torque is imposed at the knee, the extension force is measured and the muscles are

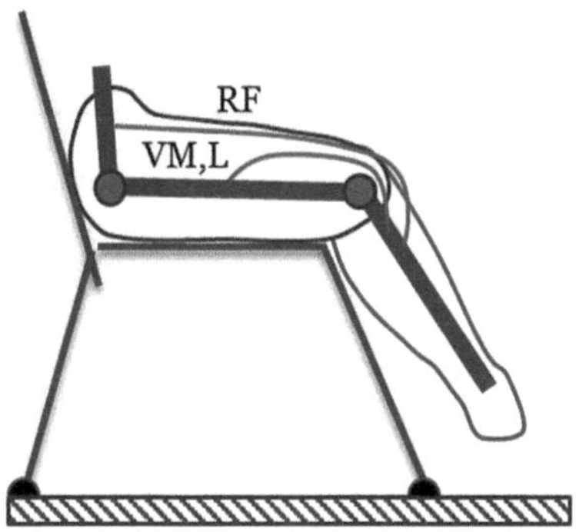

Fig. 8 Muscle recruitment for knee extension

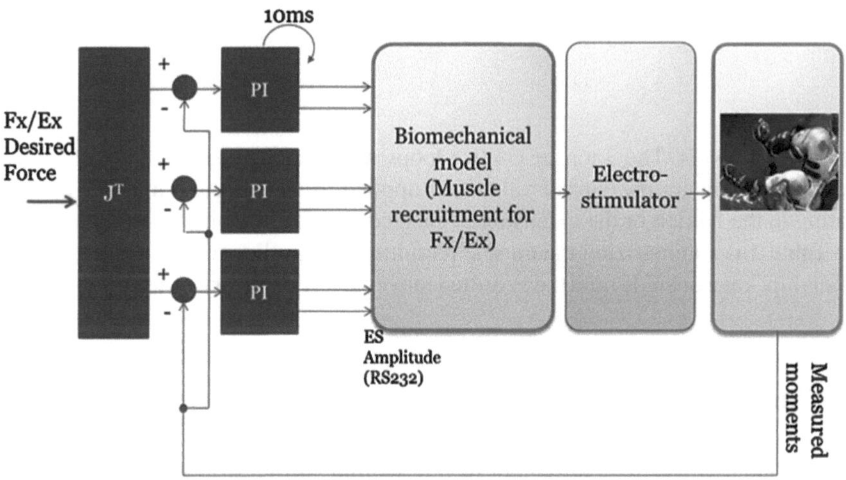

Fig. 9 The academic prototype of MotionMaker developed at EPFL and its commercial version

electrostimulated through a PI controller to reach the targeted torque. Meanwhile, extension movements (Green) are carried out by the motorized orthosis.

The recruited muscles are the RF (Rectus Femoris), the VM and VL (Vastus Medialis and Lateralis). The obtained results have proved the possibility to follow an isotonic torque command during an isokinetic knee extension by closed loop electrical stimulation (Fig. 8).

The MotionMaker has been used for the implementation of the strategy. This device allows flexion/extension movements for each leg. Each joint is equipped with a force sensor. The foot force is hence measured thanks to the Jacobian matrix J (Sciavicco and Siciliano 2000).

Figure 9 illustrates how the closed loop force control works. First, a flexion or extension target force at the foot is set. This force corresponds to the desired torques

Table 1 Muscle recruitment

Joint	Flexion movement	Extension movement
Hip	Rectus Femoris (RF)	Gluteus Maximus (GM)
Knee	Hamstring (HA)	Vastus Medialis and Lateralis (VM + L)
Ankle	Tibialis Anterior (TA)	Gastrocnemius (GA)

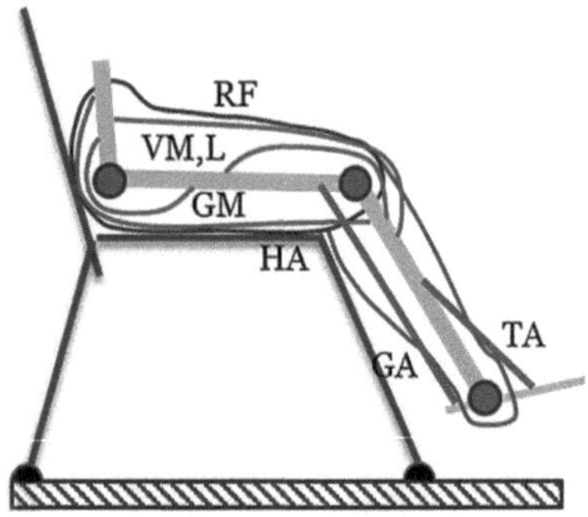

Fig. 10 The total of 7 muscles have been used in the loop: *RF* Rectus Femoris, *VM, L* Vastus Medialis and Lateralis, *GM* Gluteus maximus. *HA* Hamstring, *GA* Gastrocnemius, *TA* Tibialis Anterior

at the joint levels. The 3 torque control loops work independently and the PI (Proportional + Integrator) current values are applied to the recruited muscles participating to the flexion or the extension of each corresponding joint (Metrailler 2005).

Table 1 is summarizing the muscle recruitment regarding to both corresponding joint (hip, knee or ankle) and the executed movement (flexion or extension) (Fig. 10).

3 Clinical Studies

Two clinical studies are presented in this section. In the first one, the academic MotionMaker has been used with 5 paraplegic subjects to evaluate the voluntary force progress and the reduction of the spastic behavior. The second study concerns the clinical results obtained by the commercial MotionMaker provided by the Swiss company Swortec during the last 5 years.

3.1 Clinical Study 1

In collaboration with the CHUV[4] hospital and the CRR,[5] the first clinical trials were performed in the year 2005 (Stauffer et al. 2007) using the first prototype of

[4] CHUV, University Hospital of Canton of Vaud.

[5] CRR, Rehabilitation Clinic Of Swiss Romande (www.crr-suva.ch).

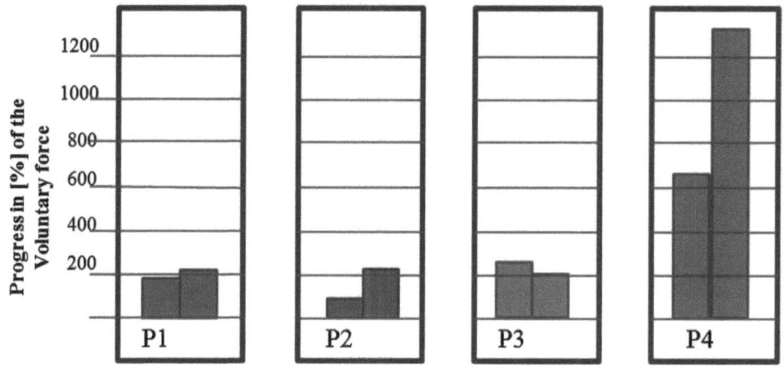

Fig. 11 Progress, in % between the first and the last session of the mean force voluntarily developed by the 4 incomplete paraplegic subjects (P1-P4) (*left bar* corresponds to the left leg)

MotionMaker developed at EPFL-LSRO (Fig. 6). In these trials the patient's leg was flexed and extended by the MotionMaker. This study aimed to assess the progress of the voluntarily developed force by the subject and the reduction of the spastic behavior.

Five patients took part in the experiment, four of which were incomplete paraplegics and the last one was complete (ASIA-A). This clinical study was conducted during 2 months with 2 or 3 sessions of 60 min per week.

Before starting the closed loop electrostimulated exercises, the patient was asked to perform predefined flexion extension movements in his range of mobility as best as he could without any external help. This test assesses the non-electrostimulated voluntary force. The bar diagram (Fig. 11) shows the progress of the voluntary force exerted by the patients compared between the first session and the last one. The considered force was computed as a mean value of the 3 last movements.

One can easily observe that in all cases the muscles are stronger and can exert larger forces after the therapy.

During the therapeutic exercises, combined the flexion extension movements the muscles of the subjects were electrostimulated to reach the desired predefined force in each cycle. For the sake of having a clear understanding of the role of the therapy in strengthening the muscles of the subjects, the electro-induced force exerted by the leg of the subject before and after the set of therapy sessions is also measured. The following diagram (Fig. 12) shows the results of this measurement for all the five participated subjects. The increase in the electro-induced force means that the muscles response has increased during the therapy.

Figure 13 also shows the progress of the average power expended for one subject during the clinical study. The subject power increases as well with or without the electrostimulation.

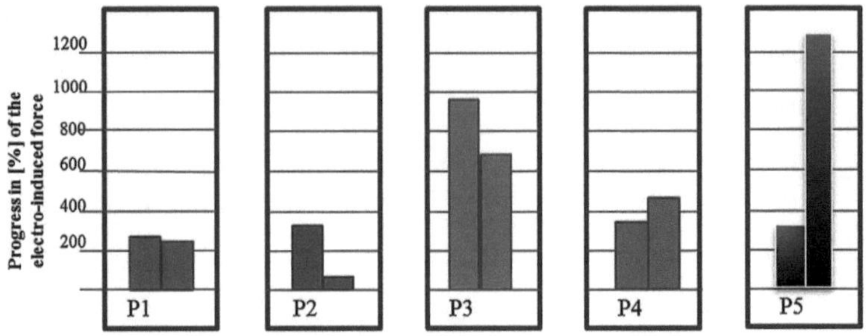

Fig. 12 Evaluation, in % between the first and the last session, of the mean electro-induced force developed without voluntary participation, for the left and right legs

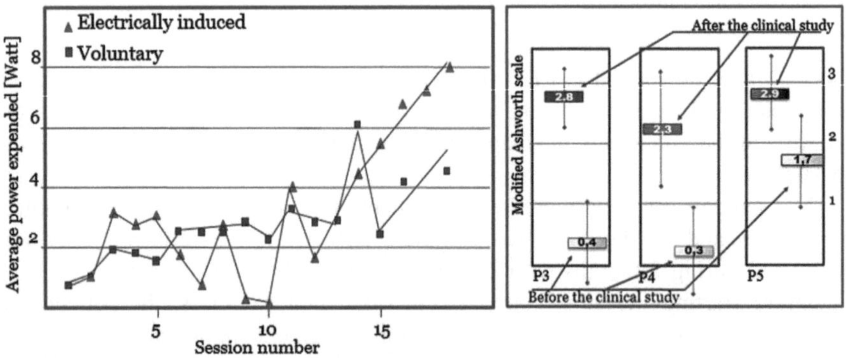

Fig. 13 *left*: Progress of the Voluntary and electrically induced expended power for one subject, *right*: Progress of the mean and standard deviation of spasticity

One of the main problems of these patients is the spasticity of their muscles. The spasticity decreases, as the muscles get stronger during the therapy treatment. This can be seen in the diagram which shows the case for three of the subjects.

3.2 Clinical Study 2

This study considered more than 24 subjects who have used the commercial MotionMaker (Fig. 5) between the years 2008 and 2012 in the CRR-Sion. The results show that almost all the subjects benefit from the therapy sessions and only few of them have not achieved any improvement (Table 2).

The diagrams in Fig. 14 show the voluntary and voluntary plus electro-stimulated forces during the therapy sessions for a sample subject.

Table 2 summarizes the progress of 24 paraplegic subjects who used the MotionMaker. The mean progress of the exerted forces is positive for practically

Table 2 List of the subjects and their progress by using the MotionMaker at the CRR

Id patient	MM use (h)	Progress (%) left leg extension	Progress (%) left leg extension	Averaged progress (%)	Appreciation
15	52	2,380	675	1,527.5	Very strong
14	6	1,460		1,460	Very strong
11	3	1,233	790	1,011.5	Very strong
12	12	1,545	258	901.5	Very strong
24	30	680	800	740	Very strong
5	24	327	863	595	Very strong
26	18	927	198	562.5	Very strong
8	36	550	130	340	Strong
27	3	77	575	326	Strong
1	22	183	243	213	Strong
37	17	191	176	183.5	Strong
2	4	137	168	152.5	Strong
10	45	107	168	137.5	Strong
46	15	97	57	77	Good
35	14	84	47	65.5	Good
31	10	−31	112	40.5	Average
53	7	20	45	32.5	Average
16	10	18	39	28.5	Average
23	9	40	15	27.5	Average
42	13	21	23	22	Average
41	16	18	7	12.5	Average
6	9	−1	14	6.5	Average
32	24	29	−29	0	NAI
19	11	−73	−67	−70	NAI

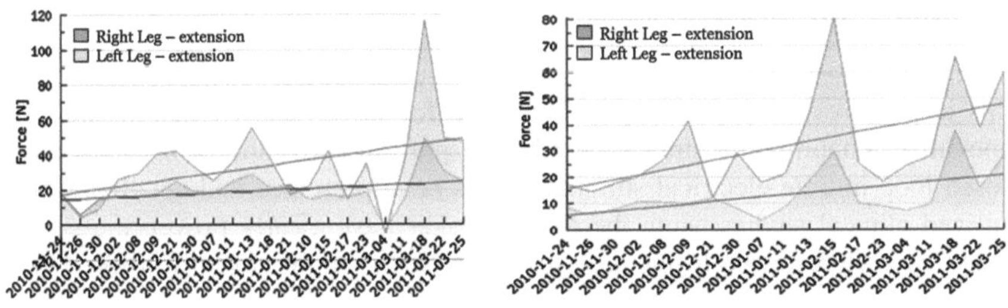

Fig. 14 Force exerted by *right* and *left legs* in sequential therapy sessions—(*left*) voluntary force (*right*): voluntary plus electrostimulated force

all the patients. Figures 15, 16 confirm that by showing the force evolution among the sessions the subjects used the MotionMaker.

The 2 subjects P19 and P32 have not registered any progress. The reasons have been evaluated as follows:

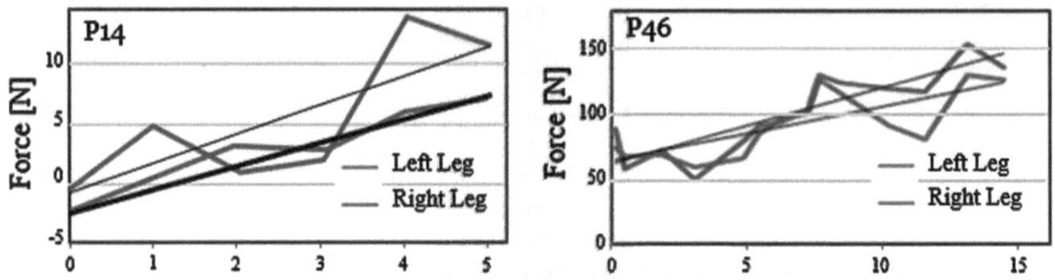

Fig. 15 Force exerted by *right* and *left* legs function of the number of sessions

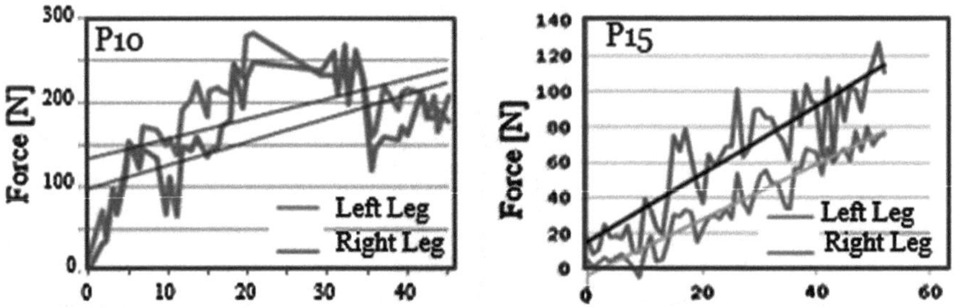

Fig. 16 Force exerted by *right* and *left legs* function of the number of sessions

- P32 is tetraplegic with a Tumor
- P19 is also a tetraplegic and had a trouble with understanding the objectives (not a French native subject).

4 Conclusion and Outlines

This chapter reviewed the usage of robotics for lower limbs rehabilitation. An innovative rehabilitation strategy combining pure mobilization of the legs and a closed loop muscle electrical stimulation has been presented and detailed. The 2 outlined clinical studies using the MotionMaker have clearly proven the contribution of such a device to increase the voluntary available extension force. The muscle electrostimulation does strengthen the muscles. Increasing the number of treatment sessions will improve the growth of the voluntary force exerted by the patient. Having stronger muscles, the spastic effects are reduced and the quality of the daily life of the paraplegics is improved.

Tetraplegia is an important topic and must be particularly considered when using the MotionMaker. The measurement of the voluntarily developed force is not necessarily the correct metrics to qualify the use of the bi-therapy offered by this device. This aspect has not been considered in this clinical study.

Another clinical study with the same set of data gathered at the CRR-SUVA during this period (2008–2012) is in progress to evaluate the correlation between the type of motion (flexion or extension) and the muscle recruitment. The importance of joint based mobilization with respect to foot based mobilization is also evaluated.

References

Bernhardt, M.F., M.; Colombo, G.; Riener, R. *Hybrid Force-Position Control Yields Cooperative Behaviour of the Rehabilitation Robot LOKOMAT.* in *9th International Conference on Rehabilitation Robotics*. 2005. Chicago, IL, USA.

Bouri, M.S., Y.; Schmitt, C.; Allemand, Y.; Gnemmi, S.; Clavel, R.; Metrailler, P.; Brodard, R., *The WalkTrainer (TM): A robotic system for walking rehabilitation.* 2006 IEEE International Conference on Robotics and Biomimetics, Vols 1-3. 2006, New York: IEEE. 1616–1621.

Brodard, R., Clavel, R., *Therapeutic and/or training device for a person's lower limbs*, U.P.U. A1, Editor. 2004.

Brodard, R., Clavel, R., *Dispositif de reeducation et/ou d'entrainement des membres inferieurs d'une personne*, E.P.E. B9, Editor. 2002.

Colombo, G.J., M.; Dietz, V. *Driven gait orthosis to do locomotor training of paraplegic patients.* in *Eng. Med. Biol.* 2000. IEEE.

Koenig A, O.X., Novak D, Riener R. *A review on bio-cooperative control in gait rehabilitation.* in *Rehabil Robot.* 2011. IEEE.

M. Bouri, R.C., *Le robot Lambda, l'innovation au service de la remise en forme*, in *ROBIO*. 2009.

Metrailler, P., *Système robotique pour la mobilisation des membres inférieurs d'une personne paraplégique*. 2005, EPFL.

Metrailler, P.B., V.; Perrin, I.; Brodard, R.; Frischknecht, R.; Schmitt, C.; Fournier, J.; Bouri, M.; Clavel, R., *Improvement of rehabilitation possibilities with the MotionMaker (TM)*, in *2006 1st Ieee Ras-Embs International Conference on Biomedical Robotics and Biomechatronics, Vols 1-3*. 2006, Ieee: New York. p. 626–631.

Riener, R., Lünenburger, L., Jezernik, S., Anderschitz, M., Colombo, G., Dietz, V. *Patient-cooperative strategies for robot-aided treadmill training: First experimental results.* in *Neuronal Systems and Rehabilitation Engineering*. 2004. IEEE.

Schmitt, C.M., P.; Al-Khodairy, A.; Brodard, R.; Fournier, J.; Bouri, M.; Clavel, R. *A Study of a Knee Extension Controlled by a Closed Loop Functional Electrical Stimulation.* in *9th Annual Conference of the International FES Society*. 2004. Bournemouth, UK.

Sciavicco, L.S., B., *Modelling and Control of Robot Manipulators*. 2000: Springer.

Stauffer, Y., *Verticalized Rehabilitation control strategies: Application to the WalkTrainer*. 2009, EPFL.

Stauffer, Y.A., Y.; Bouri, M.; Fournier, J.; Clavel, R.; Métrailler, P.; Brodard, R.; Reynard, F., *Pelvic motion measurement during over ground walking, analysis and implementation on the WalkTrainer reeducation device*, in *Intelligent Robots and Systems*, I.R.I. Conference, Editor. 2008: Acropolis Convention Center, Nice, France.

Stauffer, Y.A., Y.; Bouri, M.; Fournier, J.; Clavel, R.; Metrailler, P.; Brodard, R.; Reynard, F., *The WalkTrainer-A New Generation of Walking Reeducation Device Combining Orthoses and Muscle Stimulation.* Ieee Transactions on Neural Systems and Rehabilitation Engineering, 2009. **17**(1): p. 38–45.

Stauffer, Y.R., F.; Allemand, Y.; Bouri, M.; Fournier, J.; Clavel, R. *Pelvic motion implementation on the WalkTrainer.* in *Robotics and Biomimetics*. 2007. Sanya, China: IEEE.

Stauffer, Y.B., M.; Schmitt, C.; Allemand, Y.; Gnemmi, S.; Fournier, J.; Clavel, R.; Métrailler, P.; Brodard, R., *Cyberthèses, Mise en œuvre d'un nouveau concept de rééducation pour paraplégiques et hémiplégiques*. Journal Européen des systèmes automatisés, 2007. **41**(2): p. 261–278.

www.thera-trainer.de.

www.yaskawa.co.jp.

www.swortec.ch.

Robot-Assisted 3D Medical Sonography

P. B. Petrovic, N. Lukic and I. Danilov

Abstract This chapter presents the conceptual framework of humanoid robot application in the field of non-invasive medical diagnostics based on interactive ultrasound scanning and spatial visualisation of sonograms. Humanoid robots appear in this context as intelligent assistants which enable acquisition of 3D sonograms using the conventional ultrasound probe for 2D manual scanning through collaborative work with humans–slave mode, or through machine precision execution of the kinematic motion primitives–autonomous mode. In this way a qualitatively new technology can be created, opening the door for the development and application of new ultrasound examination techniques, which a sonographer cannot apply through conventional approaches based on free-hand 2D scanning. From the engineering aspect, the key technological step forward is the development of an anthropomorphic robotic humanoid which will enable safe and collaborative work (Co-X robotics) in a complex physical and cognitive sonographer–robot–patient interaction.

Keywords Medical ultrasound · 3D sonography · Soft robotics · Human–robot interaction

1 Introduction

Two-dimensional ultrasound sonography (2D US) is a flexible and cost-effective medical visualization technology, most widely used since the discovery of radiography. It allows the sonographer to acquire and record in real time a large number of various thin anatomical sections of the human body in the arbitrarily

P. B. Petrovic (✉) · N. Lukic · I. Danilov
Faculty of Mechanical Engineering, Belgrade University, Belgrade, Serbia
e-mail: pbpetrovic@mas.bg.ac.rs

A. Rodić et al. (eds.), *New Trends in Medical and Service Robots*,
Mechanisms and Machine Science 20, DOI: 10.1007/978-3-319-05431-5_4,

chosen plane. Also, if used correctly, 2D US has no known risks to the human health (no harmful ionizing radiation involved) and that is why it has practically unlimited diagnostic application.

However, conventional 2D US technology has several weaknesses (Downey et al. 2000). The first and the most important is strong operator dependency. The operator determines the conditions under which the ultrasound probe comes in contact with the patient's body, i.e. the intensity of the contact force and probe orientation. Especially critical is the need to memorise a large number of local sections based on which the operator reconstructs in his mental space the abstract spatial model of the observed organ. Additionally, this process is inherently time-consuming and inefficient since the operator is forced to perform multiple scans (sweeps) of the observed organ in order to gradually complete its spatial impression.

Conventional 2D US technology generates anatomical cross-sections without the exact information of their location relative to the patient's body. It is therefore impossible to accurately compare the results of sonographic examinations performed over a long period of time. This prevents adequate monitoring of pathology, i.e. the intensity of the changes on the organ under observation, or long-term effects of the treatment during the follow-up. Moreover, the recorded 2D cross-sections are static, frozen in time, which reduces the potential for subsequent analysis, especially in terms of viewing the biological structures of the organ from a more favourable plane, or eliminating the effects of organ movement due to respiration and similar dynamic processes, or inadequate patient position during the examination. The phrase 'this was missed by ultrasound' is nothing more than a choice of an inadequate scanning plane.

It is also important to mention that the quality of the generated data depends on the intensity of the contact force between the ultrasound probe and the patient's body. Generating and precisely maintaining appropriate contact force requires significant physical effort from the operator. Freehand US examination is physically challenging.

Previously mentioned weaknesses can be partially resolved by the volume imaging technology, i.e. three-dimensional sonography (3D US). Although the first three-dimensional recording was practically demonstrated in 1970, and the first commercial system of this type came to life in 1989 (Kretztechnik AG, COMBISON 330), the development of 3D US technology was not as explosive as computed tomography (CT) and magnetic resonance imaging (MRI) technologies. The reality is that 3D US is in the early stages of clinical assessment and validation, and it is gradually leaving the laboratory environment and becoming commercially available for routine clinical application (Elliott 2008). Recent technological breakthroughs in the domain of silicon ultrasonic transducers are speeding up this process. Contemporary semiconductor and microelectromechanical system (MEMS) technologies enable the construction of high-resolution large area 2D matrix arrays of micromachined ultrasound transducers integrated with application-specified integrated circuit (ASIC) processing module, which enables effective work in real time (Khuri-Yakub and Oralkan 2011; Wagner

2006). Also, semiconductor micromembranes enable reconfigurability (geometrical and functional) and variable performance of US transducers and US probes altogether (Lin et al. 2013), which gives this technology new clinical value, while the reconstructed spatial models/images became photorealistic.

Simultaneously, with the breakthroughs in research and development of a new generation of 3D US transducers, research is focused on the new, notably more complex and medically more valuable concept of robot-assisted 3D US sonography, which emerges from the convergence of 2D/3D US technology and contemporary robotic technology. As stated in (Elliott 2008), ultrasonography is, and probably always will be, a skilled profession, with that skill applied almost entirely during the stage of image acquisition, i.e. the examination. A good ultrasound practitioner will operate a complex scanning system as if playing a musical instrument, while at the same time making diagnostic decisions based upon interpretation of the displayed dynamic images. The essence of robot-assisted 3D US technology is to transfer a part of that skill to the robot by diverse implementation of the robot co-worker concept (Co-Robot), which means automating the examination, carrying it out quickly and with machine precision. In this new concept, the Co-Robot executes routine and repeatable tasks, the computer processes 2D/3D US sensory data and uses them to reconstruct spatial models of the scanned biological structures, while the sonographer and/or doctor carries out complex analyses and takes diagnostic decisions based on the processed data. In that way a new real-time imaging technology is founded, which is clinically highly valuable, and comparable to, but also with a series of advantages over CT and MRI.

This chapter presents an overview of the research activities and the basic conceptual framework of robot-assisted 3D US technology, with a focus on the physical and cognitive human–robot interaction in performing various clinical tasks which are based on the application of ultrasonography. The aim of this chapter is to identify the key research issues which are related to acquisition of specific skills and knowledge of sonographers in order to enable the Co-Robot to partially or even completely replace them in US examination or similar clinical applications. Another issue of the highest practical importance is related to the problem of the inherently non-well structured and dynamic environment, which significantly increases the complexity of the tasks performed within the robot-assisted US. This issue is also discussed in this chapter.

2 Conceptual Framework

The idea of using robotic technology to address the challenges and limitations of 2D US manual (free hand) examination goes back to the early 1990s and the first use of industrial robots configured as medical tool holders. Among the few ultrasound robots that have actually been tested in clinical environments, none have been commercialized so far. Regardless of this fact, the conceptual

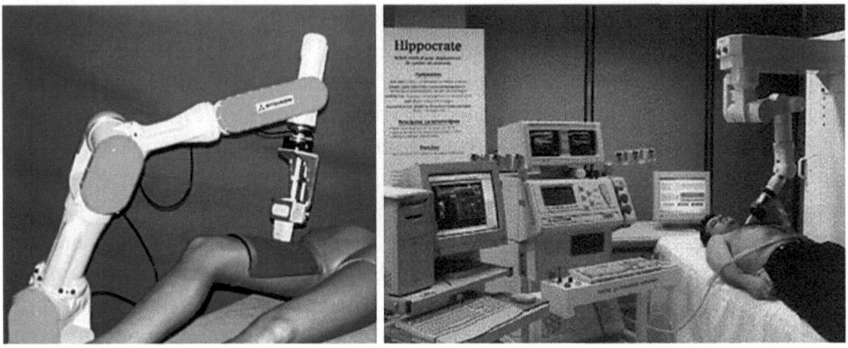

Fig. 1 The Hippocrate project: test table with force controlled Mitsubishi PA-10, 7 d.o.f. robot (*left*), and dedicated 6. d.o.f. Hippocrate robot in the environment for 3D US rendering of major blood vessels geometry (*right*)

framework of robot-assisted 3D sonography is gradually developing and maturing through a series of research projects. Evolution of this technology is illustrated by three specific robotic systems which are developed for experimental purposes in a laboratory environment.

2.1 Evolution

Probably the first system dedicated to robot-assisted 3D US was developed within the Hippocrate project. This project was initiated in 1994, with the aim of preventing cardiovascular diseases on a regular basis. The task was detection and precise analysis of atheromatous plaque using ultrasonography, where accuracy and repeatability are of tremendous importance, (Pierrot et al. 1999). The feasibility study used a 7 d.o.f. anthropomorphic robot PA-10 from the Mitsubishi Heavy Industry, which was modified to meet a good level of safety requirements (Fig. 1). The contact force between the US probe and the patient's body is directed at an interval of 1–5 N through the application of the so-called external force control scheme, (De Schutter and Van Brussel 1988), which has been proven to be the best solution regarding safety constraints. The force feedback sensor is installed on the robot tip and maximum robot speed is reduced by reconstructing its actuation system. Moreover, each individual measurement, i.e. each tomographic section acquisition, was synchronised with the heartbeat to avoid the variation of the artery diameter during the cardiac cycle. In the second stage of the project, during 1997, an intrinsically safe robot was developed in order to comply with safety constraints of robots intended for hospital use. The robot was anthropomorphic in configuration, with 6 d.o.f., suspended above the bed since this was proven to be more efficient. In essence it was a mini robot (links 2 and 3 are about 30 cm long, which was enough for both the carotid and femoral zones to be

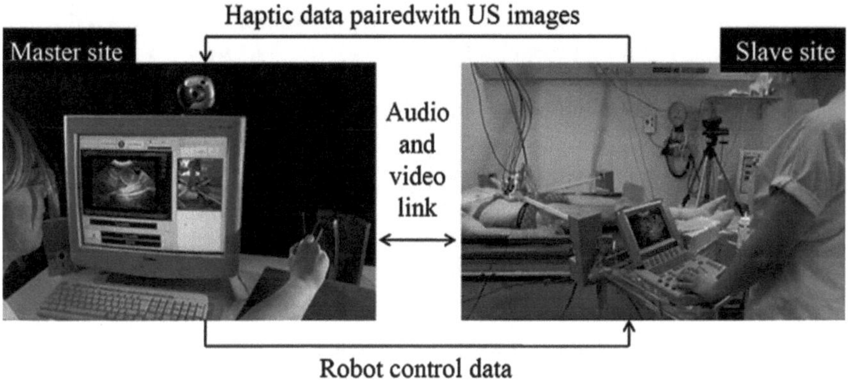

Fig. 2 Architecture of the master-slave TER robotic system for remotely operated 3D abdominal ultrasonography, (Vilchis et al. 2001)

reachable), driven by a low power stepper motor, with external 6 d.o.f. force sensor mounted on the robot tip and maximum contact force limited to 30 N (Fig. 1). The Hippocrate project was ended in a clinical validation at the Broussais Hospital in Paris in 1999.

Research which has taken place in the domain of robot-assisted tele-ultrasound examination is significant from the aspect of concept development. Unlike the Hippocrates project, their goal was to develop a teleoperated robotic system which operates the US probe in contact with the patient's body and is able to give control of those motions to the remotely located expert operator. In that way, the remote expert both acquires images and interprets them. According to the results achieved within this kind of robot-assisted US, the TER project draws special attention (Banihachemi et al. 2008). The architecture of the TER robot-assisted tele-ultrasound examination system is presented in Fig. 2.

The TER system is based on the Master-Slave concept, whereby the doctor and the patient are physically/spatially separated, and the only contact is made through a two-way audio-video connection. Using an appropriate haptic unit, the sonographer controls the motion of the probe which is placed at the tip of a cable driven parallel robot (robot tip is equipped with a specially designed mechanical interface in the form of an annular platform). Robot motion in a horizontal plane is driven by two antagonistic pairs of actuators, which move and pretense the annular platform, Fig. 3. The first version of TER robots was driven by pneumatic muscles, but they were not capable of achieving the required kinematic and positioning performances. Therefore, the second version of the TER cable robot was driven by electromotors and reducers, (Banihachemi et al. 2008). The annular platform carries a motion module with two additional degrees of freedom, dedicated to orientation of the ultrasound probe carrier. The orthogonal component of the contact force between the US probe and the patient's body was controlled within an interval of 30–270 N. The robot measuring system provides information on the

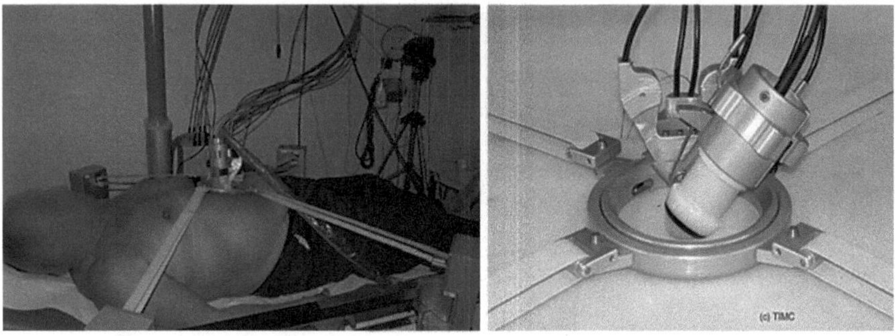

Fig. 3 Details of the TER dedicated, cable driven robot shown in contact with the patient's body (*left*) and the ultrasound probe annular interface with two additional degrees of freedom for probe orientation (*right*), (Vilchis et al. 2001)

coordinates of the probe workspace, i.e. the haptic data, which allows the formation of 3D US images. The robot repeatability was 4 mm, resolution on the working surface was 2 mm for the main translation and 1° for orientation. Such performances were quite satisfactory since the primary project goal was not to reach the given absolute location but to explore remotely an anatomical environment with continuous image feedback. The clinical validation of the second prototype was started in June 2003. VTHD optical connection (IPv6 embedded Internet protocol) between Brest and Grenoble hospitals (1,125 km) is used for remote sonographic examination of patients with abdominal aortic aneurysms.

As reported in (Vilchis et al. 2001), in its later development phases, the TER system was used for performing the first global feasibility experiments of cardiac and abdominal US exploration located in an isolated hospital of North Morocco and a satellite communication platform was employed for this purpose.

The TER project is not unique by its contents. Research in the domain of robot-assisted tele-ultrasound examination is taking place in a number of laboratories simultaneously, and as a rule of thumb, they are based on dedicated robots of different configurations, for example, the UMI robot at The University of Tokyo, (Hong et al. 2004), or the lightweight robot with parallelogram structure which allows a remote-centre-of-rotation, developed at the University of British Columbia, (Lessard et al. 2006).

From the aspect of evolution and consolidation of the general concept of robot-assisted sonography, the research delivered within (Conti et al. 2010) has high significance. It is a project based on the KUKA/DLR LWR IV universal robot with anthropomorphic configuration (Albu-Schaffer et al. 2007). As shown in Fig. 4, the robot is controlled via a haptic unit, i.e. remotely operated, as is the case with the TER system. The control system is designed to mimic the sonographer's movement, without direct physical contact with the patient and the US probe.

The LWR robot has 7 d.o.f., like a human hand. Each joint is compliant and equipped with a torque sensor which measures the driving torque delivered by the actuator to the driven segment and to the rest of the kinematic chain towards the

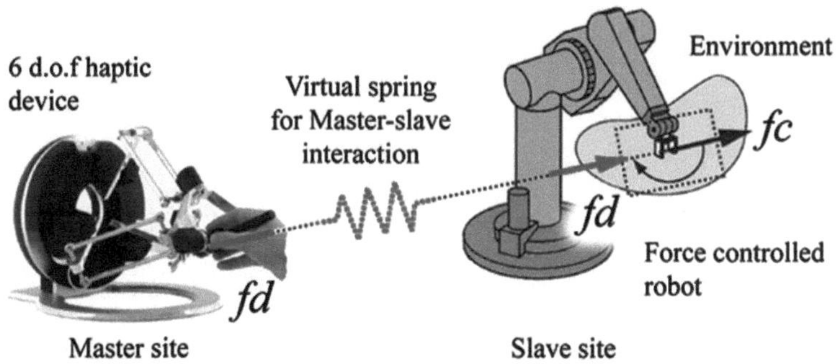

Fig. 4 Mechanical coupling of the robot arm and the haptic device achieved through the virtual spring and force control concept, as proposed in (Conti et al. 2010)

robot tip. The robot has position and torque control, it is intrinsically compliant, and includes the backdrive functionality. Payload is 15 kg, which means that the robot is capable of delivering 15 daN contact force on the environment. The robot is lightweight compared to its payload capacity (overall mass of the robot arm is 15 kg), which is important for enabling mobility and minimizing the risk of injury. This robot has high technological value for application in the field of robot-assisted US, and in general, it falls into the domain of soft robotics (Albu-Schaffer et al. 2011).

The haptic unit used to remotely control the movement of the robot-tip, and thereby the ultrasound probe, generates resistance in its motion which is proportional to the contact force between the robot and the patient's body. This allows the sonographer to feel the physical interaction between the probe and the body of the patient and to control this interaction. In order to avoid physically overloading the sonographer while performing the examination procedure, the contact force with the environment is reduced by the appropriate scaling factor. Force feedback enables mechanical coupling of the robot arm and the haptic device in the form of a virtual spring, as presented in Fig. 4. The robot has the ability to operate in 3 standard modes: floating, haptic and automatic.

Figure 5 presents the architecture of this robotic system using the phantom foetus as an example. A 3D model generated in real time is also presented in Fig. 5, bottom right.

2.2 Application Scenarios and Concept Definition

The essence of robot-assisted 3D sonography is the collaborative work of humans and robots, which in a generic sense falls into the domain of Co-X technology, i.e. Robot Coworker scenario of human–robot teamwork. Within the Co-X concept, the human has the role of the tutor, and the robot the role of the assistant, which,

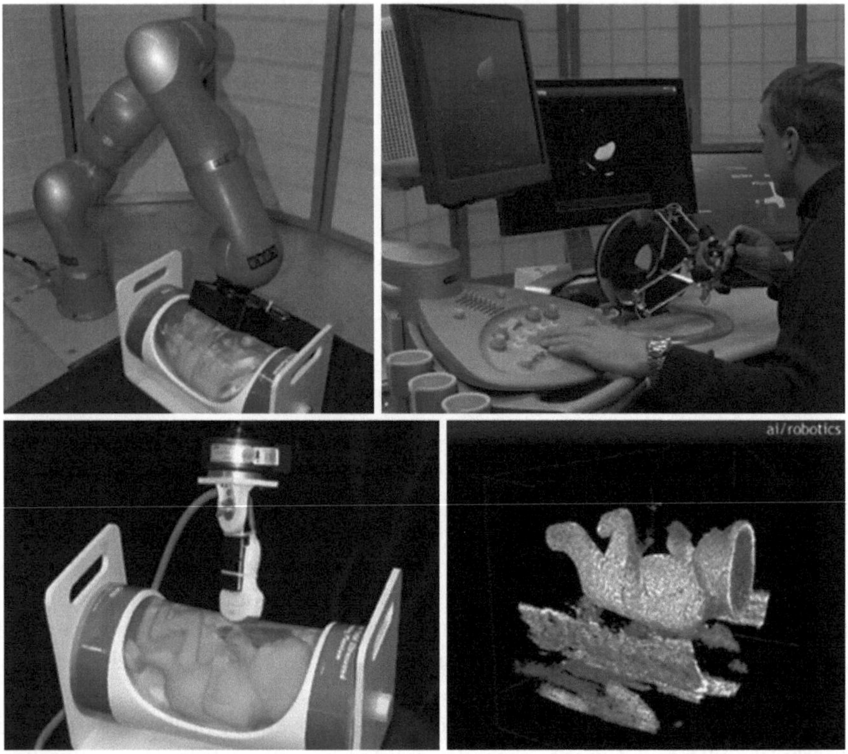

Fig. 5 The concept of robot-assisted 3D tele-operated sonography which is developed through the application of the KUKA/DLR LWR IV soft anthropomorphic robot arm, (Conti et al. 2010)

teamed up with a human or autonomously, performs certain sequences of a complex task. The concept considered here excludes tele-operation.

In general, there are two basic scenarios for clinical application of robot-assisted 3D US. The first scenario, given in Fig. 6, relates to the case of human–robot–human system with direct physical interaction. The operator (sonographer) establishes direct physical contact with the US probe, and, via the probe, physical contact with the patient.

Within the first application scenario, the robot has the role of an intelligent and mechanically flexible US probe driver. The robot has several work modes which enable various forms of behaviour during its performance of an ultrasound examination. The generated US tomographic cross-sections are synchronously paired up with the spatial coordinates of the US probe, thereby generating inherently 3D data, a factual spatial pixel cloud, regardless of whether the robot is using a linear or matrix (3D) probe. This series of tomographic recordings with added data on their spatial coordinates is sent to the acquisition system in the form of a time series. The acquisition system further processes this data and generates two basic outputs: sequential stream of 2D/3D sonograms, or reconstructed 3D

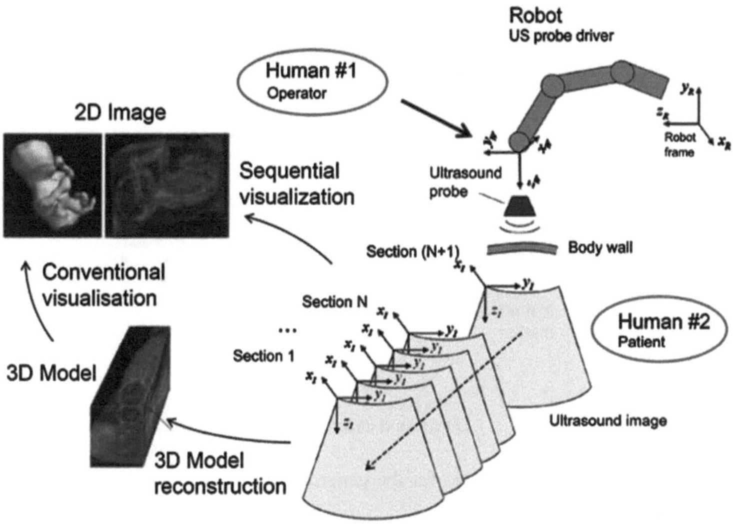

Fig. 6 The first application scenario for the generic concept of robot-assisted 3D US

surface or volume model. An appropriate human–machine interface enables visualisation and manipulation of the generated sonographic cross-sections/ models.

The second application scenario is significantly more complex and it implies multiple human and multiple robot physical interaction in the execution of a generic task of surgical instrument/needle insertion under 3D ultrasound guidance in real time. This type of application is significant for guiding minimally invasive surgical interventions when direct vision is not possible. For example, in beating heart intra-cardiac surgery the surgeon must work inside the heart while it is filled with opaque blood, thus precluding the use of an endoscopic camera (Stoll et al. 2006). The second example is a two-handed experimental system in which robot arms manipulate both the ultrasound and needle placement devices in the surgical context of liver cancer biopsy and ablation, (Boctor et al. 2004).

In the specific case shown in Fig. 7, two robots are interacting with a team of people, i.e., the surgeon, the sonographer and others, whereby one of the robots performs the function of the US probe driver and the other of the instrument/needle driver. Both robots have the role of robot co-assistant, where the US driver robot provides anatomic visual feedback so that the entire robotic system, including certain members of the human team, is in a visual servoing functional configuration. In such a system, the 3D US vision system plays a vital role by recognising the location of the instrument in relation to the target organ in the human body as it enables the surgeon to track its position with high precision and perform the surgical procedure based on the information on the actual situation in the anatomical environment.

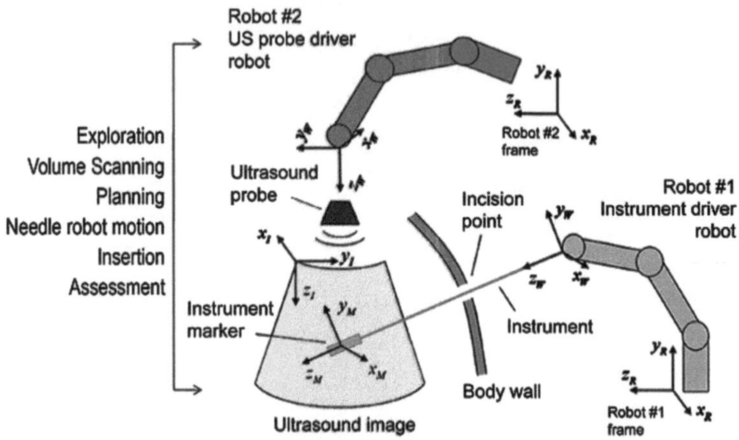

Fig. 7 The second application scenario for the generic concept of robot-assisted 3D US guided surgery

3 Building Blocks

As stated in (Conti et al. 2010), due to limited force sensing capabilities of the robots used, early systems often failed to offer sufficient compliance, dexterity and control performance. In both scenarios robot has the key role equally shared between its mechanical system, control system, as well as its higher control layers which contain cognitive functions for robot behaviour modulation in interaction with the environment, adaptation, learning and autonomy. In the past decade new robot designs were developed to better match the force requirements and back-drivable capabilities often absent in highly geared industrial robots. Especially interesting for robot-assisted 3D US application scenarios is soft robotics, (Conti et al. 2010). The notion of soft robotics in this chapter refers to anthropomorphic humanoid robots which have intrinsic compliance and backdrivability, and they are not to be mistaken for soft robots which have deformable structures that can morph between different shapes. The concept of such robots is still in the development stage and closer to laboratory than practical implementation.

From the aspect of performing the task of ultrasound examination/visualisation, the robot must encompass the following capabilities:

1. Controlled active mobility—conventional robot position control;
2. Controlled passive mobility—backdrivability, and
3. Controlled flexibility (reactive interaction with the environment) and the ability of generating and following the trajectory of the set contact force/admittance in its interaction with the environment, i.e. the patient body.

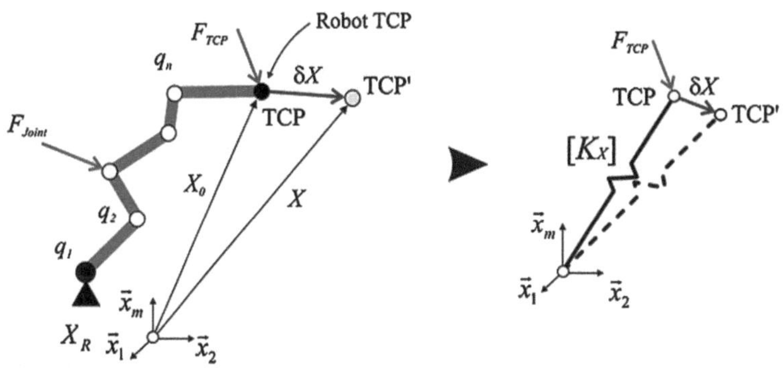

Fig. 8 Reduction of multidegrees of freedom soft robotic arm to 6 d.o.f. generalised elastic system (virtual spring) with variable and programmable stiffness

This requirement becomes more complex with the fact that the overall work environment is not entirely deterministic or a priori known. On the contrary, it is inherently non-well structured.

Such definition makes the control task significantly more complex than in conventional robots used for performing industrial tasks which include physical interaction with the environment.

Fortunately, requirements for the contact task control in robot-assisted sonography are relaxed by the fact that interaction is performed with an environment which has very low stiffness and high damping. Such a context guarantees stability in achieving the given motion command and the given contact force.

3.1 Compliance and Backdrive Control Architecture

The starting point in control system design in this specific context is understanding robots as a nonlinear elastic structure, with compliance which is concentrated in its joints.

The basic relation between the force and the geometrical domain is derived based on the model presented in Fig. 8:

$$F_{TCP} = K_X \delta X \tag{1}$$

where: F_{TCP} is the vector of the contact force with the environment, δX is the displacement vector of the robot tip, and K_X is the generalised stiffness matrix expressed in robot task coordinate system. The generalised stiffness matrix is the basic control variable which is used to shape the robot behaviour in interaction with the environment during the execution of the ultrasound examination task.

The matrix of generalised stiffness can be transformed into the actuation system matrix. This sets the task which is to be completed by joint actuators in order to

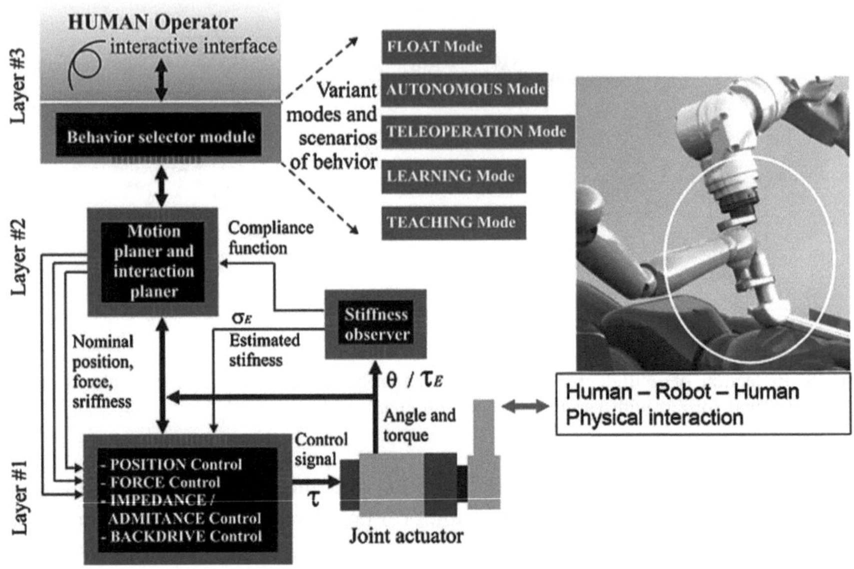

Fig. 9 General architecture of the robot control system

achieve the desired robot behaviour defined by the given generalised stiffness (1). Congruent transformation of the generalised stiffness matrix leads to:

$$K_q = J^T(q) K_X J(q), \quad K_q \in R^{n \times n} \tag{2}$$

where: $J(q)$ is the Jacobian matrix and K_q is the matrix of generalised robot stiffness in joint coordinates, i.e., the stiffness matrix of the robot actuating system. In general, K_q matrix is a nonlinear function of robot joint coordinates. Therefore, control of the generalised robot stiffness requires variable stiffness actuators (VSA). Moreover, actuating stiffness matrix K_q is non-diagonal. Physical realisation of non-diagonal stiffness members requires actuation and kinematic redundancy. VSA, kinematic and actuation redundancy, among other aspects, are one of the most important building blocks which define soft robots as a specific technological entity.

Soft robot control system has stratified architecture with three basic layers (Fig. 9). At the bottom of the hierarchy is the executive layer which is used for position and force control, as well as other more complex control primitives such as impedance/admittance and backdrive control. Great efforts have been made in the previously mentioned projects to synthesise control laws which would adequately meet the very specific conditions of controlling ultrasound probe compliant movement in contact with the human body. As part of the research activities conducted in the Cyber-Manufacturing Systems Laboratory at Belgrade University

(CMSysLab), a dedicated impedance control law has been developed with explicit control of the contact force:

$$\begin{aligned} \tau &= H(q)\Big[\ddot{q}_o + M_q(q)^{-1}\big(-B_q(q)\delta\dot{q} - K_q(q)\delta q + J^T(q)(F_{TCP} - F_o)\big)\Big] \\ &\quad + h(q,\dot{q}) - J^T(q)F_{TCP} \\ M_q(q) &= J^T(q)M_X J(q), \quad B_q(q) = J^T(q)B_X J(q) \\ K_q(q) &= J^T(q)K_X J(q), \quad \delta q = (q - q_0) \end{aligned} \tag{3}$$

This control law was originally developed for controlling robots in performing part-mating tasks in robotic assembly. The meaning of the symbols used in (3) is as follows: $H(q)$ is the robot inertia matrix, $h(q, dq/dt)$ is the nonlinear function vector, Fo is the nominal contact force which in general case function of time, $Mq(q)$ is the nominal inertia tensor, $Bq(q)$ is the nominal damping matrix, and $Kq(q)$ is the nominal stiffness matrix. The specificity of this approach lies in the fact that highly nonlinear dynamics of manipulating robot joint mechanism is reduced to the equivalent 6 d.o.f. mechanical system with concentrated mass whose dynamic behaviour in interaction with the environment is governed by the generalised inertia tensor M_X, generalised damping B_X, and generalised stiffness K_X, i.e., the parameters of the given generalised impedance. The control law is intrinsically dynamic and can be derived from the estimated dynamic robot model by using feedback linearization method for solving the problem of nonlinearity. This approach is also specific due to the fact that a single control law is used to simultaneously control position and force while at the same time enabling a change of its internal structure by changing the parameters of the given generalised impedance. This allows the control system to be transformed into various forms which, for instance, enable only position, only stiffness or combined force and position control.

The second hierarchical level of the multilayered control system contains the module for motion and interaction planning, as well as the stiffness observer module, whose basic function is to recognise the properties of the environment the robot interacts with.

Bidirectional human-operator interface which contains the robot behaviour mode selector is at the highest control level. The behaviour mode selector enables the operator, i.e., sonographer to establish complex interactions with the robot and, indirectly, with the patient, during the US examination or medical procedures (biopsies or non-invasive surgical interventions, for example). This is the key component of the control system that enables practical implementation of the Co-X concept, i.e., Robot Coworker in this specific robotic application. Behaviour mode selector and motion/interaction planner make the cognitive core of the control system in robot-assisted ultrasonography.

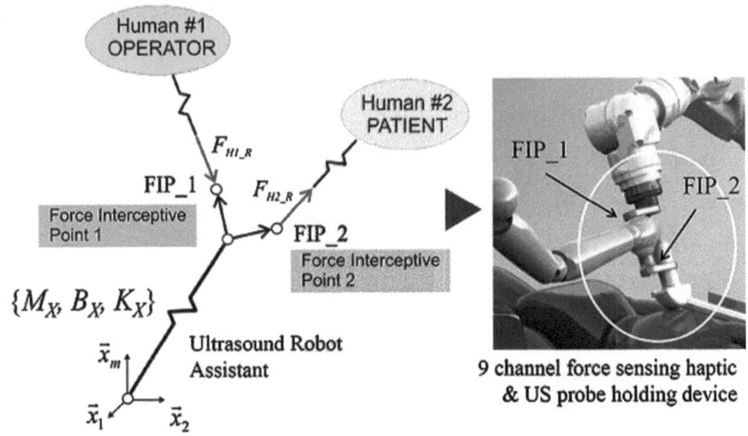

Fig. 10 The general model of simultaneous multiple human–robot interaction achieved through a dedicated haptic interface with 9 sensory channels with appropriate force interceptive points

3.2 Modes of Human–Robot Interaction in 3D US

Within the Robot Coworker scenario of human–robot teamwork in a 3D sonography system, the sonographer has the role of the tutor, while the robot performs the role of the assistant. In this specific context, the robot establishes twofold interaction with humans, as, besides the interaction with the sonographer, the robot also interacts with the patient, who, unlike the sonographer, has a passive role. Therefore, the robot must be capable of establishing complex physical and cognitive interaction with more than one human simultaneously. Figure 10 shows a generic robot model with multiple human–robot interaction. CMSysLab is working on developing a special haptic interface with two interceptive channels which enable simultaneous acquisition of the contact force with the sonographer and the patient based on the redundant force sensing system.

Generally, the following robotic system modes are relevant for robot-assisted sonography:

1. Float mode—Robot behaves as a passive assistant
   - Robot compensates for the gravitational forces only and allows the operator to freely move the robot by hand in order to place the US probe in the desired position and orientation. It also enables the operator to manually acquire US data.
   - Robot applies contact force generated by the operator hand using 9 ch. force sensing haptic and US probe interface. The force applied by the operator can be augmented and limited for patient safety.
   - Robot maintains nominal contact force.

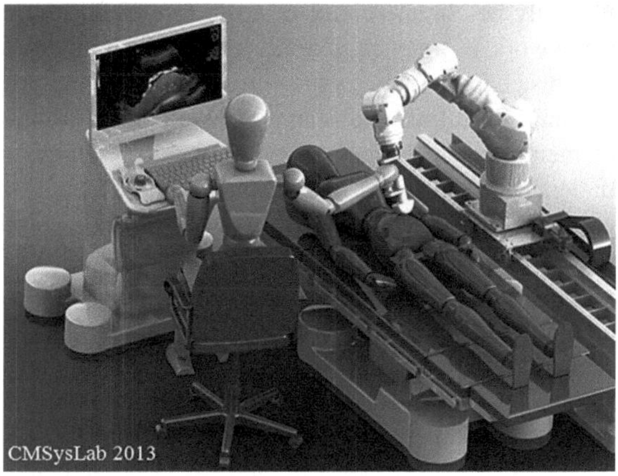

Fig. 11 Virtual model of a robot-assisted 3D medical sonography system, which is under development in the CMSysLab: active flexible humanoid arm—robot Yaskawa SIA 10F carries the ultrasound probe and, through various modes of interactive operation, enables a wide range of behaviours in a cooperative sonographer–robot–patient system

- Robot maintains nominal orientation of the US probe relative to the patient's body.

2. Autonomous mode—Automatic 3D sweep scans, or repetition of previously recorded and validated (learned) scanning paths together with recorded and postprocessed contact force patterns.
3. Learning (passive) mode—Acquiring and generalizing behaviour of the operator, i.e., operator skill transfer to the robot.
4. Teaching (active) mode—Education of the unskilled operator.

As needed, the operator can freely choose one of the previously listed modes and in that way change the behaviour or the role of the robot in performing ultrasound examination.

Figure 11 shows a virtual model of a robot-assisted 3D medical sonography system which is currently under developed at the CMSysLab. The system is based on the 7 d.o.f. anthropomorphic robot arm Yaskawa SIA10F, with 10 kg payload and 810 mm reach, which was adapted to this type of application using the MotoPlus open control development system. The concept which is being developed within this project is based on direct human–robot interaction and excludes tele-operation.

4 Conclusion

The technology of ultrasound sonography has remarkable clinical potential and a number of advantages in comparison to the alternative methods of medical anatomic imaging. The shortcomings of conventional 2D ultrasonography can be reduced by introducing 3D sonography and applying robotic technology. In time, 3D ultrasound will supersede 2D ultrasound, and robot-assisted ultrasonography will become a competitive alternative to CT or MRI technologies, and it will probably be commercialized in the foreseeable future. In order to implement this framework in practice, extensive multidisciplinary research is needed.

This chapter analyses the current research and proposes the concept of a robotic assistant for ultrasound scanning based on soft robots (industrial humanoids), with elements of intelligent robot behaviour, which is aware of the context and understands the needs of the sonographer. Such a robot features general compliance, selective compliance, backdrivability, ability to generate appropriate impedance/admittance of the ultrasound probe and to generate and maintain the given contact force.

Our future activities will be focused on: (1) Generic issues in VSA and soft humanoid robotics, (2) Building a multidisciplinary team for conducting research in parallel engineering and the medical domain, (3) Development of open architecture experimental robotic platform for 3D US imaging based on 7 d.o.f. Yaskawa SIA10F robot arm, and (4) Development of time- and computationally-effective algorithms for ultrasound data processing, recognition, spatial model building/reconstruction and imaging.

Acknowledgments This research work is supported by the Serbian Ministry for Education, Science and Technology Development through the project titled Smart Robotics for Customized Manufacturing, grant No: TR35007.

References

Albu-Schaffer A., at all, “The DLR lightweight robot: Design and control concepts for robots in human environments”, Industrial Robot: An Int. J. 34/5, pp: 376–385, 2007.

Albu-Schaffer A., at al., Anthropomorphic Soft Robotics – From Torque Control to Variable Intrinsic Compliance, Robotics Research: The 14th Int. Symp. ISRR, pp 185–207, 2011.

Banihachemi J.J., at al., TER: A Robot for Remote Ultrasonic Examination: Experimental Evaluations, Telesurgery, Springer Verlag (Ed.)), pp: 91–99, 2008.

Boctor E. M., Fischer G., Choti M.A., Fichtinger G., Taylor R.H., A dual-armed robotic system for intraoperative ultrasound guided hepatic ablative therapy: a prospective study, ICRA ‘04 IEEE Int. Conference on Robotics and Automation, pp 2517–2522 Vol.3, 2004.

Conti F, Park J., and Khatib O, Interface Design and Control Strategies for a Robot-assisted Ultrasonic Examination System, Proc. of the International Symposium on Experimental Robotics, New Delhi, India, December 2010.

De Schutter J. and Van Brussel, H., (1988) Compliant robot motion - II – a control approach based on external control loop, The Int. J. of Robotic Research, Vol. 7(4), pp. 18–13.

Downey, D., Fenster A., Williams J.C., Clinical Utility of Three-dimensional US, Imaging & Therapeutic Technology, March-April 2000, Volume 20, Number 2, pp: 559–571.

Elliott, S.T., Volume ultrasound: the next big thing?, The British Journal of Radiology, 81, pp 8–9, 2008, DOI: 10.1259/bjr/13475432.

Hong J., et al., An Ultrasound-driven Needle Insertion Robot for Percutaneous Cholecystostomy,” Phys. Med. Biol., Vol. 49, issue 3, pp 441–455, 2004.

Khuri-Yakub, B. T. and Oralkan, O., Capacitive micromachined ultrasonic transducers for medical, imaging and therapy, J. of Micromech. Microeng., vol. 21, No. 5, (11 pp). 2011.

Lessard S. et al. Parallel Robot for Medical 3D-Ultrasound Imaging, IEEE International Symposium on Industrial Electronics, 2006.

Lin D.S., et al., Packaging and Modular Assembly of Large-Area and Fine-Pitch 2-D Ultrasonic Transducer Arrays, Ultrasonics, Ferroelectrics and Frequency Control, IEEE Transactions on, vol. 60, no. 7, pp.1356–1375, Jul. 2013.
Pierrot F., et al., Hippocrate: A safe robot arm for medical applications with force feedback, Med. Image Anal., vol. 3, no. 3, pp. 285–300, 1999.
Stoll J., Novotny P., Howe R., Dupont P., Real-time 3D ultrasoundbased servoing of a surgical instrument, IEEE Int. Conf. on Robotics and Automation, pp 613−618, 2006.
Vilchis A., et al., TER: A system for robotic tele-echography, in Proc. 4th Int. Conf. Medical Image Computing and Computer Assisted Intervention, 2001, pp. 326–334.
Wagner P. Silicon Ultrasound — Technology for the Future, Medical Solutions RSNA: Siemens Medical Solutions; 2006.

Innovative Approaches Regarding Robots for Brachytherapy

D. Pisla, N. Plitea, B. Galdau, C. Vaida and B. Gherman

Abstract This chapter presents an overview of the most important innovative approaches in Brachytherapy. Brachytherapy is an advanced cancer treatment technique, where radioactive seeds are delivered directly in the tumor without damaging the proximal healthy tissues. A medical protocol for the robotized brachytherapy procedure is described. Latest achievements in robotic assisted brachytherapy provided by several worldwide research centers are presented. Their critical analysis has shown that the already developed structures are built for specific organs and moreover almost all are targeting the prostate In order to overcome the limitations of current robotic systems for brachytherapy and to make possible an universal technique for cancer treatment on several organs of human body within brachytherapy, a new family of modular parallel robots is presented.

Keywords Brachytherapy · Robotic assisted brachytherapy · Parallel robot · Kinematic analysis

1 Introduction

> The purpose of medicine is to prevent significant disease, to decrease pain and to postpone death. Technology has to support these goals-if not, it may even be counterproductive.
>
> —Joel J. Nobel.

Cancer (Wikipedia Dictionary, http://en.wikipedia.org/) (scientific name: Malignant neoplasm) is a class of diseases characterized by the uncontrolled division of a group of cells that have the ability to invade other tissues in the body,

D. Pisla (✉) · N. Plitea · B. Galdau · C. Vaida · B. Gherman
Research Center for Industrial Robots Simulation and Testing,
Technical University of Cluj-Napoca, Cluj-Napoca, Romania
e-mail: Doina.Pisla@mep.utcluj.ro

A. Rodić et al. (eds.), *New Trends in Medical and Service Robots*,
Mechanisms and Machine Science 20, DOI: 10.1007/978-3-319-05431-5_5,

either by direct growth into adjacent tissues (invasion) or by cell migration to distant places in the body (metastasis). An uncontrolled cell division is triggered by abnormal DNA of cancer cells.

Research centers from all over the world focus their work on developing advanced robotic solutions for various medical applications (Tarnita and Marghitu 2013) by studying new solutions or by improving existing ones (Talaba 2012; Ottaviano et al. 2011).

There are many cases where the treatment options for cancer are scarce (Ottaviano et al. 2011; Tornes and Eriksen 2009; Podder et al. 2010a), but at the same time there are many therapeutic approaches in the fight against cancer like: surgery, irradiation, chemotherapy or a combination of them, followed by rehabilitation in strong dependence with the specific patient needs: inversion therapy (Kacso 2005), robotized massage beds and so on. In radiation therapy high-energy rays are used to damage cancerous cells. It can be used as single therapy or in combination with cancer treatments (Mateescu 2010). The traditional radiation therapy affects the entire body damaging also healthy tissue, but the researchers developed alternative therapies, aiming to concentrate the radiation in the tumor area with higher dosage, to increase the treatment positive effects while minimizing the adverse ones. One of the advanced techniques is the brachytherapy (BT). This involves the placement of the miniaturized radioactive sources very precisely in the tumor area, delivering high dosage of radiation in the cancerous cells. Its positive results are demonstrated, and its side effects are reduced to a minimum, but it requires very high positioning precision and a clear linear path to the tumor (Shah et al. 2010). BT is used for the treatment of tumors located in areas proximal to the skin, such as cervical (Davidson et al. 2008), lung (Shah et al. 2010), breast but many studies showed its positive results in other body sites (Oudard et al. 2009). The widest spread BT application is the treatment of prostate cancer (Jiang et al. 2010; Carpenter et al. 2011).

As a clear limitation in the use of BT stand its accuracy requirements for the radioactive seeds placement inside the tumors (Buzurovic et al. 2010). For that, many research institutes focused on the development of robotic devices aiming to increase the placement precision of the BT devices, but most of them are dedicated only for prostate therapy. Yu et al. (2006) present a modular robot for ultrasound guided robotic prostate BT, consisting of a ultrasound probe drives and a 3 DOF gantry robot. Fischer et al. (2006) present a 4 DOF hybrid robot for real-time control transperineal prostate needle orientation under MRI guidance and perform the insertion motion manually. Jiang et al. (2010) developed a prototype and 3D model of a 5 DOF hybrid robot for prostate needle insertion surgery under continuous MRI guidance. As a conclusion to the state of the art reference is made to the study (Podder et al. 2010a) published by the American Association of Physicists in Medicine (AAPM) in 2010 where the 13 robotic systems developed for prostate cancer were analyzed. This study clearly points out that until now, research has been focused on the brachytherapy treatment of the prostate (due to the much simpler imagistic feedback) emphasizing the need of additional robotic devices capable to guide the brachytherapy needles in other body locations.

This work presents a possible solution for this request, proposing a family of brachytherapy robotic systems for general BT working under real-time CT guidance, including the treatment for internal organs like: liver, lungs, paravertebral areas, etc.

The chapter is organized as follows: Sect. 2 presents modern methods for cancer treatment. Section 3 illustrates the latest achievements in robotic assisted brachytherapy. Section 4 deals with a new family of innovative structures of parallel robots for BT, developed based on the medicals specifications. Some conclusions are presented in the last section.

2 Modern Methods for Cancer Treatment

Cancer is treated in several ways (Fig. 1), depending on each person's medical condition and the type of cancer (Mateescu 2010).

Laser therapy uses light to treat cancer cells. Lasers are used to remove very small tumors without affecting the surrounding tissue. **Radiation therapy** represents therapeutic radiology or radiant oncology, which uses special kinds of energy waves or particles to fight cancer and sometimes non-cancerous diseases. **Chemotherapy** is one of the most common treatments for cancer, which uses drugs to treat cancerous cells. **Hormone therapy**. Hormones are chemical substances produced by glands such as the ovaries and testes; it helps to certain types of cancer cells to grow, such as breast cancer and prostate cancer. **Biological therapy** uses the body's immune system to fight against cancer. The immune system may be also able to determine differences between healthy cells and cancer cells in the body, and to eliminate cancer cells. **Therapy with angiogenesis inhibitors** is a process controlled by certain chemicals produced in the body. Sometimes called antiangiogenic therapy, this experimental treatment can prevent the development of cancer by blocking the formation of new blood vessels. **Hyperthermia** is based on heat treatment and it was used for centuries as a treatment. **Surgery** is the oldest form of cancer treatment according to the American Cancer Society (ACS). Another treatment is **Brachytherapy**.

2.1 Brachytherapy (BT)

Brachytherapy is an **innovative option** called also **internal radiation**, which enables the physician to deliver higher doses of radiation to more-specific areas of the body, compared with the conventional form of radiation therapy that projects radiation from a machine outside the body.

BT involves the placement of tiny radioactive miniaturized sources very precisely in the tumor area, delivering high dosage of radiation in the cancerous cells. The major difference in comparison with conventional methods refers to the fact

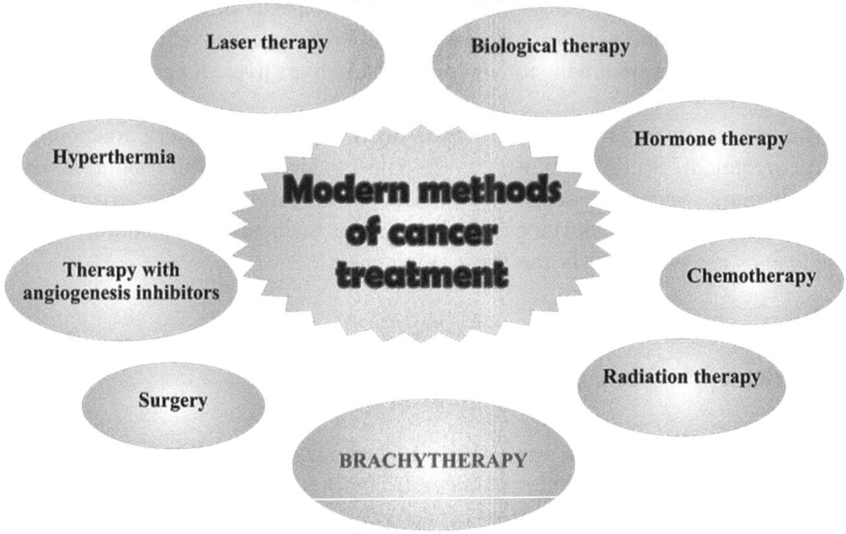

Fig. 1 Modern methods of cancer treatment

that the radiation source is placed in or in close proximity to the body region to be irradiated. Radiation effect is felt only on a very limited region, thus maximizing the impact on the target area without affecting the entire patient body. It is an efficient therapy, being currently used for cancer treatment in: cervical area, prostate, breast and on skin level but major efforts are done to extend the BT use in many other body sites.

Its effectiveness is clearly demonstrated, its side effects are reduced to a minimum but it involves several **important conditions**: the catheters delivering the radioactive sources **must be placed precisely**, as the radiation dose decreases abruptly from the base and an incorrect positioning causes the necrosis of healthy tissue without affecting the tumor; the radiology therapist needs to find out a way **to place the catheters inside the tumor**.

Advantages of brachytherapy: the risk of local side effects is limited; acute or subacute side effects are reduced normally within a few days or a few weeks; it depends on the clinical presentation of the disease and may be combined with other forms of therapy, for example, an operation, an external radiation therapy or chemotherapy; greater effect; good compatibility; protection of neighboring tissue and nearby organs.

Besides the above mentioned advantages, BT has some **limitations**: the doctor should introduce into the tumor a number of needles with a 1.6 mm diameter, through that radioactive seeds will be introduced later. These needles are straight, rigid and must be placed on a linear trajectory which can be defined easily on the basis of imaging data obtained by CT / MRI, but especially for deeply located tumors the needle placement is impossible without visual feedback; the accuracy required by the medical procedure is 1 mm from the target point, which is very hard to achieve due to tissue and needle elasticity, a recent study (Strassman et al. 2011) showing that manual placement is limited to around 3 mm (2.7 ± 0.7 mm).

There are two possible options for the minimally invasive brachytherapy:

Echo-guided manually insertion of needles. The solution is simple but limited to visible areas with ultrasound. The most common brachytherapy treatment technique is for **prostate**, where an ultrasound probe is inserted through the anus, allowing very precise control of the needles position in the prostate. In the case of manual technique, is also used an auxiliary element, that is a sieve having a pattern of holes which is mechanically attached to the patient skin (being sewn), which ensures to a large extent the correct trajectory of the needle. However, geometrically is shown that at a distance of 200 mm, an error of more than 0.3° from the point of insertion, generates positioning error over 1 mm, which makes it impossible to apply this technique in the proximal area of blood vessels or organs sensitive.

Achievement of a precise and rigid positioning device, which can target any area of the body, enabling also the visual monitoring of the positioning trajectory (real-time or interim positions). It results that the development of a robotic assisted brachytherapy system is a necessity. The main objectives for a robotic assisted brachytherapy device are to improve accuracy of needle placement and seed delivery, consistency of seed implant, avoidance of critical structures (blood vessels, nerves, and neighboring organs) and to reduce the learning curve.

Functional requirements: quick and easy disengagement in case of emergency; provision for reverting to conventional manual brachytherapy at any time; method for the clinician to review and approve the motion plan before needle placement; visual feedback during needle insertion using a CT scan device; visual confirmation of each seed deposition or the needle tip at the resting position; ease of cleaning and decontamination; compatible for sterilization of the required components; ease of operation in the OR (Operating Room) environment; robust and reliable; safe for the patient, clinician, and the OR environment.

3 Robotic Assisted Brachytherapy

Definition of the medical application. The robotic structure should introduce, based on radiologic data, rigid needles of diameter varying from 0.6 mm up to 2 mm and a length from 50 mm up to 250 mm inside the patient body following a linear trajectory. Due to the long distances, the variable tissue density it is compulsory to ensure constant precision for the entire displacement and to avoid any deviations from the predefined trajectory (Fig. 2).

Based on the definition of the medical application it was developed a protocol for the robotic brachytherapy procedure (Plitea et al. 2014).

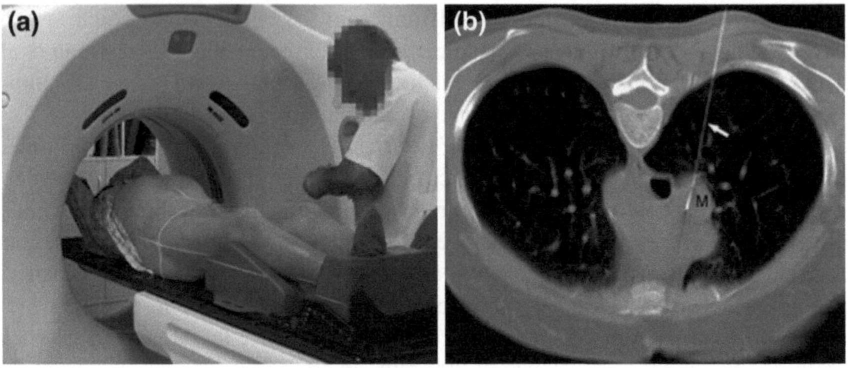

Fig. 2 Brachytherapy procedure: **a** Placement of external markers on the patient body for calibration, **b** Validating the correct needle insertion by CT scan control (Gupta et al. 2005)

1. The medical data is received from the physicians defining the target points locations and the desired linear trajectories.
2. The patient is placed in the CT device and immobilized in a predefined position, then calibrated with respect the laser system of the machine (Fig. 2a).
3. The robot frame is rigidly fixed near the CT table and calibrated with respect to the laser system. After this step the robot must remain fixed until the procedure ends.
4. Based on the medical data provided, the needle is oriented parallel with the linear trajectory to be achieved.
5. The needle is superposed over the imposed trajectory.
6. The needle is driven along the trajectory.
7. The correct needle position is checked by scanning the patient with the CT machine (Fig. 2b). If needed, corrections are applied.
8. If multiple needles must be inserted, if the trajectories are pure parallel, steps 5–8 are repeated, otherwise steps 4–8 must be performed.

3.1 Past and Present Development in Robotic Assisted Brachytherapy

Due to the tremendous therapeutic potential of brachytherapy, many research centers in the world have tried to provide solutions for the enhanced placement of BT devices inside the patient body, thus developing into a special category of "positioning devices", namely brachytherapy robotic systems (Fig. 3).

Yu et al. (2006) develop a robotic system Endo–Uro Computer Lattice for Intratumoral Delivery, Implantation, and Ablation with Nanosensing (EUCLIDIAN). The prototype robotic system comprised of a 9 DOF Positioning Module and a 7

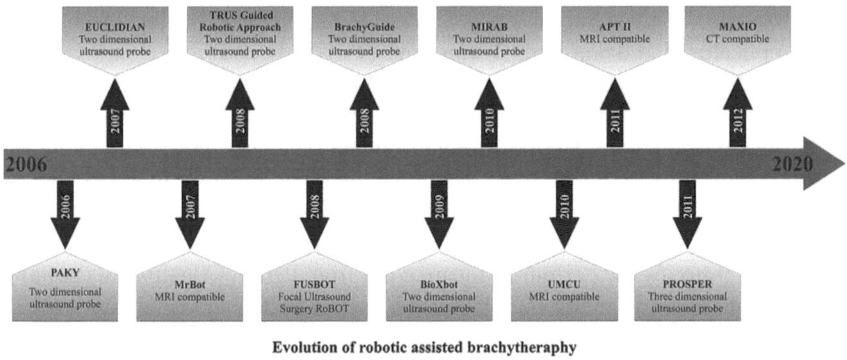

Fig. 3 Evolution of robotic assisted brachytherapy

DOF Surgery Module. Positioning module consists of: Cart (3 DOF), Supporting Platform (6 DOF) and the Surgery module of: ultrasound probe driver (2 DOF), gantry (3 DOF), needle driver (2 DOF), seed pusher, teach pendant.

Stoianovici et al. (2007) construct **MrBot**, the first fully-actuated MRI robot, in the form of a platform supported by articulated linear actuators in a 5 DOF parallel link structure. All components are designed of nonmagnetic and dielectric materials that have been successfully tested for MRI. MrBot is customized for transperineal needle insertion.

Another brachytherapy robotic system designed by Fichtinger et al. (2007) is **TRUS** Guided Robotic Approach. The robot consists of two 2D Cartesian motion stages arranged in a parallel configuration. The xy stage provides planar motion relative to the mounting posts, in the plane that corresponds to the face of the template. The workspace of ±4 cm in each direction is sufficient to cover the prostate with a generous margin. The $\alpha\beta$ stage rides on the xy stage, with a workspace of ±2 cm.

BrachyGuide by Septimiu et al. (2008). A two-axis wrist is positioned by a translation stage consisting of two stacked nickel-plated aluminum. The first translation stage in the Y (vertical) axis is mounted to the brachytherapy stepper. The slider of the X axis Unislide is mounted to the slider of the Y-axis Unislide.

Chauhan et al. (2008) provided a robotic system called **FUSBOT** (Focal Ultrasound Surgery Robots) developed for several clinical applications, such as breast surgery (FUSBOT BS), urological (FUSBOT U.S.) and neurosurgery (FUSBOT NS). Their common features include: use of image-guided, interactive control and supervision of the surgeon. Once they decide surgical protocol, the robot positions accurately all transducers at the locations specified so that the focus coincides with the position of the lesion once planned on a 2D image.

Podder et al. (2010b) designed **MIRAB**. The MIRAB is a 6 DOF robot capable of inserting and rotating 16 needles concurrently and depositing seeds autonomously according to the dosimetric plan. The MIRAB consists of five modules:

Rotary Needle Adapter, Surgical x–y Carrier, Mounting and Driving Mechanism, Seed Applicator, and Transrectal Ultrasound (TRUS) Driver.

PROSPER presented by Hungr et al. (2012). It consists of two primary elements: a 5 degrees of freedom (DOF) needle positioning module and a 2 DOF needle insertion module. The positioning module positions the needle along the appropriate insertion axis, allowing needle inclinations in the sagittal and coronal planes. The insertion module drives the needle to a given depth and can rotate the needle during insertion if necessary. The clinician inserts the seed manually.

MAXIO (http://www.perfinthealthcare.com) from Perfinth Healthcare (India) is a 5 DOF robotic arm for use in ablation, biopsy, drug delivery, drainage, robotic assistance for placing the probe. Positioning module is fixing each side of the CT table on the floor of stainless steel and a robotic arm. MAXIO robotic arm has movements with accuracy of less than 1 mm and less than one degree. This ensures that the procedures can be performed at different table heights, reach difficult lesions that require more angulation focusing on patient demographics.

4 New Modular Parallel Robots for Brachytherapy

The Research Center for Industrial Robots Simulation and Testing (CESTER) developed a family of modular parallel robots for brachytherapy. The kinematic scheme of the first robotic solution is illustrated in Fig. 4, with two 3D models illustrated in Fig. 5. The robot has a modular architecture, consisting of a parallel module with M = 3 DOF and family F = 1, of type 2CRRU with three active joints and a second parallel module with M = 3 DOF and family F = 1, of type CRU with two active joints (Podder 2010b).

The BR1 structure, has a modular architecture, the first module, type 2CRRU, integrating 4 revolute passive joints which connect the mobile platform of the module 2CRRU to the first Cardan joint. The second module, type CRU, uses two additional revolute which connect to the second Cardan joint of the robot. These joints are illustrated in the scaled model presented below (Fig. 6).

The second structure uses two modules working in cylindrical coordinates, its kinematic scheme being illustrated in Fig. 7. The two modules are positioned vertically on the lateral sides of the fixed frame with respect to the CT table, one having three active joints while the second one only two. Two 3D models are presented in Fig. 8.

Each module has two active translational joints consisting ball-screws actuated by motors 1, 2 respectively motors 4 and 5 (Fig. 7) (Plitea et al. 2014). For the first module, with three actuated joints, the translational active joints move two bushings on the grooved shaft which represents an active revolute joint actuated by the motor 3. The bushings move linear with the translational joints and rotate with the grooved shaft. For the second module, which has only two active joints, the grooved shaft is replaced by a cylindrical shaft which acts as a passive, driven, revolute joint. Both modules work in cylindrical coordinates.

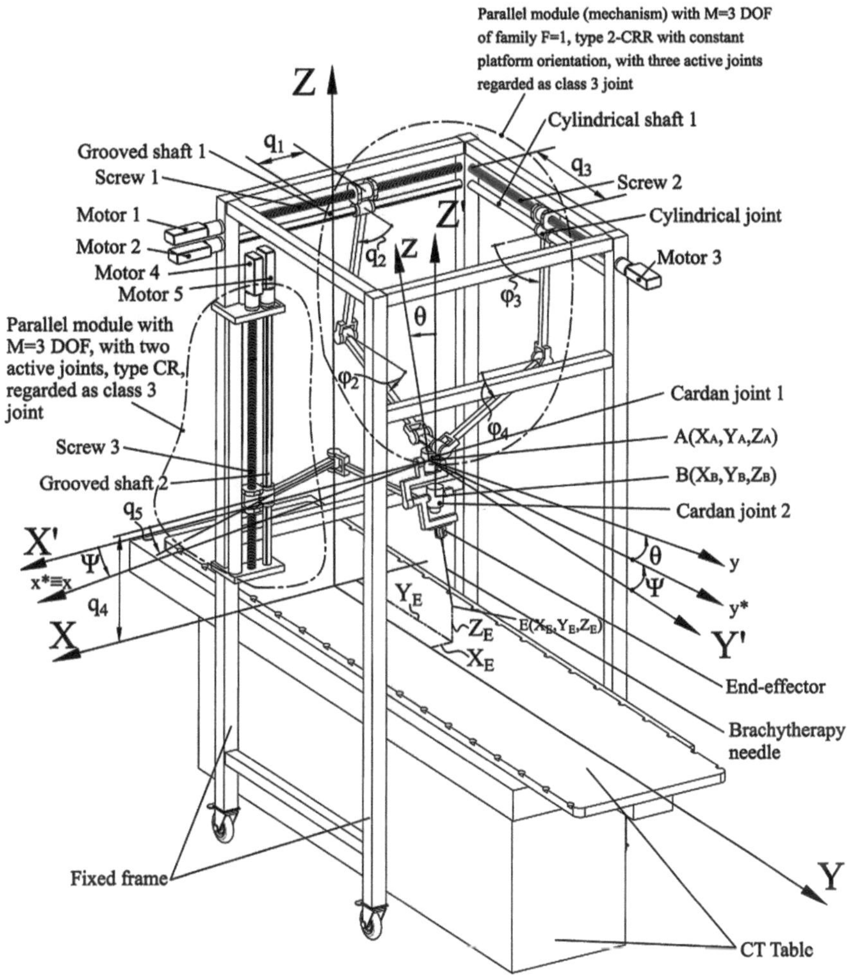

Fig. 4 Parallel robot, BR1, with M = 5 DOF and family F = 1 with modular construction having two kinematic chains for the platform guidance of type 2CRRU and CRU using rotary motors (Plitea et al. 2013a)

The kinematic scheme of the BR3 cylindrical parallel robot consists of two modules, the first one having 3 DOF and 3 active joints and a second module with 3 DOF and 2 active joints. The first two joints of each cylindrical module are translational joints, while the third motion is a rotational one around the axis of the first joints, whereas the first module has an active joint while the second one a passive joint. A scaled model of this structure is illustrated in Fig. 9.

Based on the simulation results of all the 3D models developed, after a thorough analysis conducted together with a team of oncology specialists the model presented in Fig. 9 has been selected for further developments. Thus an experimental

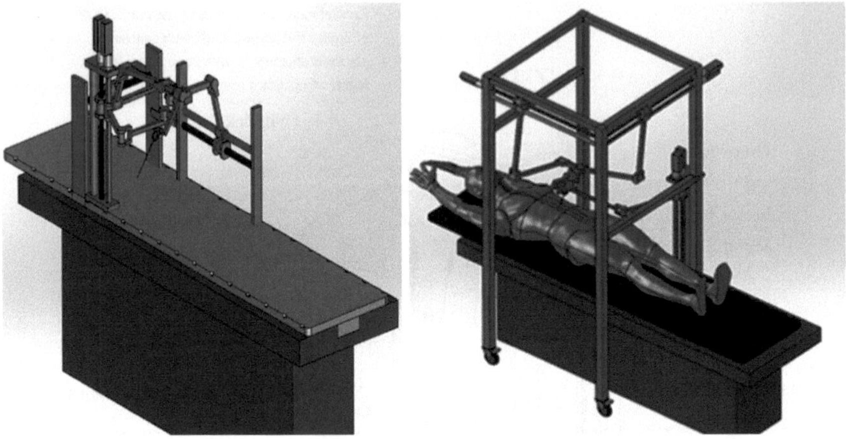

Fig. 5 The two 3D models of the parallel robot with M = 5 DOF type 2CRRU-CRU

Fig. 6 The scaled model of the BR1 robotic structure

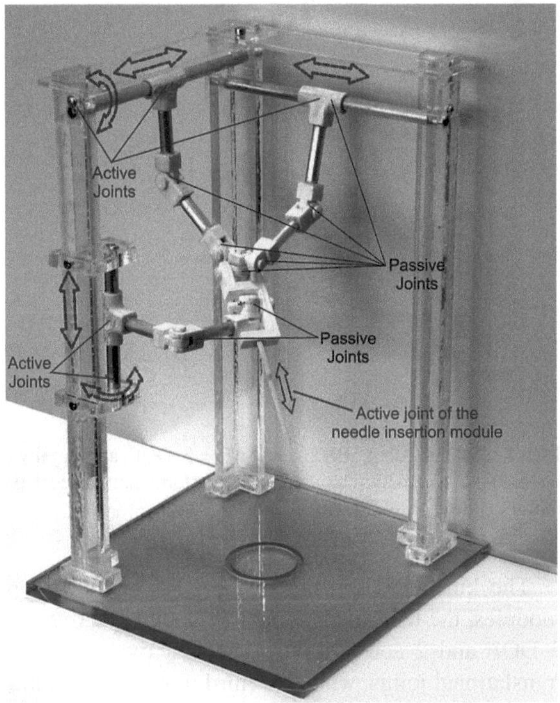

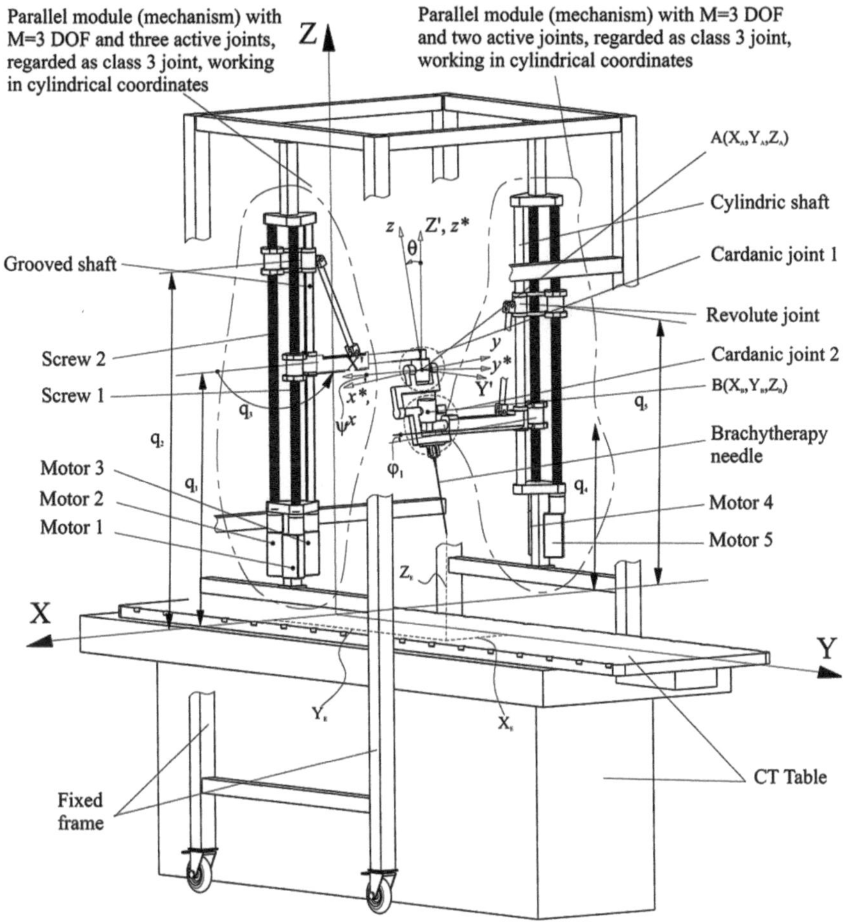

Fig. 7 Parallel robot with M = 5 DOF and family F = 1 with modular construction having two kinematic chains for the platform guidance working in cylindrical coordinates (Plitea et al. 2013b)

model is currently under construction. The constructive solution, entitled PARA-BRACHYROB has been tested in a virtual environment which includes a CT-Scan type GE Lightspeed 6RT specially designed for BT use. Figures 10 and 11 illustrate the robot capacity to target liver tumors (Fig. 10) and neck tumors (Fig. 11).

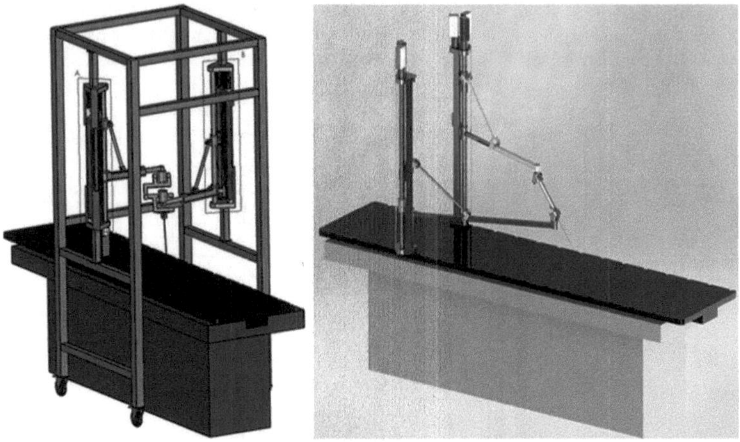

Fig. 8 The two 3D models of the parallel robot with M = 5 DOF working in cylindrical coordinates

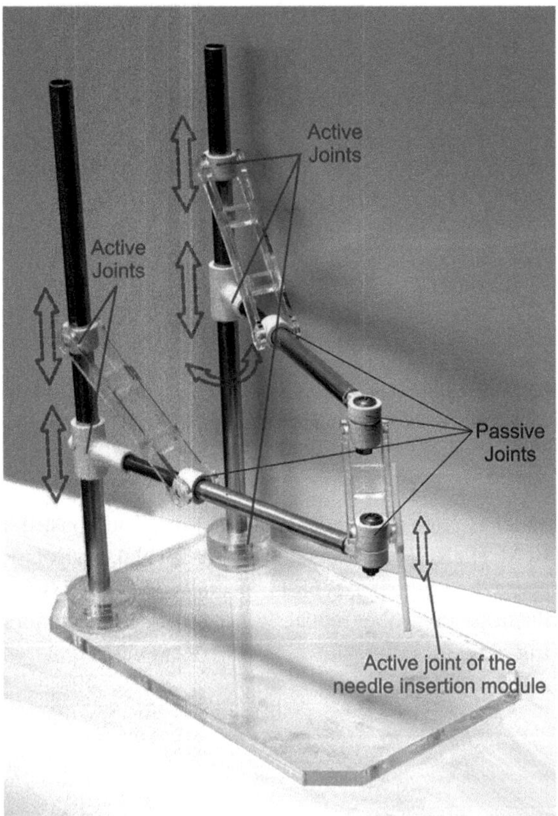

Fig. 9 The scaled model of the BR3 robotic structure which eliminates the fixed frame

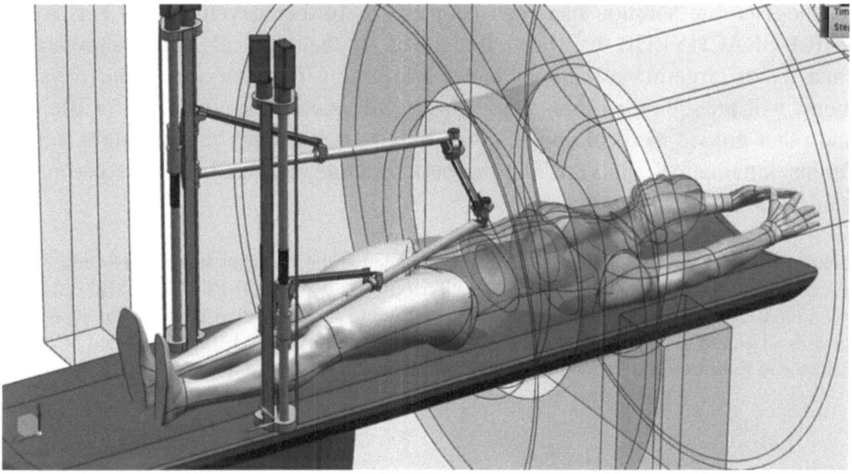

Fig. 10 PARA-BRACHYROB targeting a liver tumor under CT guidance

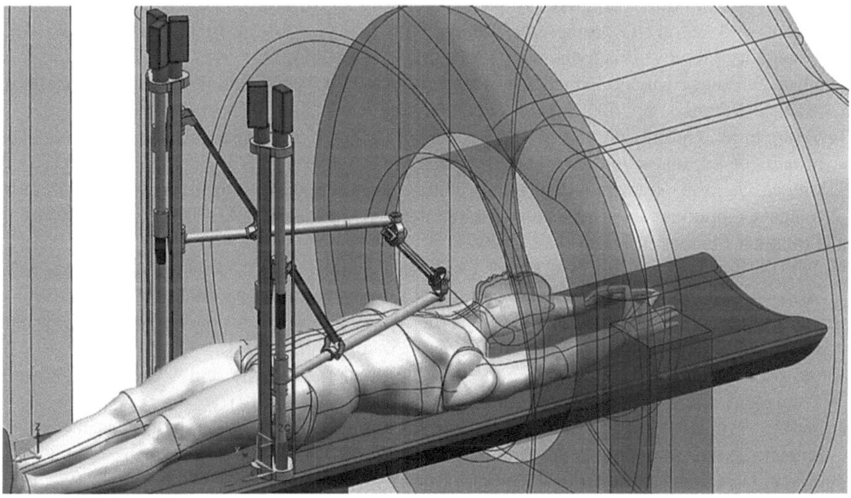

Fig. 11 PARA-BRACHYROB targeting a neck tumor under CT guidance

5 Conclusions

Robotic assisted brachytherapy is an efficient approach for cancer treatment. A new protocol for robotic assisted brachytherapy is presented. Innovative robotic solutions for brachytherapy systems have been presented, emphasizing the advantages of parallel robots which provide several solutions capable of targeting any area of the patient body. Based on a thorough analysis, together with a team of oncologists one solution has been adopted for further development. This robot, PARA-BRACHYROB has been integrated in the medical arena, showing its capacity of targeting any tumor under real-time CT guidance. Further developments will broaden the robots field of use, with possible applications for Biopsies and other guided medical applications. Based on this study the structures will be further kinematical analyzed and the best structure will lead to the experimental model for brachytherapy.

Acknowledgments The authors gratefully acknowledge the financial support provided by the research grant financed by the UEFISCDI national project code PN-II-PT-PCCA-2011-3.2-0414, no. 173/2012 entitled "Robotic assisted brachytherapy, an innovative approach of inoperable cancers—CHANCE" and by the Scopes International Grant IZ74Z0_137361/1 entitled "Creative Alliance in Research and Education focused on Medical and Service Robotics CARE-Robotics".

References

Buzurovic, I., Podder, T. K., Yu, Y.: Prediction Control for Brachytherapy Robotic System. Journal of Robotics, Vol. 2010, 10 pages, doi:10.1155/2010/581840 (2010)

Carpenter, T. J., et al.: Outcomes for patients with extraprostatic prostate cancer treated with trimodality therapy. Brachytherapy, 10(4): 261–268 (2011)

Chauhan, S.: Image Guided Robotic Systems for Focal Ultrasound Based Surgical Applications. Medical Robotics, pp. 526, I-Tech Education and Publishing, Vienna (2008)

Davidson, et al.: Optimization of high-dose-rate cervix brachytherapy applicator placement: The benefits of intraoperative ultrasound guidance. Brachytherapy, 7(3):248–253 (2008)

Fichtinger, G., et al: Robotic Assistance for Ultrasound Guided Prostate Brachytherapy, Medical Image Computing and Computer-Assisted Intervention—MICCAI 2007 Lecture Notes in Computer Science, 4791:119–127, (2007)

Fischer, G. S., et al: Design of a Robot for Transperineal Prostate Needle Placement in MRI Scanner, Mechatronics Conference on Digital Object Identifier, pp. 592–597 (2006)

Gupta, S. et al: Imaging-guided percutaneous biopsy of mediastinal lesions: different approaches and anatomic considerations, RadioGraphics, 25, 763–788, (2005)

Hungr, N., et al: A 3D Ultrasound Robotic Prostate Brachytherapy System with Prostate Motion Tracking, IEEE Transactions on Robotics, 28: 1382–1397, (2012)

Kacso, G.: Permanent iodine 125 brachytherapy as curative local monotherapy for organ confined prostate cancer (T1–T2)—a new option." PHD thesis, UMF "Iuliu Hatieganu" Cluj, (2005)

Mateescu, D.: Ghidul pacientului oncologic, Bucureşti, ISBN 978-973-87129-7-3 (2010)

Ottaviano E., Vorotnikov S., Ceccarelli M., Kurenev P.: Design improvements and control of a hybrid walking robot, Robotics and Autonomous Systems, 59, pp. 128–141, 2011

Oudard, S., Banu, E., Medioni, J., Scotte, F., Banu, A., Levy, E., Wasserman J., Kacso G., Andrieu JM.: What is the real impact of bone pain on survival in patients with metastatic hormone-refractory prostate cancer treated with docetaxel? 103(12):1641–6 (2009)

Plitea, N., et al.: Parallel robot for brachytherapy with two kinematic guiding chains of the platform (the needle) type 2CRRU and CRU, Patent pending, A/10004/2013a

Plitea, N., et al.: Parallel robot for brachytherapy with two kinematic guiding chains of the platform (the needle) type CYL-U, Patent pending, A/10006/2013b

Plitea, N., Vaida, C., Gherman, B., Szilaghyi, A., Galdau, B., Cocorean, D., Covaciu, F., Pisla, D.: Structural Analysis and Synthesis of Parallel Robots for Brachytherapy, New Trends in Medical and Service Robots. Mechanisms and Machine Science, 16: 191–204, (2014)

Podder, T.K., et al.: Robotic Brachytherapy—of robotic brachytherapy approaches and synergistic applications. In: AAPM Annual Meeting (2010a)

Podder, T.; Buzurovic, I.; Huang, K.; and Yu, Y.: MIRAB: An Image-Guided Multichannel Robot for Prostate Brachytherapy, Bodine Journal, 3(1), 39, (2010b)

Salcudean, S. E., Prananta, T. D., Morris, W. J. Spadinger, I.: A Robotic Needle Guide for Prostate Brachytherapy. Robotics and Automation, 2975–2981 (2008)

Shah, A.P., et al.: A dosimetric analysis comparing electron beam with the MammoSite brachytherapy applicator for intact breast boost. Physica Medica, 26–2, 80–87 (2010)

Shan Jiang, Jie Guo, Shen Liu, Jun Liu, Jun Yang,: Kinematic analysis of a 5-DOF Hybrid-Driven MR Compatible Robot for minimally invasive interventions in the prostate, Robotica, (2010)

Stoianovici, D., et al.: "MRI Stealth" robot for prostate interventions. Minim Invasive Ther Allied Technol. 16(6):370 (2007)

Strassman, G., et al.: Advantage of robotic needle placement on a prostate model in HDR brachytherapy, Strahlenther Onkol. 187(6), (2011), 367–272

Talaba D.: The angular capacity of spherical joints used in mechanisms with closed loops and multiple degrees of freedom, Robotics and Computer-Integrated Manufacturing 28(5), pp. 637–647, 2012

Tarnita D., Marghitu D.: Analysis of a hand arm system, Robotics and Computer-Integrated Manufacturing, 29(6), pp. 493–501, (2013)

Tornes, M. Eriksen,: A New Brachytherapy Seed Design For Improved Ultrasound Visualisation, Ultrasonics, 2:1278–1283 (2009)

Yu, Y., Podder, T., Zhang, Y. D., Ng, W. S., Misic, V., Sherman, J., Fu, L., Fuller, D., Rubens, D. J., Strang, J. D., Brasacchio, R. A., and Messing, E. M.: Robot-Assisted Prostate Brachytherapy, International Conference on Medical Image Computing and Computer-Assisted Intervention 9(1):41–9 (2006)

Markerless Vision-Based Skeleton Tracking in Therapy of Gross Motor Skill Disorders in Children

B. Karan, Š. Golubović and M. Gnjatović

Abstract This chapter presents a research towards implementation of a computer vision system for markerless skeleton tracking in therapy of gross motor skill disorders in children suffering from mild cognitive impairment. The proposed system is based on a low-cost 3D sensor and a skeleton tracking software. The envisioned architecture is scalable in the sense that the system may be used as a stand-alone assistive tool for tracking the effects of therapy or it may be integrated with an advanced autonomous conversational agent to maintain the spatial attention of the child and to increase her motivation to undergo a long-term therapy.

Keywords 3D sensing · Skeleton tracking · Computer-aided therapy · Human-machine interaction

1 Introduction

From the early stages of their development children have a desire to move and learn about the environment by exploring their physical surroundings. These experiences represent a foundation for future learning. Every learning process essentially includes the same stages: information acquisition, processing, association, cognition and response (Buccino and Riggio 2006). Learning and child

B. Karan (✉)
Institute of Technical Sciences of the Serbian Academy of Sciences and Arts, Belgrade, Serbia
e-mail: branko.karan@itn.sanu.ac.rs

Š. Golubović
Faculty of Medicine, University of Novi Sad, Novi Sad, Serbia
e-mail: spela@uns.ac.rs

M. Gnjatović
Faculty of Technical Sciences, University of Novi Sad, Novi Sad, Serbia
e-mail: milangnjatovic@yahoo.com

A. Rodić et al. (eds.), *New Trends in Medical and Service Robots*,
Mechanisms and Machine Science 20, DOI: 10.1007/978-3-319-05431-5_6,

development are based on development and regulation of basic mechanisms: sensor modulation and integration, motor planning and sequencing, visuospatial processing, auditory processing and emotional modulation. Children with motor development impairments can experience problems at any stage of the learning process or mechanism regulation, which affects their general functioning.

From a therapeutic point of view such a complex issue requires a range of interventions which should begin in early childhood. Early stimulations sometimes need to start immediately after birth in order to efficiently harness high plasticity of the brain, thus encouraging reorganization of nerve structures, where intact areas of the brain take over the function of the affected areas (Joković-Turalija et al. 2002). When planning rehabilitation programs for children with motor disabilities, it seems wise to start the treatment by stimulating basic emotional reactions, perceptuo-motoric abilities and communication using movement and body as the basis for intervention. This is a specific type of rehabilitation which, through the use of structural motor activities, influences the development of functions and abilities that form the basis for learning. Movement therapy aims to remediate or improve incorrect motor activities, and develop compensatory abilities and functional cognitive mechanisms in order to improve the child's performance in the domains affected by impairment. Treatment strategies involve exercises through which children acquire new motor knowledge, develop motor skills (Schmidt 1991) and develop perceptive and gnostic abilities, cognitive function and communication.

Treatment of motor and cognitive deficits requires long and painstaking work on the part of the child and his or her environment. To help direct inappropriate forms of behavior and movement into appropriate motor reactions we can use modern computer technology (Calderita et al. 2013; Dias et al. 2011; Moreno et al. 2013). It provides opportunities for the child to be involved in treatment in a more interesting manner. Furthermore, it helps implement individual treatment plans with an emphasis on more frequent repetition of specific activities and movements, their correction, better record keeping and thus more precise evaluation of treatment outcomes.

Computer vision technologies may play an extremely important role in implementation of environments for computer-aided therapy. A notable example of a virtual reality rehabilitation system that uses the Microsoft Kinect to enable children with hemiparesis to improve their affected hand is reported in (Yamaguchi et al. 2012). In the rehabilitation application, the patient controls the virtual avatar and attempts to touch a virtual object. A specialized algorithm is introduced to aid a Kinect sensor to recognize the paralyzed arm's limited field of movement, and to penalize the use of the unaffected arm (Yamaguchi et al. 2012). In contrast to this research, we do not involve a prescripted motion-based video game tailored to a particular gross motor skill disorder, but propose an avatar-based conversational agent whose role is to facilitate the interaction between the child and the therapist (cf. Sect. 4).

The research presented in this chapter aims at developing a scalable vision system that could provide assistance in different aspects of therapy of gross motor skills of pre-school to lower grade school children. From the technical aspect, the vision system could be used to make recordings of therapeutic sessions, and to extract clinically relevant quantitative measures related to the child's movements, postures, etc. From the motivational aspect, it may provide feedback for a simple graphical system to present visual stimuli to engage children's attention. From the interactional aspect, the vision system may be incorporated with a more complex intelligent autonomous agent (e.g., a robotic system, a conversational agent, a computer game, etc.) whose role is either to be the child's playmate or an independent actor in interaction between the child and the therapist.

2 Therapy Practices

Motor impairments usually emerge relatively early in childhood. These impairments appear as a result of brain damage caused by a set of factors that affect brain maturation. The symptoms manifest as deviations in the area of sensory, motor, verbal, cognitive and social development of a child. Impaired motor abilities and skills range from mild motor disability to severely impaired movement, balance and coordination. Impaired motor functioning is characterized by slower execution of movement, difficulties in planning and organizing movement, difficulties in learning new motor skills and combining basic motor activities, as well as in motor response itself.

Children with developmental disabilities experience problems when identifying parts of the body, difficulties with spatial and time orientation, rhythm, lateral awareness. This means that rehabilitation programs should structure activities which would integrate motor and cognitive aspects of learning, thereby developing sensory differentiation, perception and thinking, enhancing memory, attention, concentration, and promoting acquisition of new concepts and communication (Bojanin 2006; Krstić 2006). Exercises should be structured to meet the needs and abilities of every individual child; starting from the level that presents no difficulties for the child, then gradually changing and combining different activities. Initially, the activities should have a relaxing influence on the child, creating the basis for fluid execution of new movements, correction of uncoordinated movements, execution of more complex movements, awareness of the body parts involved and the body as a whole.

When doing the exercises there is no predefined method or order. By using simple movements, experiences acquired earlier are revised, reintegrated, and communication between child and therapist is established. This enhances motivation and encourages the child to participate. If the child experiences feelings of anxiety, insecurity or is emotionally immature, this can hinder fluid execution of movements and interfere with communication. In such cases, the therapist needs to create situations and develop activities which would ensure the child receives more attention, and allow the child to actively participate in the activities, thus enhancing communication with the therapist.

Communication encouraged when doing the exercises can be verbal or non-verbal. The former includes identifying movements and body parts, describing activities, spatial and time relationships, expression of emotions; while the latter is achieved through gesture, mimicking, movement and images. The first communication is usually established through modeling movement, starting with the command: "Now, do this". Thus initiated dialogue continues with the child imitating the therapist, and therapist following the child's lead. Some behavioral studies have shown that observation of movements can affect their execution, because it involves motor observation, motor imagery and movement execution (Brass 2000; Craighero et al. 2002).

Through movement children acquire awareness of themselves, their body and other individuals, which forms a basis for personal development. Becoming aware of its body, the child becomes aware of its own existence in physical environment, acquires and consolidates spatiotemporal relationships, develops a need for socializing and communication (Bojanin 2006; Krstić 2006). These are simple activities which are easily recognized, and in which certain parts of the body are identified, shown and touched. "Let's put our hands on our head, now on our stomach, now on our back, and now on our legs." This is followed by movement of larger joints, which enhances awareness of own body; while using proprioceptive and vestibular systems allows control of movement. Exercises include movement in all directions: crawling, walking, running, moving upper part of the body, moving the head, arms, legs, hands and feet in all directions—stretching, bending, rotating, lifting, side bending, throwing and catching. The most common exercises are focused on: body scheme perception, differential laterality, equalizing muscle tone, achieving independent movement, coordination of movement to rhythm, spatial orientation and relaxation activities.

Both group and individual exercises take place in non-competitive atmosphere and without assessment according to the plans developed after the children's abilities have been evaluated. Group exercises promote communication between children, whereby they establish social contact and are motivated for group work. Individual exercises implement plans tailored to meet individual abilities and needs. Irrespective of the type, group or individual, activities are carefully planned and aim to meet set objectives. Objective can be directed at mastering certain motor skills, or at learning the characteristics of a certain object, space, etc.

3 Vision-Based Skeleton Tracking

The vision system is expected to achieve efficient tracking of full-body motion. Having in mind the actual functionality to be supported, we distinguish 3 different levels of functions, in increasing order of complexity:

1. Recognition of movement/gestures: at this level, the vision system should be able to answer whether the patient has made a move pattern belonging to a

specific class (or at least that he or she attempted to make such a move). This information is a basic input to automatic interactive agent. Besides, from the standpoint of overall therapy tracking, this information provides a basis to build an indicator of number of times that the specific exercise has been repeated.

2. Estimation of quality of the movement, expressed e.g. as a function of differences of specific motion parameters with respect to the pre-specified "golden criterion." This information can be used to improve system interaction by providing different levels of interactive feedback (e.g., audio/visual rewards or praises) in dependence to estimated level of patient efforts.
3. Estimation of improvements or generally changes in quality of performed movements. This level of functionality is similar to (2) and the difference stem from the amount of details to be recognized by the system. Whereas in (2) it is enough to provide course categorization, here it is necessary to sense more subtle differences. This level of details might be critical for successful tracking of long-term effects of the therapy.

Further, it is highly desirable that the system is implemented without wearable artificial markers so that it would minimally interfere with normal therapy exercises.

Bearing in mind the cost aspects, it is decided to build the system using a low-cost 3D sensor for recording therapy sessions. The text to follow contains details on the chosen sensing technology and initially obtained results.

3.1 3D Sensing Technology

Last few years witnessed appearance of a new generation of low cost 3D sensors. They all employ IR projectors to illuminate environment and therefore are effectively limited to indoor applications. According to involved measurement technology, two types of sensors are dominant: structured light sensors and time of flight sensors (Fig. 1). With structured light sensors, a pattern of pixels is projected on external objects and the sensor infers the distance on the basis of disparity between reflected and reference patterns. With time of flight sensors, depth is determined on the basis of measurement of the total travelling time for a light pulse emitted from the IR laser projector, reflected from an external object, and returned back to the sensor. The time of flight method is considered more advantageous, because in principle it allows achieving a more compact design and faster response. However, the actual implementations of both technologies share the similar characteristics: the depth sensor is accompanied by a visible light camera, field of view is on the order of 60 degrees, and working distances are on the order of 1–4 m (some sensors allow switching the operating range to near-range distances of 0.15–1 m). Thanks to mass production, price is low, on the order of 250€.

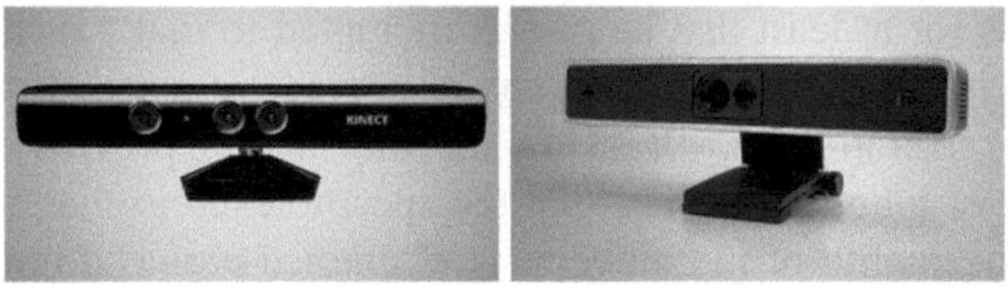

Fig. 1 Sample 3D sensors for indoor applications: *left* Microsoft Kinect for Windows (Microsoft Corporation 2013), *right* Softkinetic DepthSense 311 (SoftKinetic 2013)

Accuracy and precision are generally low (Dutta 2012; Karan 2013b) and the errors increase with distance. In the middle of the working range (2 m), typical errors are on the order of 35 mm with standard deviation of 10 mm, but they can be reduced by calibration (Karan 2013a, b; Khoshelham 2012). Such level of accuracy can be regarded as satisfactory from the standpoint of whole body motion tracking (Clark 2012; Obdržálek 2012).

3.2 Skeleton Tracking Data Set

To verify ability of chosen sensing technology to record 3D motion, track trajectories, and classify/evaluate performed exercises, a set of measurements has been organized in Milan Petrović School for children with special needs, Novi Sad, and University Children's Hospital Novi Sad. The measurements encompassed acquisition of depth maps and motion sequences for therapy sessions involving nine types of activities performed by children between the ages of 5 and 8 that were affected by mild motor disorders, such as mild intellectual disabilities, hemiparetic form of cerebral palsy and autism. All children understood the instructions and were motivated for work.

Measurements were made using Microsoft Kinect for Xbox 360 sensor and OpenNI/NiTE software (OpenNI Consortium 2013; PrimeSense Ltd. 2013). The obtained data set contains video clips, depth maps, and 3D motion sequences for fifteen tracked points (see Fig. 2). Collected sequences contain nine types of exercises:

1. Standing at attention;
2. Lateral weight transfer: (a) shifting body weight laterally from left to right and vice versa; right leg lunge with weight shift to the right leg (repeated afterward with left leg);
3. Step forward with weight transfer: right leg step back with lunge with weight shift on the right foot (repeated afterward with left leg);
4. Step backward with weight transfer: right leg step back with lunge with weight shift on the right foot (repeated afterward with left leg);
5. Standing on one foot: One legged stand 3–5 seconds;
6. Crouch;

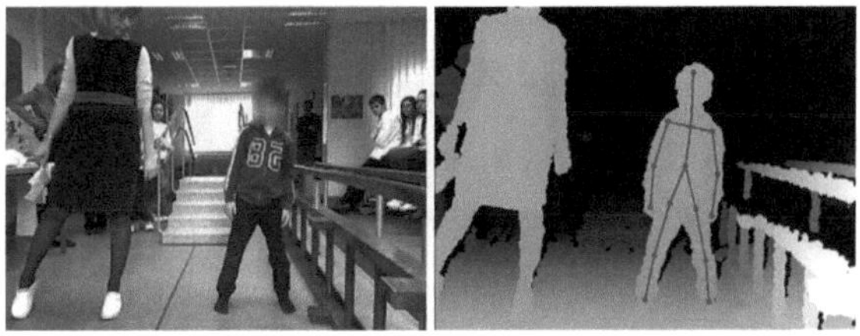

Fig. 2 Therapy session recording: *left* therapy setting; *right* recorded depth map with annotated tracked joints

7. Horizontal walk: forward gait on a horizontal flat surface;
8. Walking up/down stairs;
9. Shoulder movements: arms in front, arms up, arms down, arms back, arms to the sides.

In all cases the collected depth maps appeared satisfactory. However, the inferred trajectories were of low quality.

An illustration is given in Fig. 3 that shows a part of measurements recorded for an exercise involving lateral steps with weight transfer performed by two patients: one (Fig 3a) with very light motion disorders and the other (Fig 3b) having significant problems to keep balance during motion. The first row for each patient contains an outline of a sequence of depth maps. The sequence is accompanied below by corresponding trajectories of the left (red lines) and right shoulder (green lines). The trajectories were obtained in two manners:

1. Manually, by selecting joint positions from depth maps (solid lines) and
2. Automatically extracted by NiTE skeleton tracking software (dashed lines).

Looking at the red-green pair of solid lines at the diagram of lateral movement for the first patient, one could easily see the part between 1 and 2.5 s, when the patient performed a lateral movement of shoulders, and the second part, beginning at 4.5 s, when he started the second movement. Moreover, the trajectories are smooth, and the diagram of vertical movements clearly shows that the line between the shoulders is always maintained horizontal, implying a good balance. Trajectories obtained by the skeleton tracking software display similar behavior. However, their dynamics is not appropriate. With fast position changes of tracked joints, direction of registered movement may even become opposite with respect to the actual movement (see crossings of solid and dashed lines in the upper diagram at Fig. 3a). The trajectories obtained for the second patient (Fig. 3b) reflect a rather different behavior: here, the lateral transfer of weight is performed between 1 and 5 s and it is characterized by zigzagging with one large overshoot at 4 s. Additionally, the diagram of vertical movements shows the characteristic time-varying slope of the line between the shoulders. Here, an important feature to emphasize is that this motion is left unseen by the tracking software: the dashed trajectories are always smooth and they do not show the disparity between the vertical positions of the shoulders.

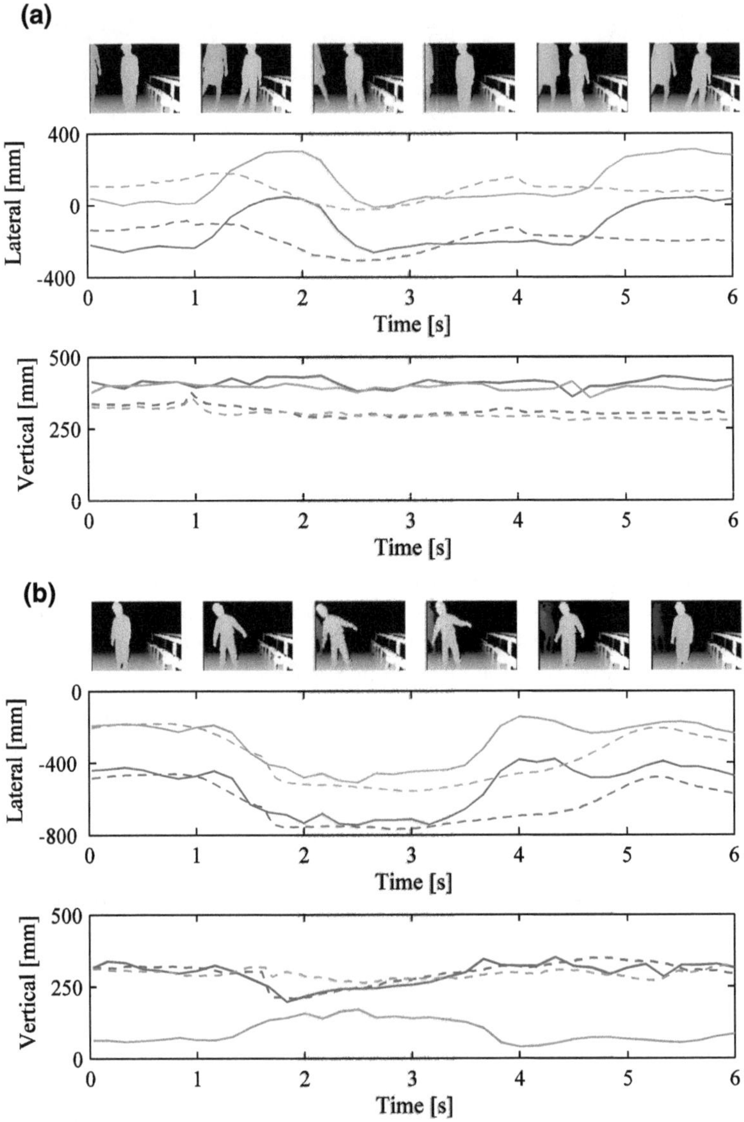

Fig. 3 Recorded trajectories for **a** patient with light balance disorders and **b** patient with heavy balance disorders *red lines*—left shoulder, *green lines*—right shoulder; *solid lines*—manually extracted from recorded depth maps, *dashed lines*—automatically extracted by the skeleton tracking software

Such behavior of the trajectory tracking software can be explained by the fact that it is optimized for recognition of the motion and not for evaluation of motion parameters. Furthermore, the software is optimized to run on hardware with modest abilities (alternative Microsoft Kinect SDK software is built using the same motion recognition principles, so that it is expected to display the similar performance).

In conclusion, the tested automatic tracking system could only be used in registering the number of conducted exercises and possibly in very coarse categorization of movements. A more subtle parameterization would require better tracking performances and possibly ability for fine-tuning of the tracking algorithm to the set of tracked exercises. Works on such software exist, e.g. (Buys et al. 2014; Rocha 2013), and it is worth to explore them.

4 Motivational and Interaction Aspects

As explained in Sect. 2, the goal of the therapy is to improve children's awareness and functional control of their own bodies. During the conventional two-party interaction between the therapist and the child, the therapist instructs and guides the child to perform different movements, e.g., to raise an arm, to make a step forward, etc. Related to the types of the exchange commodity, the interaction includes both verbal (e.g., repetition or reformulation of commands, encouragement, etc.) and nonverbal (e.g., physical demonstrations, gestures, etc.) means of communication. In our envisioned system, this general therapeutic scenario is extended to a three-party interaction between the child, the therapist and the animated avatar-based conversational agent, whose role is to facilitate the interaction, cf. (Gnjatović and Delić 2014). To achieve this, the system must implement two separate but related functionalities:

- *Dialogue competence*: the system should be able to engage in and manage natural language dialogue with the therapist, e.g., to recognize and interpret the therapist's verbal instructions, apply adaptive dialogue strategies, generate appropriate dialogue acts, etc.
- *Spatial awareness*: the system should be able to identify the relevant entities in the spatial context and to determine their positions. For this interaction domain, it means that the system should be able to detect the therapist's and the child's movements and postures.

The research question of the system's dialogue competence is already addressed in previous work in detail (Gnjatović and Rösner 2010; Gnjatović et al. 2012, 2013; Gnjatović and Delić 2014). Special attention was devoted to the research problems related to the given computer-aided therapeutic settings: robust processing of spontaneously produced therapist's linguistic inputs (e.g., elliptical or context-dependent instructions that instantiate different frames of spatial reference, etc.), and design of (emotion-)adaptive dialogue strategies for therapeutic purposes. The introduced approaches to these research problems are demonstrated to be appropriate through several prototypical dialogue systems with diverse interaction domains, such as: supporting users while they solve problems in a graphics system, a verbal user interface for the visually impaired, spatial context-aware interaction with the robot, etc.

In this chapter, the focus is on the spatial awareness in the context of computer-aided therapy of gross motor skill disorders in children. Thus, the discussion is intentionally dedicated to the vision system, abstracting away from details of the conversational agent. In the text to follow, we elaborate details of engaging the markerless vision-based tracker of human skeleton: (i) to maintain the spatial attention of the child and to increase her motivation to undergo a long-term therapy, and (ii) to support the therapist to keep track of the child's progress.

4.1 Therapeutic Settings

The dedicated therapeutic settings are given in Fig. 4. The motion sensor uses skeletal tracking to detect the therapist's and the child's movements and postures. Therefore, both the child and the therapist are expected to be within the range of the motion sensor (this area is marked in gray in Fig. 4), and they may take different spatial perspectives with respect to each other. It should be noted that this technical requirement is not restrictive for the purpose of the therapy. From the child's point of view, both the therapist and the monitor are situated in her social space and may easily come in the focus of attention.

4.2 Motivating the Child

One of the main goals of the system is to maintain the spatial attention of the child and to increase her motivation to undergo a long-term therapy. To achieve this, the system includes an animated avatar-based conversational agent. The vision system uses skeletal tracking to detect the therapist's movements and postures, and to map them in real-time onto the companion avatar displayed on the screen. The intention is to shift the spatial attention of the child form the therapist to the avatar that reflects the movements of the therapist. From the child's point of view, the avatar should be perceived as a companion. We expect that an appropriately designed avatar (both in terms of visual appearance and dialogue behavior) may be a strong motivational factor for the child to engage in the interaction and try to mimic the avatar's movements. This is in line with research in the field of robot-aided therapy for children with autism (Belokopytov and Fridin 2012; Colton et al. 2009; Dautenhahn et al. 2009; Ricks and Colton 2010; Thill et al. 2012; Vanderborght et al. 2012) and cerebral palsy (Calderita et al. 2013; Huber et al. 2008) showing

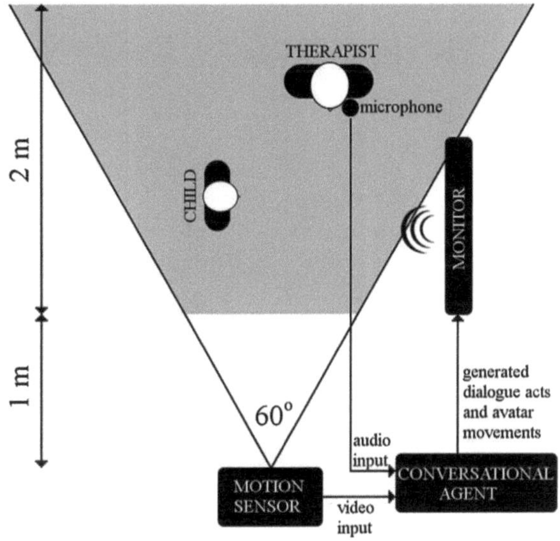

Fig. 4 Therapeutic settings

that the robot may induce positive social behavior in children, such as imitation, eye gaze, joint attention and increased motivation.

Avatar's appearance. Children's preferences for the avatar's appearance may vary depending on various factors such as their age, gender, current emotional state, etc. Therefore, a set of interchangeable, visually different, but functionally equivalent avatars have to be designed. There are two general requirements for the visual appearance of an avatar. First, it should be appealing to the child in order to enable the development of emotional attachment. Second, the avatar should have an anthropomorphic appearance, and the therapy-relevant parts of its body (i.e., arms, legs, head, etc.) should be easily perceivable by the child. In other words, the level of visual details must not be distracting for the child (Vanderborght et al. 2012). Figure 5 provides two prototypical avatars.

Avatar's behavior. One of the possible approaches to developing virtual-reality rehabilitation systems for children with gross motor skill disorders (e.g., cerebral palsy) is to implement a motion-based video game aimed to motivate and encourage the child to use, e.g., the affected limb (Kelleher et al. 2011; Yamaguchi et al. 2012). However, children with cerebral palsy are very different, and the therapy is always adapted to the particular child. In contrast to this fact, therapeutic games address only a specific motion and can be applied only to a small subset of children (Kelleher et al. 2011). Therefore, in our approach, we do not presuppose a preset interaction scenario or a therapeutic game. Instead, the therapist is free to organize the interaction according to his own discretion, and may interact with the avatar in two ways:

- Nonverbal interaction: The therapist is demonstrating moves that the child should perform, and the avatar reflects these moves in real-time.

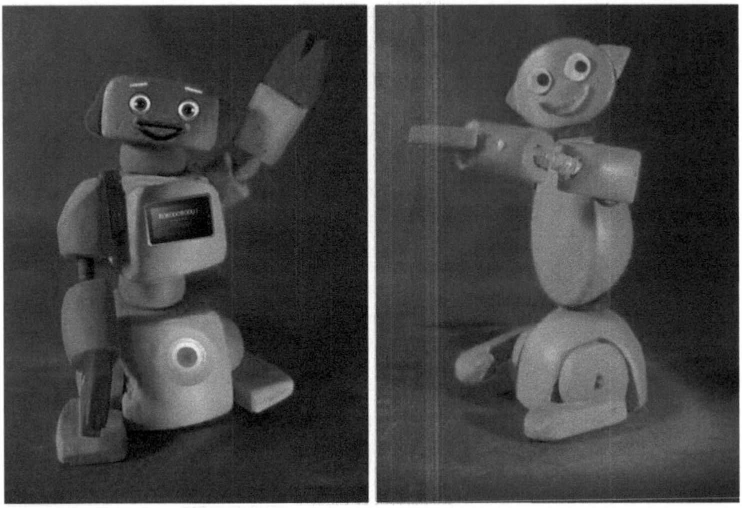

Fig. 5 Examples of female (*left*) and male (*right*) prototypical avatars (courtesy of D. Matić and D. Živančević)

- Verbal interaction: The therapist utters a command to the avatar to perform a non-verbal action (e.g., to raise an arm, etc.). The conversational agent recognizes and interprets the given verbal command, and instructs the avatar to perform the requested move. Please note that the conversational agent is discussed in (Gnjatović et al. 2013) and further references given there.

In both cases, the avatar occasionally displays simulated manifestations of its own intentionality according to its adaptive dialogue strategy (e.g., it makes an encouraging comment to the child, or complains that the exercise is hard, etc.)

4.3 Supporting the Therapist

Additional purpose of the overall system is to support the therapist to keep track of the child's progress. The conversational agent can interpret the therapist's instruction, i.e., it extracts information on the movement instructed by the therapist. On the other hand, the vision system can provide information on the child's actual movements and postures. Thus, by fusing these sources, the overall system may infer, in real-time, whether the child performed the therapist's instruction correctly. In addition, it may keep track of the child's performance over a number of therapeutic sessions, which supports the therapist to access the long-term progress of the child.

5 Conclusions

This chapter has presented initial steps conducted towards implementation of an advanced system for computer-aided therapy of children. Its most critical component is a system for markerless visual tracking of motion performed by children and it is envisioned as a scalable system built upon a low-cost 3D sensor. To provide a proof of concept, a set of recordings of therapy sessions has been made and the results have confirmed the feasibility of the approach. Additionally, scenarios of possible operation of the system within the framework of an autonomous conversational agent have been elaborated thus setting the directions for further work.

Immediate steps following this study should be focused on specific algorithms for full human body tracking in the context of not only the recognition, but also the evaluation of conducted moves. Here, two main and interrelated areas of research are tracking algorithms and motion evaluation algorithms.

A complementary task is related to motivational aspect of the therapeutic interaction. In this field, our future work will be focused on the integration of the vision system with the existing conversational agents, and the design of the agent's adaptive dialogue strategies for therapeutic purposes, cf. (Gnjatović and Delić 2014).

Acknowledgments This research is funded in part by the Ministry of Education, Science, and Technological Development of the Republic of Serbia under the contracts III44008 and TR32035. The research is complementary supported by the project *Inclusive physical education in Vojvodina schools: challenges and perspectives,* co-financed by the Provincial Secretariat for Science and Technological Development of AP Vojvodina. The pictures given in Fig. 5 are produced by Dragan Matić and Dragan Živančević, affiliated with the Academy of Arts at the University of Novi Sad, and are not published before. The authors thank D. Matić and D. Živančević for allowing them to include these pictures in the chapter.

References

Belokopytov, M. and Fridin, M.: Motivation of children with cerebral palsy during motor involvement by RAC-CP fun. In: Proc. of the Workshop on Motivational Aspects of Robotics in Physical Therapy, IEEE/RSJ Int. Conf. Intelligent Robots and Systems, (2012).

Bojanin, S.: Reedukacija psihomotorike ili tretman pokretom. Psihijatrija danas, 38(1), 11–27 (2006).

Brass, M. et al.: Compatibility between observed and executed finger movements: comparing symbolic, spatial and imitative cues. Brain and Cognition, 44, 124–143 (2000).

Buccino, G. and Riggio, L.: The role of the mirror neuron system in motor learning. Kinesiology, 38(1), 5–15 (2006).

Buys, K. et al.: An adaptable system for RGB-D based human body detection and pose estimation. Journal of Visual Communication and Image Representation, 25(1), 39–52 (2014).

Calderita, L. et al.: THERAPIST: Towards an autonomous socially interactive robot for motor and neurorehabilitation therapies for children. In: Proc. 2013 7th Int. Conf. Pervasive Computing Technologies for Healthcare, PervasiveHealth 2013, pp. 374–377 (2013).

Clark, R. A. et al.: Validity of the Microsoft Kinect for assessment of postural control. Gait & Posture, 36, 372–377 (2012).

Colton, M.B. et al.: Toward therapist-in-the-loop assistive robotics for children with autism and specific language impairment. In: Proc. of the AISB 2009 Symposium on New Frontiers in Human-Robot Interaction, Edinburgh, Scotland (2009).

Craighero, L., Bello, A., Fadiga, L., and Rizzolatti, G.: Hand action preparation influences the responses to hand pictures. Neuropsychologia, 40, 492–502 (2002).

Dautenhahn, K. et al.: KASPAR – A minimally expressive humanoid robot for human-robot interaction research. Applied Bionics and Biomechanics 6(3-4), 369–397 (2009).

Dias, O.P., Amaral, T.G.B., and Fernão Pires, V.: Computer assisted learning in manipulative therapy education. Manual Therapy, 16(3), 270–272 (2011).

Dutta, T.: Evaluation of the Kinect sensor for 3-D kinematic measurement in the workplace. Applied Ergonomics, 43(4), 645–649 (2012).

Gnjatović, M., and Rösner, D.: Inducing genuine emotions in simulated speech-based human-machine interaction: The NIMITEK corpus. IEEE Trans. Affect. Comput. 1, 132–144 (2010).

Gnjatović, M., Janev, M., and Delić, V.: Focus tree: Modeling attentional information in task-oriented human-machine interaction. Applied Intelligence, 37(3), 305–320 (2012).

Gnjatović, M. et al.: Linguistic encoding of motion events in robotic system. In: Proc. 6th PSU-UNS International Conference on Engineering and Technology (2013).

Gnjatović, M. and Delić, V.: End-user design of emotion-adaptive dialogue strategies for therapeutic purposes. In: Proc. 23rd Italian Workshop Neural Networks, WIRN 2013 (Series: Smart Innovation, Systems and Technologies). Springer, 26, 371–378 (2014).

Huber, M. et al.: PlayStation 3-based telerehabilitation for children with hemiplegia. In: Proc. Virtual Rehabilitation Conference, Vancouver, 2008, pp. 105–112 (2008).

Joković-Turalija, I., Ivkić, D., and Oberman-Babić, M.: Neki aspekti rane dijagnostike i terapije djece sa cerebralnom paralizom. Hrvatska revija za rehabilitacijska istraživanja, 38(1), 121–126 (2002).

Karan, B.: Calibration of depth measurement model for Kinect-type 3D vision sensors. In: Proc. 21st Int. Conf. Central Europe on Computer Graphics, Visualization, and Computer Vision, Plzen, pp. 61–74 (2013a).

Karan, B.: Accuracy improvements of consumer-grade 3D sensors for robotic applications. In: Proc. IEEE 11th Int. Symp. Intelligent Systems and Informatics (2013b).

Kelleher, C., et al.: Towards a therapist-centered programming environment for creating rehabilitation games. Proc. IEEE Computer Games, 2011, pp. 240–247 (2011).

Khoshelham, K. and Elberink, S.O.: Accuracy and resolution of Kinect depth data for indoor mapping applications. Sensors, 12, 1437–1454 (2012).

Krstić, N.: Reedukacija psihomotorike kao oblik neuropsihološke rehabilitacije. Psihijatrija danas, 38(1), 51–66 (2006).

Microsoft Corporation: Kinect for Windows. Online: http://www.microsoft.com/en-us/kinectforwindows/ (2013).

Moreno, J.C. et al..: Effects of robotic guidance on the coordination of locomotion. Journal of NeuroEngineering and Rehabilitation, 10, 79 (2013).

Obdržálek, Š. et al.: Accuracy and robustness of Kinect pose estimation in the context of coaching of elderly population. In: Proc. Annual Int. Conf. IEEE Engineering in Medicine and Biology Society (EMBS), 2012, pp. 1188–1193 (2012).

OpenNI Consortium: OpenNI, the standard framework for 3D sensing. Online: http://www.openni.org/ (2013).

PrimeSense Ltd.: NiTE 2 API programmer tutorial guide. PrimeSense (2013).

Ricks, D.J. and Colton, M.B.: Trends and considerations in robot-assisted autism therapy. In: Proc. of the IEEE International Conference on Robotics and Automation (ICRA), Anchorage, AK 2010, pp. 4354–4359 (2010).

Rocha, J.: Skeltrack - A free software skeleton tracking library. Online: http://github.com/joaquimrocha/Skeltrack (2013).

Schmidt, R.A.: Motor learning and performance: from principle to practice. Human Kinetics Pub. (1991).

SoftKinetic: DepthSense cameras. Online: http://www.softkinetic.com/products/depthsense cameras.aspx (2013).

Thill, S.et al.: Robot-assisted therapy for autism spectrum disorders with (partially) autonomous control: Challenges and outlook. Paladyn. Journal of Behavioral Robotics 3(4), 209–217 (2012).

Vanderborght, B. et al.: Using the social robot probo as a social story telling agent for children with ASD. Interaction Studies 13(3), 348–372 (2012).

Yamaguchi, T. et al.: Upper-body interactive rehabilitation system for children with cerebral palsy: the effect of control/display ratios. In: Proc. 9th Int. Conf. Disability, Virtual Reality & Associated Technologies, Laval, France, 2012, pp.181–186 (2012).

Force Training for Position/Force Control of Massage Robots

V. Golovin, M. Arkhipov and V. Zhuravlev

Abstract In the chapter the force training mode for position/force control is considered. This problem is especially actual for medical robotic interacting with soft tissues during massage. The force training mode is necessary to control the deformation of human soft tissues, which have a number of features. It is proposed to extend the concept of the usual teaching geometric point with force information. This requires a sensor that measures the forces of interaction of the robot with the soft tissues. Such an approach for position/force control provides reproduction of path and forces imitating skilled physician. The psychophysiological efficiency is provided by biotechnical control circuit.

Keywords Force training · Position/force control · Medical robot · Soft tissues · Massage

1 Introduction

In 80–90s many investigations had been devoted to contact problems of a robotics. The scientific researches of robotic systems with force sensing are often left behind their practical use (Golovin et al. 2012; Vukobratovic and Rodic 1997). The practice of contact problems is the following:

- in machining (cutting, grinding) it is necessary to support the assigned power (velocity, force) at a variable allowance of work piece;
- at burrs removal on the casts or list edge on the stamped details;
- at surface polishing with constant pressing force of the polishing tool on a detail;

V. Golovin (✉) · M. Arkhipov · V. Zhuravlev
Moscow State Industrial University, Moskovsky, Russia
e-mail: medicalrobot@mail.ru

A. Rodić et al. (eds.), *New Trends in Medical and Service Robots*,
Mechanisms and Machine Science 20, DOI: 10.1007/978-3-319-05431-5_7,

- assembly problems which include the connection by a shaft insertion in the plug, and also carving connections;
- details extraction from nonoriented box with a necessary detail recognition and capture;
- force unloading of the loaded robot links;
- remote bilateral manipulators control;
- measurement and account of small deformations in aircraft designs speaking not only about robotics;
- manipulations on soft tissues and joints;
- in agriculture (plowing field).

One of the contact problems studied in lesser degree is soft tissue deformation by robots in restorative medicine. The restorative medicine includes a number of therapies including nonmedical, one of them is massage. Among a set of known means of massage the robotics possesses the greatest possibilities.

The history of massage robots occurrence in restorative medicine is the following. In 1997 the only work of robotics for restorative medicine was presented at the second forum IARP on medical robotics. That was the robot for massage (Golovin 1997). In 2002 on a web-site of the Dutch firm a Tickle robot for massage appears as a tickling small insect (Golovin et al. 2012). In 2003 there was a Russian patent of the robot for train-massage (Golovin et al. 2012). In 2005 on a Silicon Valley web-site there was a message (Jones et al. 2003) about the Puma robot usage for massage purposes. The basis of this development was the idea stated in the Russian work (Golovin and Samorukov 1998; Golovin 1998; Golovin and Grib 2002).

However, the interaction of the robot with patient's soft tissues causes new approaches to position/force control, in particular in robot training. To train the robot the force training is proposed (Golovin et al. 2005).

Despite a considerable quantity of papers in the field of contact problems, a number of problems both theoretical and practical remain unsolved. Therefore the problem of robot position/force control systems creation with easily realized regulators that allow quick and precise movements on any spatial trajectories with precise providing assigned forced influence is an actual one—whether it is possible to transfer known methods to control the medical robot performing manipulations on soft tissues.

To answer these questions we will address to the objects of manipulation. In known contact problems in industrial robotics they are rigid bodies. The interaction consists in pressing the robot to the rigid bodies (assembly, details joint definition at welding, polishing) or in pressing and cutting the rigid bodies (machining, cutting, grinding). The rigid bodies are considered as mechanical constrains which are known in advance and can be programmed.

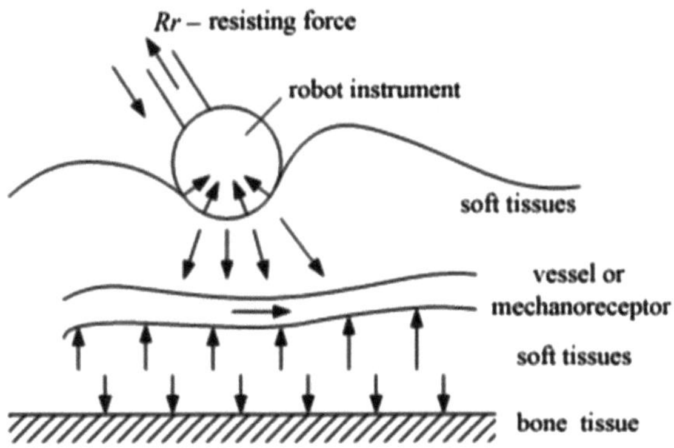

Fig. 1 Distributed character of force loading during massage

2 Soft Tissue Features

The medicine defines a soft tissue (ST) as muscles, fascias, skin, fatty layer, ligaments, cartilages and tendons. Bones are rigid tissues. The mechanical characteristics of ST, in particular elastic coefficient and deformation value, have essential differences from the mechanical characteristics of details materials in assembly or machining.

It is necessary to note the distributed character of force loading during massage (Fig. 1) excepting acupressure. But further for contact interaction models we use the equivalent concentrated environment resistance force $\mathbf{F_e}$ which is balanced by drive force.

The certain force picture of the physician's hand or the robot tool interaction with a patient's body is given as a six-component vector:

$$\mathbf{F} = \left(F_x, F_y, F_z, M_x, M_y, M_z\right)^T, \tag{1}$$

where F_x, F_y, F_z are projections of the force acting on the robot tool from patient's body,

M_x, M_y, M_z are the moments around axes x, y, z;

T is a transposing symbol.

In the most general model the ST can be presented as an anisotropic, multi-layered, viscoelastic, plastic, inertial, and non-stationary environment (Golovin et al. 2005).

In Table 1 some typical massage techniques, movements, and force loadings are resulted. The masseur's hand parts or technical devices fixed on the end link of the robot can be used as a tool.

In Table 1 the following designations are introduced:

F_e, M_e are the force and the moment of ST resistance;

F_S, F_f, F_d are the force of elasticity, the ST friction force, the drive force.

Table 1 Specific massage techniques, movements, and loadings

No.	Techniques	Resisting forces
1	Palpation, shiatsu, force training	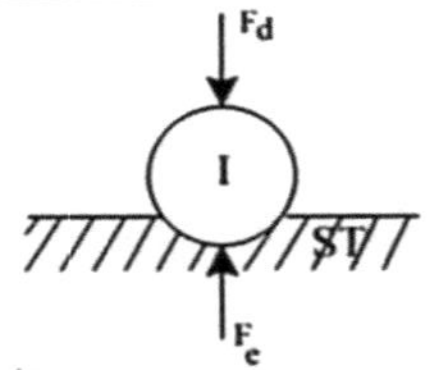
2	Pincement	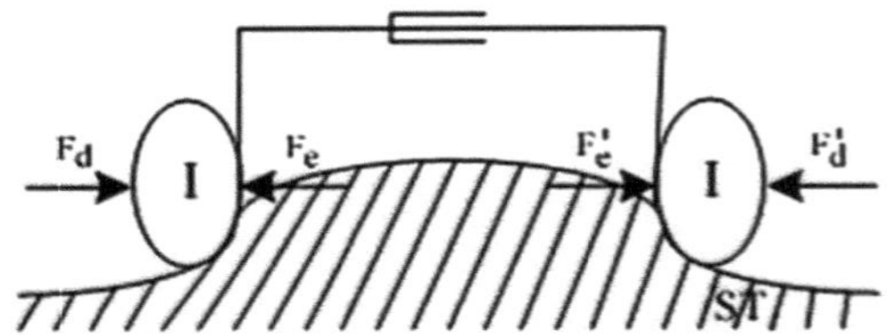
3	Traction (stretch)	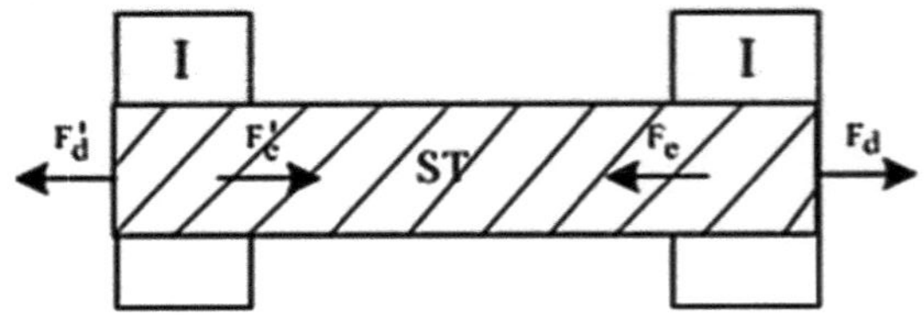
4	Vacuum massage (drawing)	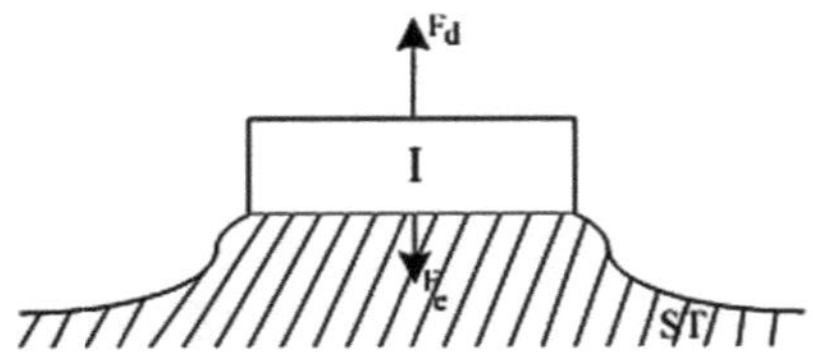

(continued)

Table 1 (continued)

No.	Techniques	Resisting forces
5	Pincement with spinning	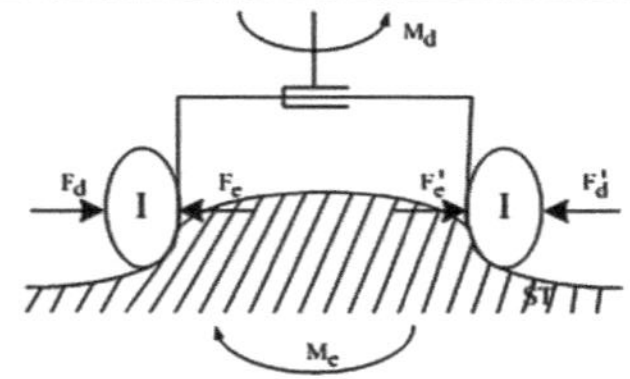
6	Pointillage with shear (without creeping)	
7	Petrissage, rubbing, squeezing (with creeping)	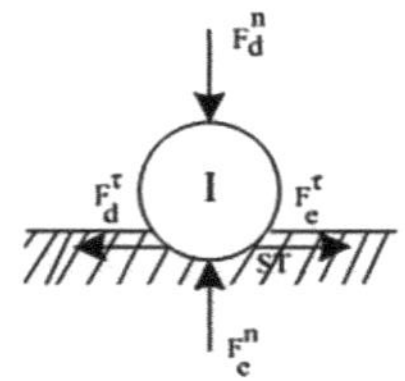
8	Ordinary petrissage (with creeping)	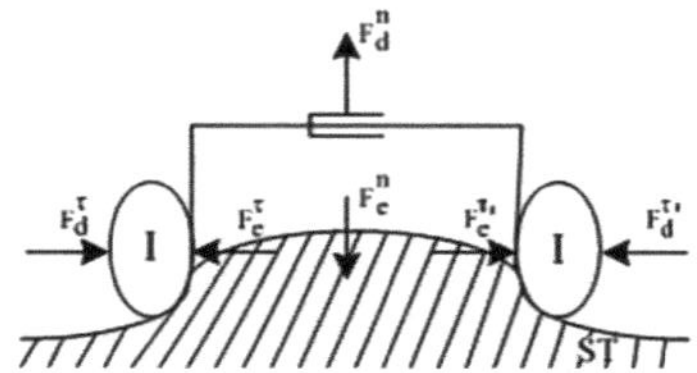
9	Vacuum massage (with creeping)	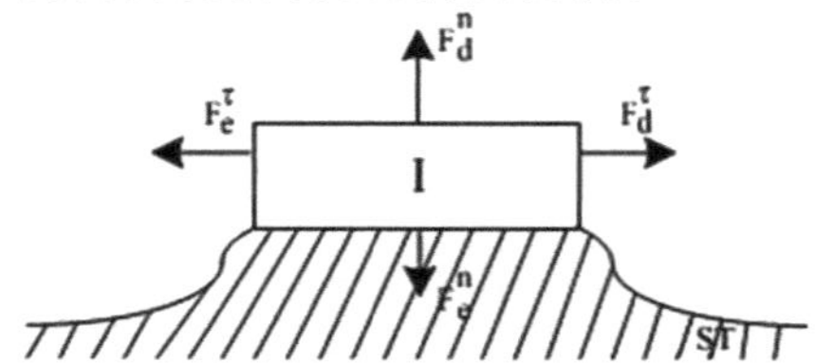

Table 2 The values of speed, strength, pressure on soft tissues developed in massage movements

	Size of part (m)	Speed (m/s)	Force (N)	Area of contact spot (m^2)	Pressure (Pa)
Stroking	0.01–1,0	0.01–0.3	<1	10^{-4}–10^{-2}	<10^2
Squeezing	0.01–1.0	0.01–0.2	1–100	10^{-4}–5 · 10–3	10^2–10^5
Pointillage	>0.02	0.01–0.3	1–30	4 · 10^{-6}–10^{-4}	10^4–10^6
Pressing kneading	(0.01–0.1)	0.01–0.3	1–100	10^{-4}–5 · 10^{-3}	10^2–10^5
Drawing petrissage	(0.01–0.1)	0.01–0.2	1–50	–	–
Traction	0.01–1.0	0.01–0.1	1–50	–	–
Pulse mobilization	–	0.1–1.0	50–200	~10^{-3}	10^5

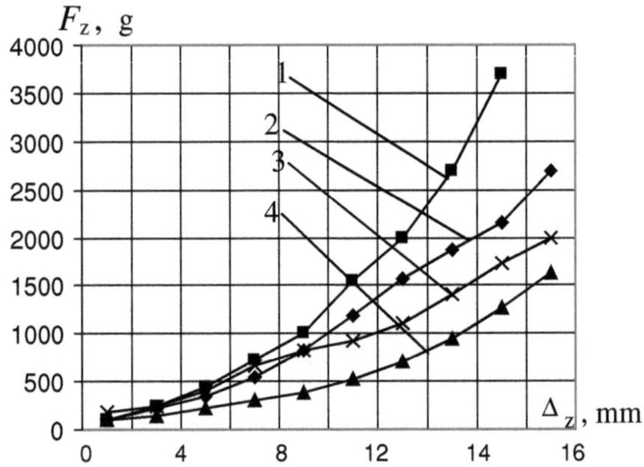

Fig. 2 Experimental curves $F_z = F(\Delta z)$, at various strain degree of muscles *1* tense forearm, *2* relax forearm, *3* tense hip, *4* relax hip

The values of speed, forces and pressures on ST during typical movements are given in Table 2. These values determine the ranges only. The forces and the torques of drives should be balanced with the support reaction. The supports are necessary during both the manual and the robot massage. The bones of the patient's skeleton are less compliant than ST and they can be used as a support for pressing and stretching methods (Golovin et al. 2012).

The ST elasticity measurement with a static method can be used not only for robot position/force control, but also to diagnose the patient's muscles state and patient's state in whole. On Fig. 2 the strain degree of forearm muscles (curves 1, 2) and hips (curves 3, 4) influence on $F_z = F(\Delta z)$, slope is shown.

The essential components of force interaction in massage are dry and viscous friction. The experimental dependence curve of the friction force on the speed is given on Fig. 3. The curve shows an increase of friction force due to viscous friction component.

We can interpret a massage as different types of force loading. For example, stroking is a wave of normal pressure on ST without shearing, rubbing is a

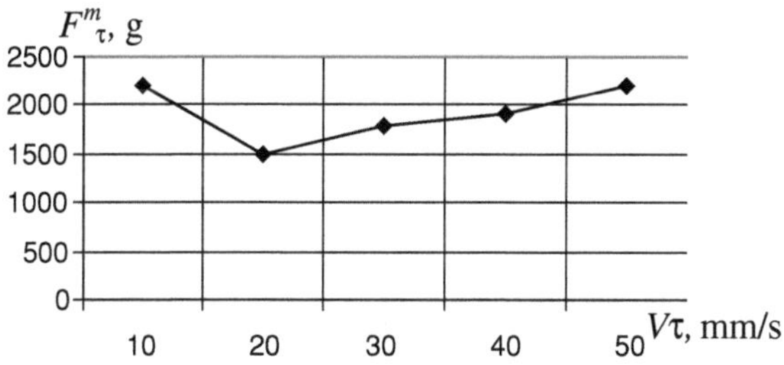

Fig. 3 Experimental dependence curve of the friction force on the speed

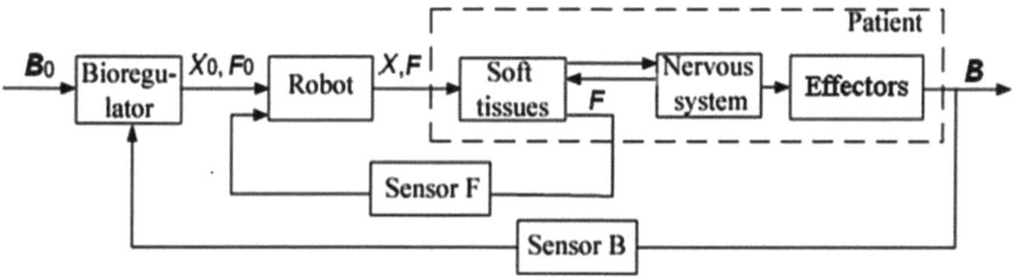

Fig. 4 Block diagram of bio-technical control system

shearing of skin and hypoderm, kneading is shearing and torsions of muscles, squeezing is a significant normal pressure on ST with shearing, squeezing by a roller is a wave of normal pressure on ST without shear.

3 Two Control Contours of Massage Robot

The main control purpose for medical robots is to lead patient's state variables to physiologically normal ones by means of robot mechanical influences (either directly on soft tissues or as manipulations on joints). Therefore it is necessary to consider two closed loop contours of force and biotechnical control, and also two basic control vectors: a vector of psycho-physiological state variables and a vector of measured forces of robot tool interaction with patient's ST (Fig. 4). The tool movement is also a control vector. In this system we consider a patient as a control object. In the contour of position/force control the patient's ST is a control object. In the contour of biotechnical control the converter of mechanical influence variables to variables of a psycho-physiological state is a control object (Golovin et al. 2012).

On Fig. 4 the following vectors are defined:

X, **F**, **B** are the vectors of real movement, force and patient's biomedical signals;

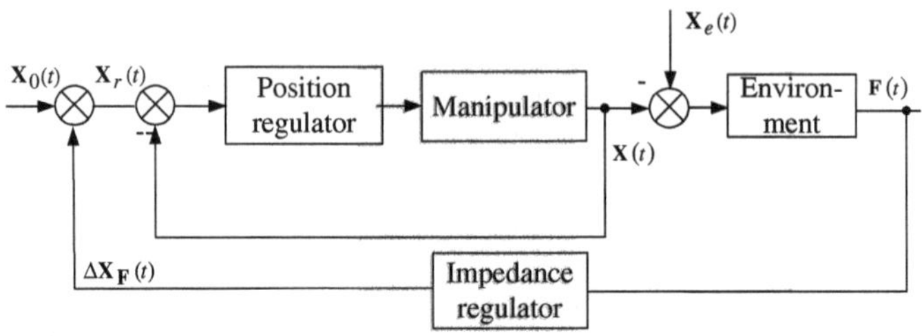

Fig. 5 Impedance control system

$\mathbf{X}_0$, $\mathbf{F}_0$ are the vectors of planned tool movement and assigned tool interaction force with the patient;

$\mathbf{B}_0 = (f, p, m, k, R)^T$, is the vector of normal biomedical signals, for example, pulse rate, arterial pressure, signals of miography, muscular tone, electric skin resistance.

The impedance approach can be the basis of the robot position/force control (Vukobratovic and Rodic 1997). An impedance control assumes providing a desirable balance between position and force errors developed on the robot end link. The block diagram of impedance control is shown on Fig. 5.

On the block diagram the following designations are introduced: $\mathbf{X}_0$, $\mathbf{X}$ are the position trajectory desirable and real values, $\mathbf{X}_r$ is the value of the position trajectory corrected by impedance regulator, $\mathbf{X}_e$ is the relief of the environment contact surface, $\mathbf{F}$ is the real force value.

4 Force Training in Position/Force Control

Though main efficiency criteria of robots for restorative medicine are indicators of the patient's phychophysiologic state, the robot as a mean of massage should control mechanical contact interaction between a human arm (robot tool) and the patient's body. The computer vision systems working in various ranges, for example in X-rays, visible and ultrasonic light are possible for control. These systems allow to see ST structure, their location concerning bone tissues. This is vast but expensive information.

There is an experience of blind masseurs with highly developed tactile sensation that allows to memorize, control and mark progress in procedure performance. Therefore we can talk about designing of robots using force information about ST relief and viscoelastic properties (Golovin et al. 2012).

For massage the controlled variables and control aims can be the follows:

- during the surface stroke and the minimum contact forces the constant velocity should be provided on a trajectory: $V = \text{const}$;

- on body parts with homogeneous properties it is desirable to support constant force: $F = \text{const}$;
- at deep massage with the high forces the masseur is compelled to reduce velocity when the hand meets the high resistance, therefore achievement of a constant power is relevant $N = F \cdot V = \text{const}$;
- to perform the long work the masseur has to save his energy, so the minimal energy expenses can be his aim;
- it should be taken into account that massage is performed using the tools or hands with various contact surfaces, therefore it is necessary to support assigned forces per unit of contact surface square that is pressure $p = F/S$.

Generally the vector $\mathbf{X}(t)$ represents spatial position and orientation co-ordinates. For example,

$$\mathbf{X}(t) = (\mathbf{n}, \mathbf{s}, \mathbf{a}, \mathbf{p})^T, \tag{2}$$

where **n**, **s**, **a** are the orientation subvectors, **p** is the subvector of tool position, or

$$\mathbf{X}(t) = (x, y, z, o, a, t)^T, \tag{3}$$

where x, y, z are the position co-ordinates, o, a, t are Euler's angles of tool orientation.

Generally force/torque vector $\mathbf{F}(t)$ is represented as a six-dimensional vector

$$\mathbf{F}(t) = (F_X, F_Y, F_Z, M_X, M_Y, M_Z)^T, \tag{4}$$

where F_X, F_Y, F_Z are the forces along axes of basic or tool co-ordinates system, and M_X, M_Y, M_Z are the moments around these axes.

Then the problem of position/force control is posed as providing the position trajectory $\mathbf{X}(t) \rightarrow \mathbf{X}_0(t)$ and the force trajectory at contact interaction of the robot tool with the patient's body $\mathbf{F}(t) \rightarrow \mathbf{F}_0(t)$ (Vukobratovic et al. 2009). The problem of force control provides $\mathbf{F}(t) \rightarrow \mathbf{F}_0(t)$ at any uncontrollable moving $\mathbf{X}(t)$.

It is necessary to note the following position/force control law of the robot interacting with the environment: in an uncertain or variable environment it is impossible to provide the assigned robot interaction force with this environment simultaneously and precisely on any assigned trajectory, i.e. to provide $\mathbf{X}(t) = \mathbf{X}_0(t)$ and $\mathbf{F}(t) = \mathbf{F}_0(t)$ simultaneously. It is possible precisely provide only one variable, either $\mathbf{X}(t)$ or $\mathbf{F}(t)$, conceding other variable.

There are several methods to define a spatial trajectory: by means of defined reference points; by means of points or continuous curves transferred, for example, from computer vision system; by means of trained points or curves from a manual control.

To assign the interaction forces on a spatial trajectory the following methods are known: assign the forces with a keyboard and using a force setting device. A diagnostic strain glove and methods of preliminary ST force scanning can be actual methods of force settings for massage problems.

The offered adaptation arranges system not only in the phase of the basic procedure execution, but in preliminary environment probing. The training procedure is interactive and it allows to take into account individual features of a patient.

Traditional for industrial robotics training assumes manual robot tool approach to a necessary point near contact or in contact. Then the position sensors measure joint coordinates and memorize them.

A trained point can have the same number of coordinates as the number of manipulator's drives. This is called training in the joint generalized coordinates $\mathbf{q}$.

$$\#A(q_1, q_2, \ldots, q_n). \tag{5}$$

As a rule the six-joint robots have an inverse kinematic task solver and can transform precision (generalized) point coordinates to the Cartesian ones:

$$\#A(q_1, q_2, \ldots, q_n) \rightarrow A(x, y, z, o, a, T), \tag{6}$$

where x, y, z, o, a, T are robot end link target position and orientation coordinates.

$\mathbf{X} = F(\mathbf{q})$ and $\mathbf{q} = F^{-1}(\mathbf{X})$ represent the direct and inverse kinematic tasks.

Further named force trained point in addition to geometrical coordinates includes components of interaction force vector between the robot tool and a patient's body. Generally vector $\mathbf{F}$ has six components.

$$\mathbf{F} = (F_X, F_Y, F_Z, M_X, M_Y, M_Z)^T. \tag{7}$$

These components can be measured by a six-component force sensor fixed on a robot end link between the flange and the tool. Therefore vector $\mathbf{F}$ components are measured in moving tool coordinates system.

The measurements are made at stop in a trained point. It is possible to calculate these components using force sensors located in joints.

$$\mathbf{F} = \left(J^T\right)^{-1}\mathbf{F}_\tau, \tag{8}$$

where $\mathbf{F}_\tau = (F_{\tau 1}, F_{\tau 2}, \ldots, F_{\tau n})^T$ is the vector of forces and moments in joints.

Then the force trained point A is represented by twelve-dimensional vector:

$$A(x, y, z, o, a, T, F_X, F_Y, F_Z, M_X, M_Y, M_Z)^T. \tag{9}$$

Training can be performed either by means of points or continuously. Usual continuous positional training assumes recording the spatial curve in time. In case of continuous force training in addition to continuous geometrical coordinates the point will contain measured force components, for example

$$A(x, y, z, o, a, T, F_Z). \tag{10}$$

At points force training before massage procedures a tool "penetrates" into a ST until the force sensor indication is equal to the assigned force. The robot drives

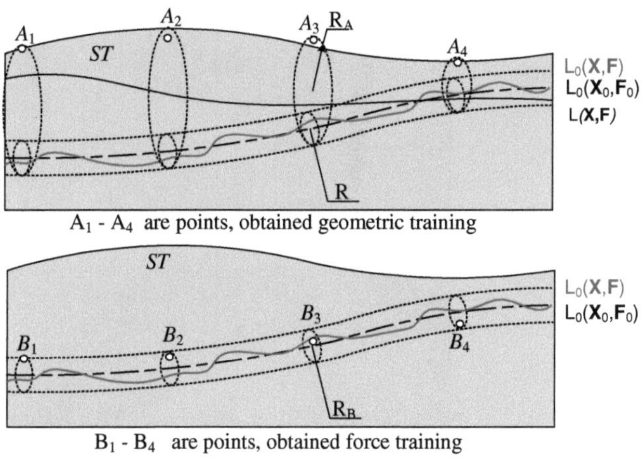

Fig. 6 The position/force control accuracy in position or force training

stop and position and orientation coordinates together with the reached forces are memorized.

At manual training a point is memorized with the tool axis orientation directed to a normal to a deformed ST surface. At automatic training of ST area by scanning a plane frame is assigned with denoting of only three point coordinates for example $A(x, y, z)$ with identical tool axis orientation without normals definition. Later with approximately calculated normals from the first automatic scanning we can repeat scanning specifying normals orientation.

Generally the force trained point can contain not only pressing forces but also forces of ST stretching, torsion, bending and tangential component.

5 Position/Force Control with Force Training Realization

Force training allows to perform the second phase of the position/force control as a positional tracking. This enables to use usual robots without force correction tracking. If a robot is able to perform the force correction then the quality of control generally increases. On Fig. 6 the curve $L_0(\mathbf{X}_0, \mathbf{F}_0)$ represents the trajectory of the robot tool when $\mathbf{X}(t) \to \mathbf{X}_0(t)$and $\mathbf{F}(t) \to \mathbf{F}_0(t)$. The curve L($\mathbf{X}$,$\mathbf{F}$) represents the trajectory of the robot tool after usual position training which depends primarily on surface relief. The curve L_0(X, F) represents the trajectory of the robot tool after force training when the required accuracy is achieved.

$$\|L_0(\mathbf{X}, \mathbf{F}) - L_0(\mathbf{X}_0, \mathbf{F}_0)\| < R \tag{11}$$

where R is the radius of the sphere, which determines the positional error.

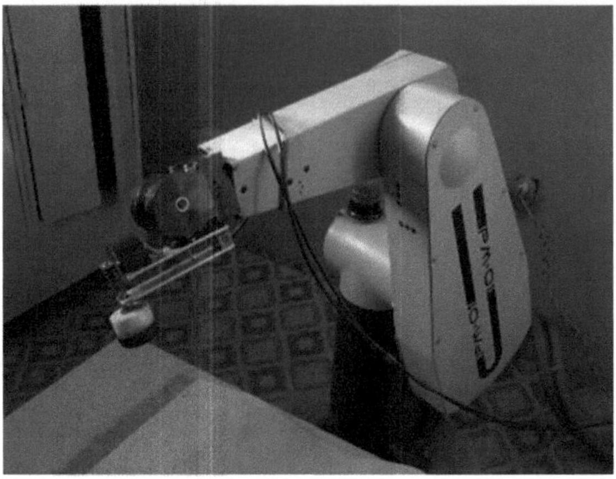

Fig. 7 Robot with position/force control for massage developed in Moscow State Industrial University

At Moscow State Industrial University the robot performing massage and extremities movements techniques is developed (Golovin and Grib 2002a, b; Golovin 2005). A basis of this robot is the industrial PUMA robot that has anthropomorphic manipulator (Fig. 7). The robot provides the contact force up to 60 N. On the end link a force module containing a strain gauge is mounted. Necessary efforts are made and supervised by position/force control system expanding possibilities of the standard robot.

The six-drive robot can perform a set of known manipulations directly on soft tissues, i.e. various massage, and also manipulations on joints in the form of passive and active extremities movements, a post-isometric relaxation (loading and unloading combinations for extremities muscles).

6 Conclusions

The soft tissues as an environment interacting with the robot have properties different from constructional materials. The force training mode as a phase of position/force control is preferred for robots deforming ST in massage. This mode was realized with the use of the modernized robot PUMA. Clinical trials of the robot performing various massage techniques on different patients have confirmed the effectiveness of the proposed force training mode.

Acknowledgments The scientific work described this chapter was supported by Grant No. 12-08-01159 of RFBR.

References

Golovin, V.: Robot for massage. Proceedings of JARP, 2nd Workshop on Medical Robotics. Heidelberg, Germany (1997).

Golovin, V.: Robot for massage and mobilization. Proceedings of workshop of AMETMAS-NoE, Moscow, Russia (1998).

Golovin, V., Arhipov, M., and Zhuravlev, V.: Robotics in restorative medicine. Robots for mechanotherapy, LAP LAMBERT Academic Publishing, GmbH & Co. KG, p. 280 (2012).

Golovin, V., Grib, A.: Mechatronic system for manual therapy and massage. Proceeding of 8-th Mehatronics Forum International Conference, University of Twente, Netherlands (2002).

Golovin, V., Grib, A.: Computer assisted robot for massage and mobilization. Proceeding. «Computer Science and Information Technologies», Conference Greece University of Patras (2002).

Golovin, V., Samorukov, A.: Massage method and device for its realization. Russian patent №2145833 from 08.05.1998 (in Russian).

Golovin, V., Zhuravlev, V., Razumov, A., Rachkov, M.: Adaptive force module for medical robots. Issues of Workshop on «Adaptive and Intelligence Robotics: Present and Future», Russia, IPM RSA, Moscow (2005).

Jones, Kenny C., Du, Winncy.: Development a Massage Robot for Medical Therapy. Proceedings of the IEEE/ASME International Conference on Advanced Intelligent Mechatronics (AIM'03), July 23-26, Kobe, Japan, pp. 1096–110 (2003).

Vukobratovic, M., Rodic, A.: Impedance control as a particular case of the unified approach to the control of robots interacting with a dynamic known environment. Journal of intelligent and robotic systems, 18, pp.191–204 (1997).

Vukobratovic, M., Surdilovic, D., Ecalo, Y., Kabic, D.: Dynamics and robust control of robot - environment interaction. Monograph series in the World scientific publishing under the title «New frontiers in robotics», World Scientific Publishing Company p. 660 (2009).

References

Flexible Bi-modal Control Modes for Hands-Free Operation of a Wheelchair by Head Movements and Facial Expressions

Ericka Janet Rechy-Ramirez and Huosheng Hu

Abstract Many kinds of head movements and facial expressions based human machine interfaces (HMIs) have been developed for hands-free control of electric-powered wheelchairs in order to assist disabled and elderly people. Most of these HMIs have a fixed configuration and do not allow users to choose a configuration suitable to their needs. It becomes necessary to provide users with different control modes and flexible configurations. This chapter presents five flexible bi-modal modes for hands-free control of a wheelchair that allow users to choose the most comfortable facial expressions and head movements. An Emotiv sensor is deployed to collect facial expressions and head movements for the bi-modal control modes. Two healthy subjects have participated in experiments, and have chosen their best configurations of the modes for controlling the wheelchair. Experimental results show that bi-modal control modes are flexible and allow users to select their preferred configurations for controlling the wheelchair reliably.

Keywords Facial expression · Head movement · Human–machine interface · Emotiv EPOC sensor · Electric-powered wheelchair

1 Introduction

Elderly and disabled people who suffer from stroke, head injury, spinal cord injury and multiple sclerosis are unable to use traditional wheelchairs that are driven by joysticks. Therefore, it is necessary to develop new human-machine interfaces

E. J. Rechy-Ramirez (✉) · H. Hu
University of Essex, Colchester, UK
e-mail: ejrech@essex.ac.uk

H. Hu
e-mail: hhu@essex.ac.uk

A. Rodić et al. (eds.), *New Trends in Medical and Service Robots*,
Mechanisms and Machine Science 20, DOI: 10.1007/978-3-319-05431-5_8,

(HMIs) for hands-free control of a wheelchair. Up to now, a number of bio-signal based HMIs have been developed for hands-free control of intelligent wheelchairs, including visual based head and hand gestures, voice, etc. For instance, certain points of the face, e.g. nose, eye and mouth, are tracked by using a camera in front of the user in order to identify his or her head movements (Adachi et al. 1998; Jia et al. 2007). In (Christensen and Garcia 2005), head movements are detected by employing infrared sensor placed behind the head of the user.

By now, electromyography (EMG) signal is widely deployed to obtain facial expressions for hands-free control of a wheelchair. In (Felzer and Freisleben 2002), only one facial expression is used for operating the wheelchair. In (Tamura et al. 2010), three facial expressions (winking left and right eyes and biting) are employed to control a wheelchair; while in (Firoozabadi et al. 2008) four facial expressions (smiling, tensing the eyebrows and pulling them up, left and right smirks) are used for giving the commands. On the other hand, (Han et al. 2003; Moon et al. 2005) have employed EMG signals for controlling wheelchairs by means of shoulder movements. Moreover, electrooculography signal (EOG) (Barea et al. 2000, 2003; Kuo et al. 2009), vision techniques (Gajwani and Chhabria 2010) and infra-red photo sensors (Crisman et al. 1991) have been used for detecting eye gaze and eye winks from the user to give the commands to the wheelchair. At the same time, electroencephalography signal (EEG) has been used for controlling a wheelchair in spite of its slow response. In (Rebsamen et al. 2007), P300 signal is employed so that the user can focus his or her attention in a desired destination from a predefined map in order to move the wheelchair from one place to another. Likewise, in (Palankar et al. 2008) a P300 signal is used for operating a wheelchair through a mounted robotic arm in a simulated environment. In (Galán et al. 2008) three mental tasks are employed for controlling a simulated wheelchair in a simulated environment.

Other works have integrated different types of techniques in order to implement HMIs for hands-free control of a wheelchair. In (Bergasa et al. 2000), head movements, lip hiding and eye winking are detected by using a 2D face tracker in order to operate the wheelchair. In (Tsui et al. 2007), EMG and EOG signals are employed to detect eyebrow tension and lateral eyes movements respectively to operate the wheelchair. In (Wei and Hu 2010), eye winking and jaw clenching movements provide the commands to the wheelchair, in which EMG signal and facial image are integrated.

With the advances in technology, there is a relative new sensor in the market able to provide potential applications in hands-free HMIs, namely Emotiv EPOC. In (Gomez-Gil et al. 2011), this sensor is deployed to recognize four fixed trained muscular events to steer a tractor, while (Carrino et al. 2011) has developed a system, namely "Virtual Move", which allows users to navigate through Google Street View (GSV) using head movements, facial expressions, thoughts and emotional states.

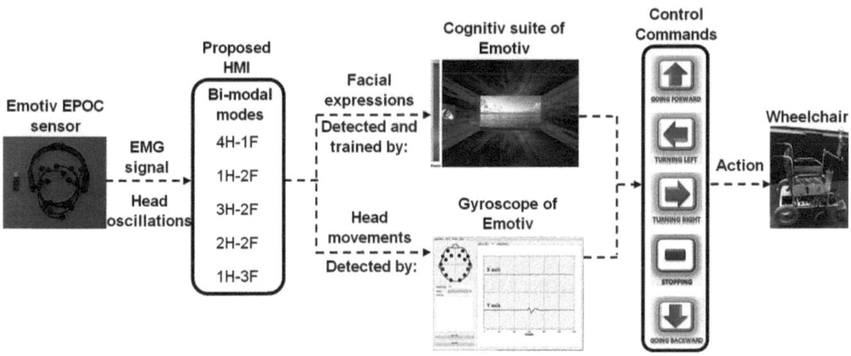

Fig. 1 Architecture of the human machine interface (HMI)

1.1 Contribution of Our Work

Taking into account the works mentioned above, to implement a HMI for hands-free control of a wheelchair is not a new topic. Looking at the HWIs that are based on vision, their common shortcoming is that their performances are likely affected by environmental noises such as illumination, brightness, camera position and background of the image; thus these HWIs cannot be used in environments with poor illumination and big noise. But, if we consider the HWIs using eye-gaze for giving the commands, these HWIs have the drawback of causing dizziness on the users during their operation because of the movement of the eye's pupil. Finally, as can be noticed, most of the existing HWIs are not flexible on the movements or expressions to be employed by the user in order to control the wheelchair. Our main contribution in this chapter can be described as follows:

> The head movements and facial expressions based bi-modal control modes are developed for hands-free control of a wheelchair in environments with poor illumination and heavy noises. The user can choose his or her preferred facial expressions and configuration for giving the commands according to his/her needs.

2 Overview of the Proposed Human Machine Interface

Figure 1 shows the Emotiv EPOC headset used in our bio-signal HMI for detecting facial expressions and head movements to generate the five bi-modal control modes. The reasons we choose it to implement the bio-control modes in this research are: (1) it is easy to wear, (2) it has suites for recognizing different facial expressions and head movements providing flexibility to the control modes, and (3) its response to the head movements and facial expressions performed by the user is fast and accurate.

2.1 Equipment

The Emotiv EPOC Headset—It is a sensing device that measures EEG activity from 14 saline electrodes (plus CMS/DRL references, P3/P4 locations). These electrodes are arranged according to the 10/20 system, and their locations are AF3, F7, F3, FC5, T7, P7, O1, O2, P8, T8, FC6, F4, F8 and AF4 (Emotiv EPOC Specifications 2012). It comes with an Emotiv Software Development Kit for research, including an API for developing applications using the three different Emotiv suites: 'cognitiv', 'expressiv' and 'affectiv' suites. Each suite has different functions as follows:

- The 'cognitiv suite' recognizes 14 conscious thoughts of the user ('neutral', 'right', 'left', 'push', 'pull', 'lift', 'drop', 'rotate left', 'rotate right', 'rotate clockwise', 'rotate anti-clockwise', 'rotate forwards', 'rotate reverse' and 'disappear'); but only a maximum of 4 actions can be used apart from the neutral action in each session.
- The 'expressiv suite' recognizes facial expressions such as 'blink', 'right wink', 'left wink', 'look right/left', 'raise brow', 'furrow brow', 'smile', 'clench', 'right smirk', 'left smirk' and 'laugh'.
- The 'affectiv suite' recognizes emotional states of the user, including engagement/boredom, frustration, meditation, instantaneous excitement and long term excitement.

Besides the suites, the Emotiv EPOC sensing device has a gyroscope with two axes, 'X' and 'Y', which give the posture data of the user's head. The 'X' axis provides data of horizontal head movements, whereas 'Y' axis gives data of vertical head movements.

The wheelchair—It is equipped with an embedded PC with the following features:

- Processor: Intel Atom CPD 525, 1.80 GHz;
- Installed memory (RAM): 4.00 GB;
- Operating system: Windows 7;
- Installed software: Microsoft Visual Studio 2010 and Emotiv research edition SDK 1.0.0.4.

The detailed description of the hardware structure of the wheelchair system can be found in (Jia et al. 2007).

2.2 Notations and Definitions

Definition 1: The facial expressions trained during the experiments involve movements of the:

- Forehead: (FB) furrow brows and (RB) raise brows;
- Eyes: LEC (left eye closed) and;
- Mouth: S (smile), LS (left smirk) and RS (right smirk).

Definition 2: The commands for operating the wheelchair provided in all the control modes are: stopping, going forward, turning left, turning right, and going backward.

Definition 3: In order to have an optimal performance of the control modes, the following rules were taken into account for choosing the facial expressions: (1) facial expressions must be different; (2) only one forehead expression can be used in the control mode; and (3) if a facial expression is smile (S), then the rest of the expressions cannot be smirk expressions (LS, RS) and vice versa. The rules (2) and (3) are used to prevent the likely false detections between expressions.

Definition 3: The bi-modal control modes are:

- **4H-1F** (facialExp1): using four head movements and two facial expressions.
- **1H-2F** (facialExp1, facialExp2): using one head movement and two facial expressions.
- **3H-2F** (facialExp1, facialExp2): using three head movements and two facial expressions.
- **2H-2F** (facialExp1, facialExp2): using two head movements and two facial expressions.
- **1H-3F** (facialExp1, facialExp2, facialExp3): using one head movement and three facial expressions.

It is important to remark that the user can choose one head movement (headMov1) in 1H-2F, 1H-3F and 3H-2F between up or down movements for stopping the wheelchair. The other two head movements of 3H-2F are already defined (right and left head movements). On the other hand, the user has to decide which head movement (either up or down) is used for going forward (headMov1) in 2H-2F, and the remaining one will be used for stopping (headMov2).

2.3 *Identifying Head Movements and Facial Expressions*

The bi-modal control modes use the gyroscope of the Emotiv sensor to recognize the head movements. A positive value of the 'X' axis corresponds to a right head movement and a negative value of 'X' represents a left head movement. On the other hand, a positive value of the 'Y' axis corresponds to an up head movement and a negative value of the 'Y' represents a down head movement.

The Emotiv sensor provides the expressiv suite for identifying facial expressions from the user, and the cognitiv suite for identifying thoughts. After doing informal experiments, we decide to deploy the cognitiv suite since it provides a faster and more accurate identification of the facial expressions than the expressiv suite. Furthermore, with the cognitiv suite, the user can train his or her most comfortable facial expressions for executing the commands, offering flexibility to the control modes. With the aim of improving the recognition of the head movements and facial expressions of the user, timers and thresholds were added to the identifications of these expressions provided by the Emotiv sensor.

2.4 The Training Process of Facial Expressions

Before using any bi-modal control mode, the user has to train the facial expressions to be employed in the control commands through the cognitiv suite. When a user is training an action of the cognitiv suite (e.g. 'right', 'left', 'push'), a cube presented in its graphical user interface will move according to the trained action. Each cognitiv action has an associated facial expression, e.g. the 'right cognitiv action' corresponds to 'right smirk'. The procedure to train the facial expressions using the cognitiv suite is as follows:

- First, the user has to train a 'neutral state' (normal pose) in which the user does nothing. The neutral action can be trained by using two modalities: one modality lasts 8 s and the other one lasts 30 s. During the training process of this action, the user has to keep a normal pose without doing any facial expression, so that action data can be recorded. This action needs more training than the other ones in order to avoid false triggered expressions. For our experiments, the subjects trained the 'neutral state' 10 times using the '8 s modality' and 3 times using the '30 s modality'.
- Then, the user has to train each facial expression during which the pose has to be kept for 8 s. Each facial expression has to be trained in a same way for several times until the action is performed easily and reliably by the cognitiv suite. One way to see whether the user is performing the same gesture is to check the skill rating of the training in the interface of the suite; it should be increasing each time. Before training a facial expression in the cognitiv suite, the sensitivity of the action associated to it has to be set as 'high'. In this way, the user can normally achieve a training rate of 80 % or more after 6 trials. For our experiments, all the expressions were trained with 6 trials by both subjects.
- Finally, if necessary, the user can adjust his or her facial expressions by decreasing the sensitivity of each action associated to each expression in the cognitiv suite at his or her convenience. In our experiments, the sensitivities of all the expressions trained by both subjects were decreased in three units below 'high sensitivity'; that is between medium and high sensitivities.

2.5 Bi-modal Control Modes

Our bi-modal control modes use facial expressions and head movements for executing the control commands. 4H-1F and 3H-2F first display the commands in their graphical user interfaces (GUI) by using head movements and then execute them by employing facial expressions; while 2H-2F and 1H-3F execute all the commands immediately. Finally, 1H-2F associates two commands to each facial expression. The manner of giving the control commands in each control mode is explained in Fig. 2.

In all the control modes, once the user had assigned either the facial expression or the head movement to a command, these cannot be changed while the mode is running. All the control modes start at the stopping control command. It is important to remark that in order to provide comfort to the user, either the facial expressions or the head movements only need to be performed by 2 s, i.e., the user does not have to maintain the movement. Therefore, the user can turn his or her head around while the wheelchair is moving without executing an undesired turning command. In all the bi-modal control modes excluding the 1H-2F, for executing the going backward command, the user has to be at the 'stopping command' and performs the head movement associated to it. In 4H-1F and 3H-2F, the reason for integrating two types of information (head movements and a facial expression) in the execution of the 'turning commands' is to allow the user to move his/her head during the operation of the wheelchair without interference.

3 Experiments and Analysis

All the bi-modal control modes have been tested by controlling a wheelchair in an indoor environment. Two healthy subjects (a female and a male) have participated in the experiments. It is important to remark that in order to evaluate how fast are the responses of the control modes during the operation of the wheelchair; none of them use obstacle avoidance function, so the control of the wheelchair only relies on the way of giving the commands in each mode.

To choose the facial expressions for controlling the wheelchair, the users deployed the 'cognitiv suite' of Emotiv. With the aim of identifying the most comfortable expressions of the users, they tested them on the HMI without moving the wheelchair. Both subjects identified various facial expressions to be used in the control modes. Due to time availability of Subject B, he only used one configuration per mode. Ten experiments were carried out by each control mode. In each experiment, the subject has to follow the route shown in Fig. 3 without hitting obstacles. Each subject did a round of ten trials per day. First Subject A did the experiments and then Subject B. The order in which the control modes were tested corresponds to the order of the modes shown in Tables 1, 2 and 3 from left to right, i.e. (1) 4H-1F, (2) 1H-2F, (3) 3H-2F, (4) 2H-2F, and (5) 1H-3F.

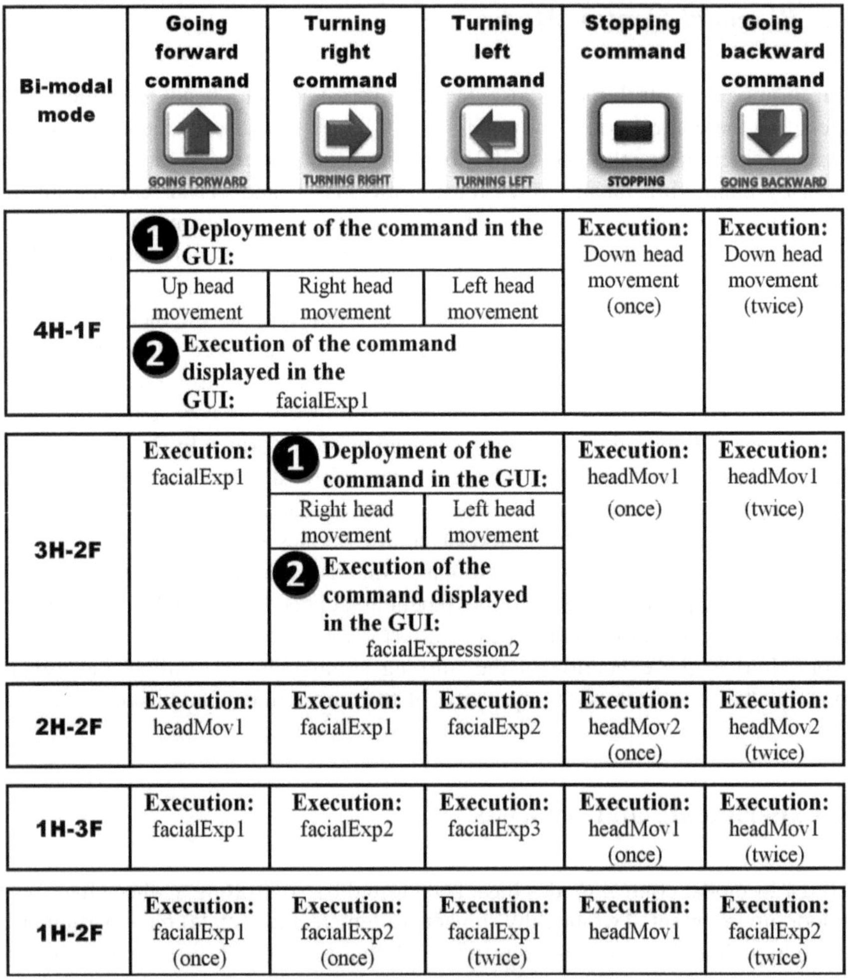

Fig. 2 Execution of the control commands of each bi-modal mode

Based on the experiences of the two subjects in controlling wheelchairs with these types of modes, it can be said that Subject A has experience in using the control modes due to her participation in the project; whereas subject B has no experience in employing these control modes. For this reason, prior doing the experiments reported in this chapter, he followed the route once (an informal trial) per each control mode.

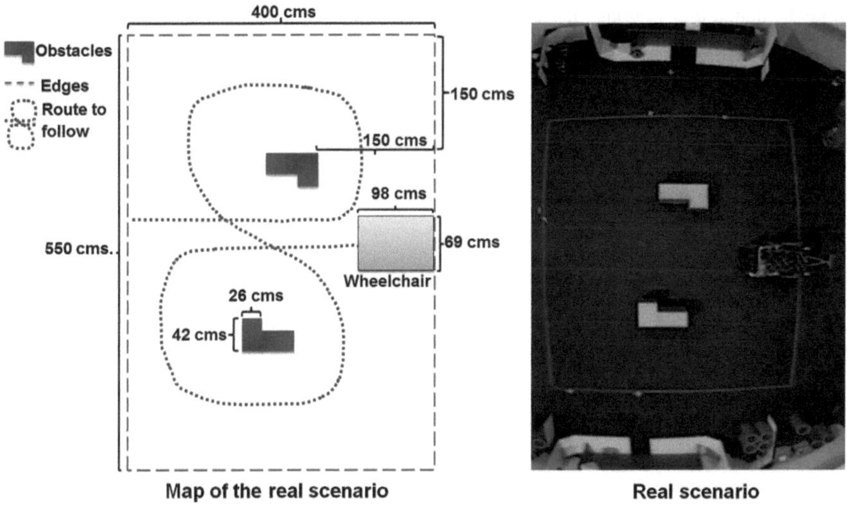

Fig. 3 The route to follow in the experiments

Table 1 Standard deviations, means, medians, minimum and maximum values of the traveling times of subject A using bi-modal control modes with different configurations

	4H-1F				1H-2F	
	(FB)	(LS)	(RS)	(S)	(LS, RS)	(S, FB)
Standard deviation	19.8	9.1	11.2	4.7	10.8	6.1
Mean	159.1	152.5	159.8	147.9	150.7	151
Median	150.5	150.5	156.5	146.5	151	149.5
Minimum value	143	138	142	147	135	144
Maximum value	205	168	156	175	168	161

Table 2 Standard deviations, means, medians, minimum and maximum values of the traveling times of subject A using bi-modal control modes with different configurations

	3H-2F			2H-2F			1H-3F
	(LS, RS)	(FB, S)	(RS, RB)	(LS, RS)	(S, FB)	(LS, FB)	(FB, LS, RS)
Standard deviation	9.2	8	9.8	8.5	8.4	10.5	7.9
Mean	144.4	149.9	153.7	152.3	147.1	144	148.1
Median	141	148	155	148.5	147	145.5	146.5
Minimum value	135	136	138	142	136	116	139
Maximum value	167	165	166	165	159	154	168

Table 3 Standard deviations, means, medians, minimum and maximum values of the traveling times of subject B using bi-modal control modes

	4H-1F (S)	1H-2F (S, RB)	3H-2F (RB, S)	2H-2F (RB, S)	1H-3F (RB, LEC, S)
Standard deviation	31.5	7.3	10.6	10.4	12
Mean	166	152.5	152.6	154.2	160.5
Median	153.5	151	149.5	152	158.5
Minimum value	145	143	143	144	142
Maximum value	240	167	176	175	180

3.1 Experimental Results

4H-1F and 3H-2F control modes use a deployment process of the commands prior to execute them, so it was expected that these modes obtained largest mean, median or maximum value of the traveling times in both subjects. As can be seen in Tables 1, 2 and 3, the experiments demonstrated the scenario that we predicted about 4H-1F. Both subjects reported the largest maximum value of the traveling times when 4H-1F was used, only that Subject B used 'S' (240 s) and Subject A used 'FB' (205 s). Furthermore, 4H-1F obtained the largest means: 159.8 s (Subject A using RS) and 166 s (Subject B). Moreover, 4H-1F presented the largest minimum values of the traveling times in both subjects when S was used (147 s for Subject A and 145 s for Subject B). Finally, Subject A reported 4H-1F using 'RS' as the control mode with the largest median (156.5 s). Nevertheless, 3H-2F obtained the smallest median in both subjects: 141 s for Subject A using LS, RS and 149.5 s for Subject B using RB, S.

On the other hand, 2H-2F and 1H-3F control modes execute the commands immediately, so it was expected that these modes reported the smallest mean, median or minimum value of the traveling times in both subjects. As we estimated, 2H-2F using LS, FB (Subject A) and 1H-3F using RB, LEC, S (Subject B) obtained the smallest minimum values of the traveling times, 116 and 142 s, respectively. Furthermore, in the case of Subject A, 2H-2F using LS, FB reported the smallest mean (144 s) and the smallest maximum value of the traveling times (154 s). On the other hand, in the case of Subject B, 1H-2F using S, RB obtained the smallest mean (152.5 s) and smallest maximum value of the traveling times (167 s).

As can be seen in Fig. 4, Subject A obtained the smallest standard deviation of the traveling times (4.7 s) when 4H-1F(S) was used, while the same mode but used by Subject B reported the largest standard deviation (31.5 s). Also, it can be noticed certain similar means between the modes used by Subject A, e.g. (1) 4H-1F (LS) and 2H-2F (LS, RS); (2) 4H-1F using FB and using RS; (3) 4H-1F (S) and 2H-2F (S, FB); and (4) 3H-2F (LS, RS) and 2H-2F (LS, FB). But only in the case ii was the same mode, as we expected. Also, 1H-2F and 3H-2F used by Subject B presented similar means. Furthermore, the modes of 4H-1F using LS (Subject A),

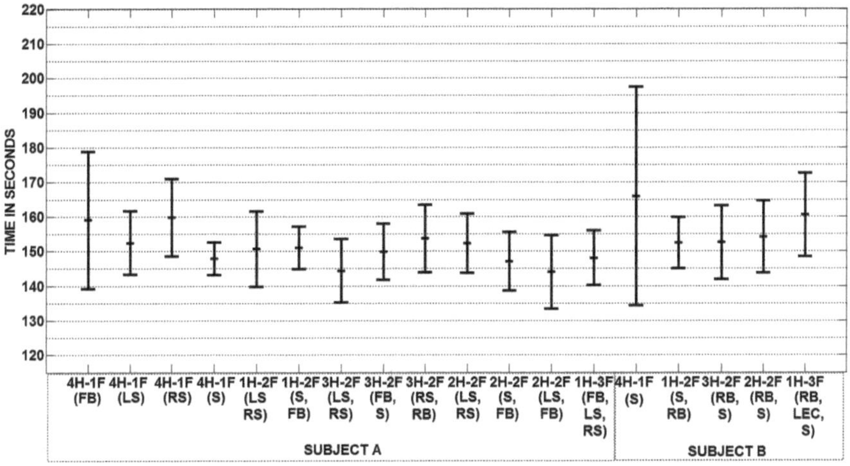

Fig. 4 Means and standard deviations of the traveling times of subjects '*A*' and '*B*' using the five bi-modal modes with different configurations

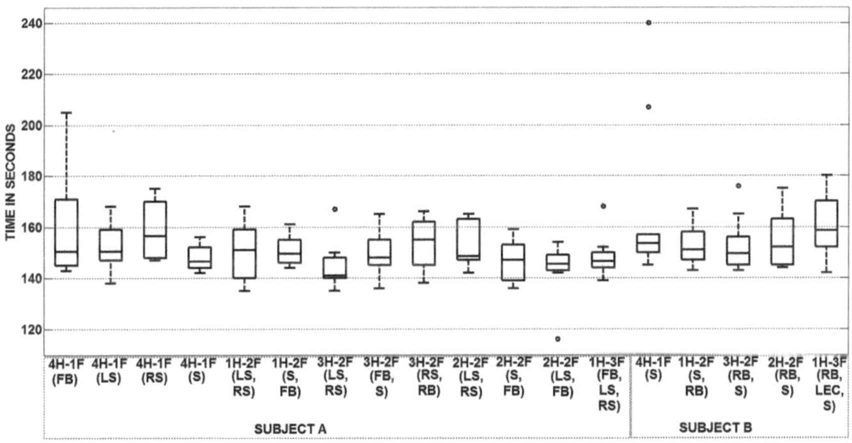

Fig. 5 Medians, minimum and maximum values of the traveling times of subjects '*A*' and '*B*' using the five bi-modal control modes with different configurations

1H-2F (Subject B), 2H-2F using LS, RS (Subject A) and 3H-2F (Subject B) have similar means (approximately 152 s).

As can be noticed in Fig. 5, although there are identical medians (two cases), minimum (four cases) and maximum values (two cases) in the traveling times between the modes used by Subject A; only in one case was the same bi-modal mode presenting identical values but using different facial expressions, i.e. 4H-1F using FB and using LS (medians of 150.5 s). Also, there were identical medians (two cases), minimum (three cases) and maximum (two cases) values in the

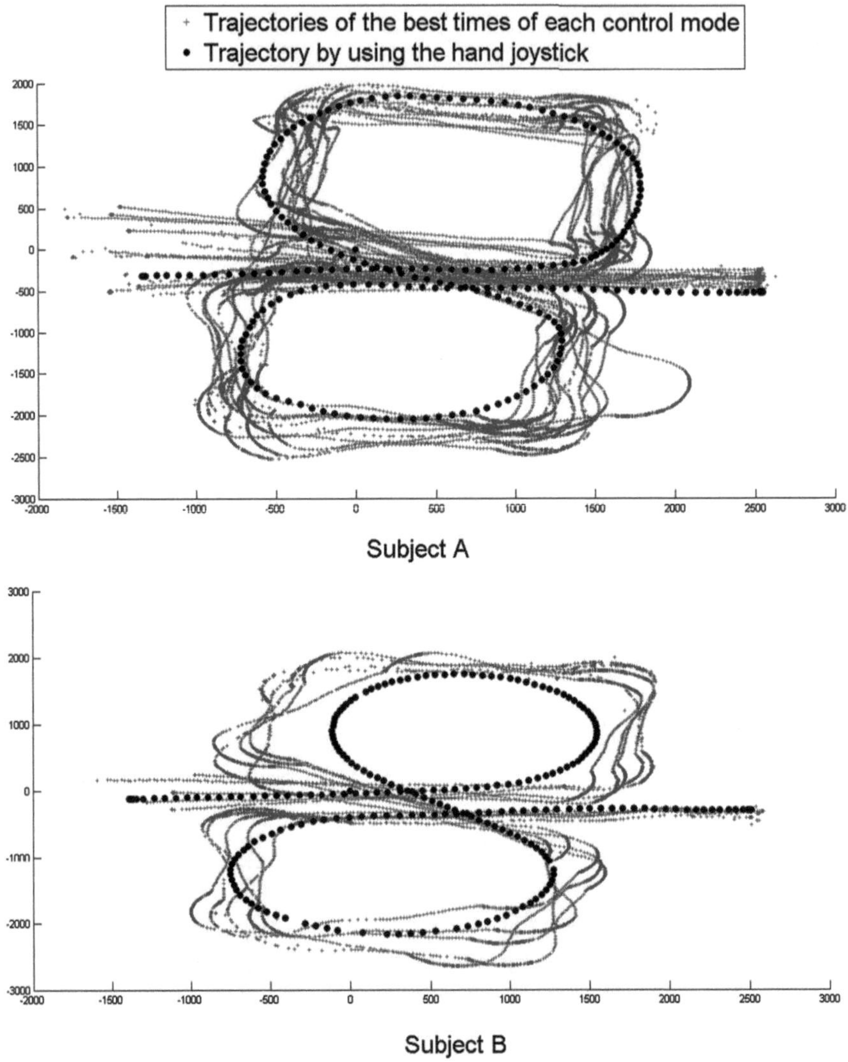

Fig. 6 Trajectories of the best times of each control mode of subjects *A* and *B*

traveling times of the bi-modal control modes between two subjects, but it was only in one case that the same mode have identical values between two subjects, i.e. 1H-2F using LS, RS of Subject A and 1H-2F using S, RB of Subject B (medians of 151 s). Finally, it can be seen that the smallest and largest medians of the modes between both subjects have a minimal difference, i.e. a gap of 17.5 s. In contrast, the differences between the smallest and largest values of the minimum and maximum values of the traveling times are considerable, i.e. gaps of 31 and 86 s, respectively.

After finishing all the experiments, both subjects agreed that their two most comfortable and favorite modes are 2H-2F, followed by 1H-3F. Moreover, Subject A mentioned that the facial expressions of LS and RS were the most comfortable ones for the mode of 2H-2F. The trajectories of the experiments were recorded by a VICON motion tracking system with five markers attached to the wheelchair. The trajectories of the best times of each control mode per each subject are shown in Fig. 6. Also, a trajectory done by each subject using the joystick was added as a reference. It is important to remark that both subjects were able to complete the route indicated in Fig. 3 without colliding with the obstacles in each experiment for each control mode.

3.2 Discussion

Although these bi-modal control modes represent alternatives for hands-free control of a wheelchair, some of them have associated limitations. The main limitation of 1H-2F is that the facial expressions have associated two control commands; therefore the execution of the commands was not very fast. Likewise, 4H-1F and 3H-2F did not provide a very fast execution of the commands because they employ a deployment process of the commands before executing them. Apart from these inconveniences, 1H-2F and 3H-2F control modes offer a fast execution of the stopping command, which can be used in environment with any illumination, i.e. good or poor. Besides, the experimental results show that the means of the traveling times between 1H-2F and 3H-2F and the rest of the bi-modal control modes have a minimal difference. Although this work only provides ten experimental results per each control mode with two healthy subjects, it represents a reliable starting point to evaluate the use of the bi-modal control modes for the hands free control of a wheelchair.

4 Conclusions

We have proposed a novel HMI that is able to provide five different control modes with different configurations for users to deploy head movements and facial expressions to operate a wheelchair. After carrying out experiments with two subjects, it can be concluded that all the control modes offer flexibility in their configurations, which allow the most comfortable facial expressions to be chosen by users to give the commands. Although the modes 4H-1F, 1H-2F and 3H-2F may not provide a fast execution of commands, experimental results demonstrated that they are usable in practice. All control modes do not require users to keep their facial expression or head movement during wheelchair operation. Finally, it is clear that the bi-modal control is safe and reliable, and represents a feasible option for implementing hands-free applications for assisting the disabled and elderly people.

Our future work will be focused on using fuzzy logic to determine better thresholds for detecting the facial expressions and testing the control modes with more subjects.

Acknowledgments The authors gratefully acknowledge the support of the EU Interreg SYSIASS project: Autonomous and Intelligent Healthcare System (http://www.sysiass.eu/), and the COALAS project: Cognitive Assisted Living Ambient System (http://www.coalas-project.eu/). The COALAS project has been selected in the context of the INTERREG IVA France (Channel)—European cross-border co-operation programme, which is co-financed by the ERDF. The 1st author has been supported by the Mexican National Council of Science and Technology (CONACYT), through the program "Becas para estudios de posgrado en el extranjero" (no. 183592) and by the Secretariat of Public Education of the Mexican Government (Secretaría de Educación Pública del Gobierno Mexicano) through the scholarship "Programa de apoyo al posgrado, beca complemento, ciclo 2013". Our thanks also go to Robin Dowling for his technical support during the research.

References

Adachi, Y., Kuno, Y., Shimada, N., and Shirai, Y.: Intelligent wheelchair using visual information on human faces. In Intelligent Robots and Systems, pp. 354–359 (1998)

Barea, R., Boquete, L., Mazo, M., López, E. and Bergasa, L.M.: EOG guidance of a wheelchair using neural networks. In Proc. of the 15th International Conference on Pattern Recognition, 4, 668–671 (2000)

Barea, R., Boquete, L., Bergasa, L.M., López, E. and Mazo, M.: Electrooculography guidance of a wheelchair using eye movements codification. The International Journal of Robotics Research, 22 (7-8), 641–652 (2003)

Bergasa, L.M., Mazo, M., Gardel, A., Barea, R., and Boquete, L.: Commands generation by face movements applied to the guidance of a wheelchair for handicapped people. In Proceedings of the 15th International Conference on Pattern Recognition, 4, 660–663 (2000)

Carrino, F., Tscherrig, J., Mugellini, E., Abou Khaled, O. and Ingold, R.: Head-computer interface: a multimodal approach to navigate through real and virtual worlds. Human-Computer Interaction. Interaction techniques and environments. LNCS: Springer, 6762, 222–230 (2011)

Christensen, H.V., and Garcia, J.C.: Infrared non-contact head sensor for control of wheelchair movements. In Proc. of the 8th European Conference for the Advancement of Assistive Technology in Europe, pp. 336–340 (2005)

Crisman, E.E., Loomis, A., Shaw, R. and Laszewski, Z.: Using the eye wink control interface to control a powered wheelchair. In Engineering in Medicine and Biology Society: Vol. 13. In Proc. of the Annual International Conference of the IEEE, pp.1821–1822 (1991)

Emotiv EPOC Specifications (2012) Retrieved August 14, 2013, from http://www.emotiv.com/epoc/download_specs.php

Felzer, T. and Freisleben, B.: HaWCoS: the hands-free wheelchair control system. In Proc. of the fifth international ACM conference on assistive technologies, pp. 127–134 (2002)

Firoozabadi, S.M.P., Oskoei, M.A. and Hu, H.: A human-computer Interface based on forehead multi-channel bio-signals to control a virtual wheelchair. In Proc. of the 14th Iranian Conference on Biomedical Engineering, pp. 272–277 (2008)

Gajwani, P.S. and Chhabria, S.A.: Eye motion tracking for wheelchair control. International Journal of Information Technology, 2(2), 185–187 (2010)
Galán, F., Nuttin, M., Lew, E., Ferrez, P.W., Vanacker, G., Philips, J. and Millán, J.R.: A brain-actuated wheelchair: asynchronous and non-invasive brain–computer interfaces for continuous control of robots. Clinical Neurophysiology, 119(9), 2159–2169 (2008)
Gomez-Gil, J., San-Jose-Gonzalez, I., Nicolas-Alonso, L.F. and Alonso-Garcia, S.: Steering a tractor by means of an EMG-based human machine interface. Sensors, 11(7), 7110–7126 (2011)
Han, J.S., Zenn Bien, Z., Kim, D.J., Lee, H.E. and Kim. J.S.: Human machine interface for wheelchair control with EMG and its evaluation. In Engineering in Medicine and Biology Society: Vol. 2. In Proc. of the 25th Annual International Conference of the IEEE, pp.1602–1605 (2003)
Jia, P., Hu, H., Lu, T. and Yuan, K.: Head gesture recognition for hands-free control of an intelligent wheelchair. Industrial Robot: An International Journal, 34(1), 60–68 (2007)
Kuo, C.H. , Chan, Y.C., Chou, H.C. and Siao, J.W.: Eyeglasses based electrooculography human-wheelchair interface. In Systems, Man and Cybernetics, pp. 4746–4751 (2009)
Moon, I., Lee, M., Chu, J. and Mun, M.: Wearable EMG-based HCI for electric-powered wheelchair users with motor disabilities. In Proc. of the IEEE International Conference on Robotics and Automation, pp. 2649–2654 (2005)
Palankar, M., De Laurentis, K.J., Alqasemi, R., Veras, E., Dubey, R., Arbel, Y. and Donchin, E.: Control of a 9-DoF wheelchair-mounted robotic arm system using a P300 brain computer interface: Initial experiments. In Robotics and Biomimetics, pp. 348–353 (2008)
Rebsamen, B., Burdet, E., Guan, C., Teo, C.L., Zeng, Q., Ang, M. and Laugier, C.: Controlling a wheelchair using a BCI with low information transfer rate. In Rehabilitation Robotics, pp. 1003–1008 (2007)
Tamura, H., Manabe, T., Goto, T., Yamashita, Y. and Tanno, K.: A study of the electric wheelchair hands-free safety control system using the surface-electromygram of facial muscles. Intelligent Robotics and Applications. LNCS: Springer, 6425, 97–104 (2010)
Tsui, C.S.L., Jia, P., Gan, J.Q., Hu, H. and Yuan, K.: EMG-based hands-free wheelchair control with EOG attention shift detection. In IEEE International Conference on Robotics and Biomimetics, pp. 1266–1271 (2007)
Wei, L. and Hu, H.: EMG and visual based HMI for hands-free control of an intelligent wheelchair. In 8th World Congress on Intelligent Control and Automation, pp. 1027–1032 (2010)

[illegible]

New Results on Classifying EMG Signals for Interfacing Patients and Mechanical Devices

G. Gini, L. Cavazzana, F. Mutti, P. Belluco and A. Mauri

Abstract In modern days the goal of rehabilitative robotics is to take advantage of robotics-inspired solutions in order to assist people affected by disabilities using physical training assisted by robots. In this way the rehabilitative exercises could be autonomously performed by the patients, with a reduced involvement of the therapist, making high-intensity rehabilitative therapy an affordable reality. Moreover high-precision sensors integrated in rehabilitation devices would allow a quantitative evaluation of the progresses obtained, effectively comparing different training strategies. That would represent a huge scientific achievement in a field where evaluations up to this day are performed only by means of subjective observations. Important results were obtained in rehabilitative robotics, but results in the field of the hand rehabilitation are poorer, due to the high complexity and dexterity of the organ. This chapter proposes to integrate the detection of the muscular activity in the rehabilitation loop. A new EMG analysis tool was developed to achieve a reliable early recognition of the movement. Experimental results confirmed that our system is able to recognize the performed movement and generate the first control variable after 200 ms, below the commonly accepted delay of 300 ms for interactive applications. This shows that it is possible to effectively use an EMG classifier to obtain a reliable controller for a flexible device, able to assist the patient only after having detected his effort.

Keywords Rehabilitative robotics · Arm rehabilitation · EMG signals · Classifiers

G. Gini (✉) · L. Cavazzana · F. Mutti
DEIB, Politecnico di Milano, Milan, Italy
e-mail: gini@elet.polimi.it

P. Belluco · A. Mauri
B10NIX, Milan, Italy
e-mail: p.belluco@b10nix.com

A. Rodić et al. (eds.), *New Trends in Medical and Service Robots*,
Mechanisms and Machine Science 20, DOI: 10.1007/978-3-319-05431-5_9,

1 Introduction

Each year 800,000 people in the U.S. experience stroke attacks, with 50 % of the survivors left with hemi paresis and 26 % unable to independently perform daily activities (American Heart Association 2011). These statistics make stroke the leading cause of physical impairment, but other pathologies such as multiple sclerosis, cerebral palsy, spinal cord injury, Parkinson disease or bones trauma and ligament degradation are cause of poor quality of life.

Tests show that significant improvement in movement ability can be achieved through proper physical training, but this leads to a strong economic pressure on the health care system. The idea behind rehabilitative robotics is to take advantage of modern robots to assist patients through physical training: from the point of view of the therapist, exercises are highly repetitive, time consuming and physically demanding, the kind of task robots are suited for. So in the last 20 years a great effort was spent in developing devices able to offer a (semi-)autonomous training and in studying better methods to help patients to regain their motor functionalities (robot-aided rehabilitation), or providing active assistance with daily activities (assistive exoskeletons). Currently, robotic therapy programs are offered by some health care centres. The ultimate goal is to make affordable domestic intensive therapy in the near future.

Tests conducted within the Veteran Affairs (VA) hospitals (Lo et al. 2010) show how patients who received high intensity therapy by a robotic device for thirty-six weeks achieved a significant gain in motor functionality, similar to the group which received a training of similar intensity from a human therapist. Both groups had a significantly greater gain if compared to a control group who received the traditional care. The cost for patient was $17,831 for the robotic therapy, $19,098 for usual care, and $19,746 for intensive non-robotic therapy. This indicates that now robotic therapy does not offer better improvements per se, but the possible drop in costs due to mass production could make high-intensity rehabilitation available on large scale. Another advantage of the robotic therapy is the ability to compare different training approaches, today left to subjective considerations of the therapist, making it possible to scientifically monitor the progresses and compare different strategies (Lo et al. 2010; Marchal-Crespo and Reinkensmeyer 2009), promoting consistency and reproducibility of the training.

A key element in rehabilitation is interactivity: the patient must not be simply dragged by the robot (Squeri et al. 2011). The rehabilitative system must promote user's effort giving assistance-as-needed, meaning only after detecting an effort, and providing no more than the force the patient needs to complete the task. This approach also makes the training exercise naturally scale with the condition of the patient, as the robot will gradually step aside as motion capabilities are regained (Wolbrecht et al. 2008).

Problems arise when the patient is unable to perform even the slightest movement, making force-triggered assist-on-need useless. For this reason EMG-triggered therapy was introduced: even if muscular tone makes the patient unable to perform any movement his intentions can still be detected if he is able to generate a minimum amount of nervous activity. Even users with better muscular conditions can exploit the EMG analysis to further anticipate their movements, or check if they are correctly performing.

Although robotic rehabilitation is rapidly developing, hand rehabilitation is relatively less dealt with if compared with the arm or the leg. This is because hand is a very complex organ, composed by 22° of freedom and actuated by nineteen muscles. Moreover muscles are tightly packed in the forearm, making signal detection pretty complex using non-invasive techniques like surface EMG, because of high interferences between muscles (cross-talk). Such complexity makes the realization of a rehabilitative device extremely challenging, both in mechanical design and control strategy.

Our goal here is to show how to improve arm, and in particular hand, rehabilitation through the EMG analysis. In the past we developed a rehabilitative device (Mulas et al. 2005), together with hand design and control strategies (Folgheraiter and Gini 2004; Folgheraiter et al. 2003; Soto Martell and Gini 2007), and an EMG-based controller for hand prosthesis (Arvetti et al. 2007; Gini et al. 2012; Lisi et al. 2011). Starting from those experiences we illustrate how the EMG classification system could meet the real time performance requirements for a smooth interaction with the patient, a key element for any EMG-triggered rehabilitative device.

The chapter is so organized. Section 2 presents an overview of the biological aspects of EMG signal generation. Section 3 gives an overview of the field of technology aided rehabilitation, and summarizes the results of the EMG signal classification for the hand movements. Section 4 discusses our EMG classifier, based on the concept of early detection. Section 5 evaluates the performances. Section 6 summarizes the results and proposes possible future developments.

2 Hand Movements and EMG Signals

The hand is one of the most complex organs, counting 22° of freedom actuated by nineteen muscles and able to perform very dexterous movements. A functional taxonomy (Bullock 2011) considers all the hand/wrist movements obtained by combination of the following basic movements.

1. Hand pronation and supination. From the neutral position with the elbow flexed at 90°, and the axis of the palm perpendicular to the floor, pronation is the rotation of the forearm that makes the palm face down, and supination is the rotation making the palm face up.
2. Wrist extension and flexion. From neutral position, wrist extension is the upward rotation of the wrist, while wrist flexion is the downward rotation.
3. Finger hyperextension and flexion. The neutral position is the open hand with fingers extended in a plane parallel to floor. Finger flexion is bending the

fingertips toward the palm, while finger hyperextension is an unusual movement where finger raises above the palm. The flexion of all fingers results in hand closing, while the motion from the close state to the neutral position is hand opening.
4. Thumb abduction and opposition. The neutral position is with the thumb extended alongside the hand, parallel to the other fingers. Abduction is the movement that moves the thumb away from the palm midline, while the opposition is the flexion on the palm.

All movements are exerted through muscles that contract when stimulated. The force they exert is unidirectional, so more than one muscle is required to perform complex movements. Most of the muscles that move the hand are located in the forearm, and move fingers by means of tendons running through sheaths and leverages (Gray 1918). In this way it is possible to transmit a large force to the fingers relocating the bulky muscles away in the forearm, the so called extrinsic muscles responsible for finger and wrist flexion. In the hand there are however intrinsic muscles.

The most relevant muscles are the flexor digitorum profundus (fdp) and flexor digitorum superficialis (fds), which originate in the proximal part of the forearm and fan out in four tendons that run through the carpal tunnel. Also relevant is the extensor digitorum communis (edc) that from the superficial part of the dorsal side of the forearm fans out in four tendons which insert in the middle and distal phalanxes, contributing to wrist and finger extension. For thumb the flexor pollicis longus (fpl) and abductor pollicis longus and brevis (apl and apb) are important.

A striated muscle, made up of a large amount of parallel fibres, is innervated by a single motor nerve; the connection of the nerve to the muscle consists of the axons of numerous alpha-Moto neurons. An important functional consequence is that the entire set of fibres innervated by an alpha-motoneuron contract in consonance.

Any voluntary movement is jointly undertaken by the motor cortex and other neural systems. The prefrontal cortex prepares the plan for the movement; the frontal cortex receives information from the parietal cortex, which is involved in spatial perception; the secondary motor areas work with the cerebellum to specify the precise time sequence of contractions of the muscles. The primary motor cortex, the brainstem, and the spinal cord produce the contractions of the muscles.

The contraction is initiated by an action potential travelling from the cell body of the alpha-motoneuron to the muscle fibres. Subsequently, the depolarization of the muscle fibre membrane causes a time-varying transmembrane electric current field that evokes potential changes in the extracellular tissue. The ionic currents flowing along the muscular fibres cause the muscle shortening.

The neuromuscular system is an association of several motor units (MUs), constituted by an alpha motoneuron and the muscle fibres it innerves. Nervous and muscular cells have electrical polarity on both sides of their cytoplasmatic membrane. The membrane potential is within -70 and -90 mV; after excitation, cells react with a transitory variation of the electrical polarity of the membrane, the action potential (AP). When a motoneuron is activated, an AP is generated and propagated to muscle fibres; each muscle fibre generates a signal, called MFAP (muscle fibres action potential). The algebraic sum of MFAPs of the single motor unit defines the MUAP (motor unit action potential). Those variations in potential generate the electro-myographic signal (EMG) (De Luca et al. 1979; Hogan and Mann 1980).

Using needle electrodes it is possible to register a single MUAP; instead, surface EMG (sEMG) techniques detect a larger number of MUAP. The problem of the single contribution detection is commonly called cross-talking.

The amplitude of the EMG signal is stochastic in nature, and can be represented by a Gaussian distribution function. The amplitude of the signal ranges from 0 to 10 mV or 0 to 1.5 mV. Signal frequency falls within 10–200 Hz: 10–30 Hz for a single motor unit, over 30 Hz for the superposition of multiple MUs.

EMG signals present two main issues that strongly influence their quality: the signal to noise ratio, and the distortion of the signal. Noise emanates from a wide range of sources, as the electronics components, the ambient, our body, movement artifacts. Most of the noise can be reduced by good electronics design and reducing signal cables length, while it is still partially unresolved how to deal with the noise generated by our body.

3 EMG Analysis and Rehabilitation

It is well known that it is possible to improve motor conditions by repetitive training: performing motions helps to improve joint plasticity, while continuous contraction and extension (even if passive) help to regain muscle tone. If the patient is affected by a neurological disorder guiding him through the exercise helps him to associate alternative pathways to help the damaged ones in performing the movement. However recent tests show how simply forcing the patient through a set of movement results in suboptimal improvements from the neuromuscular point of view: better results are achieved when there is an active user effort. So a key element in rehabilitation is the so called "assistance as needed", meaning the robot must trigger help only after detecting a concrete effort to complete the given task, thus forcing user engagement and promoting motor learning while retaining the voluntary control of the limb; moreover it should provide only the minimum force the patient needs (Dipietro et al. 2005). Another advantage in user-triggered assistance is that the pace of the exercise is determined by the patient itself.

Assistive control algorithms are based on highly backdrivable devices, able to quickly react to the force applied by the patient. Issues arise if the condition of the patient does not allow him to execute even the slightest movement, making the force-control paradigm useless. More recently new approaches based on detecting user's effort through surface EMG analysis were explored: if the patient is still able to generate some nervous activity his intentions could be detected, and some kinematic parameters could be estimated (Dipietro et al. 2005). An alternative paradigm, named impedance based, consists in letting the patient independently move through the goal, and guiding him applying mechanical impedances when he deviates from the desired trajectory. Studies showed how these strategies for robot-aided therapy can lead to a significant improvement in motor skills (Ho et al. 2011).

Historically the first field of application of EMG control was for arm prostheses. However there are some differences between rehabilitation and prosthesis control: in the first one we must restore the very same pre-accident pattern, so we are interested in a control as natural as possible. In the latter instead the level of amputation could force to map the control over other areas, so what is really important is the repeatability of the signal.

Controlling the device using the EMG signal allows implementing the aforementioned assistance as needed when user's conditions are not suitable for a force control. Plus it offers the most natural control for assistive exoskeletons or prostheses (mapping each actuator on the very same muscle it is meant to assist).

Different approaches to EMG signal analysis were proposed. The simplest technique uses signal threshold (Dipietro et al. 2005): the controller checks when the signal (or his linear envelope) exceeds a fixed value. This control paradigm has limited capabilities since the output is only binary. A more sophisticated approach is to output a continuous value roughly proportional to muscle activity. These algorithms are already employed for prostheses control, but they permits to control only few hand postures. This is due to the limited number of independent signals we can register from the forearm muscles packed in a relatively small volume.

Mixing statistical methods and machine learning provided powerful tools for automatic classification (Raez et al. 2006) and unsupervised cross-talk removal (Naik et al. 2007). A first stage of the EMG signal analysis consists in extracting the most significant features from the burst. The most common time-domain features include mean absolute value (MAV), integral absolute value (IAV), standard deviation (SD), and signal power (SP); frequency-domain features are zero crossing, power spectrum, spectrum centroids, and frequency ratio (Arvetti et al. 2007). More recently time/frequency-domain features were introduced; being the EMG a non-stationary signal, features based on classical Fourier transform can't be effectively applied because of the shifting frequencies over time. A promising technique is the wavelet analysis (Szu et al. 1996); a time-frequency representation of the signal obtained by the convolution with a finite-energy function (wavelet) obtained scaling and stretching the basic wavelet (mother wavelet). The output matrix of wavelet analysis contains a large number of elements, so dimensionality reduction should be performed.

The selected features are the input to a classifier that has to recognize the performed movement. Classification performance depends on several system parameters. The most important factor is the number of gesture under analysis; another is the number of acquired signals (Hudgins et al. 1993). Our previous works achieved 96 % accuracy rate over five gestures with one channel (Arvetti et al. 2007), and the same rate was obtained over seven gestures (grasp, hand extension, wrist flexion and extension, thumb abduction and opposition, index hyperextension) with three channels (Lisi et al. 2011).

As we anticipated, hand rehabilitation isn't very developed. However, among the few exoskeleton devices developed at various Universities we name the polimanus (Mulas et al. 2005), partially activated through EMG.

4 Our Analysis of sEMG Signals

Our project is about using a gesture classifier to control a hand rehabilitation device that assists in basic movements. Starting from our sEMG classifier for prosthesis control (Arvetti et al. 2007; Lisi et al. 2011), we focused on the real-time behaviour of the method. According to empirical analysis the maximum tolerable delay between the user command and the action of the controlled device is 300 ms (Englehart and Hudgins 2003), so the main problem is to meet this time requirement.

The first issue was to determine the number of samples needed for a successful classification. Usually the software acquires big batches of data which are later analysed to extract complete movements to classify. With this approach an online classifier is unfeasible, since it requires the movement to complete before recognizing it. So we analyzed how the movement classification depends on the length of the EMG signal so far acquired. The results have been used to define the architecture of the real time classifier (Fig. 1), implemented in Matlab 7.11:

- interface with the EMG acquisition board that outputs the parsed signal.
- analysis of the signal, designed to work with both continuous online and batch classification.
- interface to the exoskeleton.

The hardware system consists in the Eracle USB electromyograph connected to a PC (P4-2.4 GHz, 4 GB RAM). Eracle (Fig. 2) is a wearable device (Belluco et al. 2011) that provides three bipolar channels plus a common reference, used to remove the common noise between two paired electrodes. Each electrode records the voltage with respect to the common reference; each channel measures the difference between two coupled electrodes. The three resulting signals are amplified, sent through a high-pass filter with cut-off frequency at 1.5 Hz and a Sallen-Key anti-aliasing filter (double pole at 150 Hz). Finally a PIC16F688 microcontroller samples the signal at 237 Hz with 10 bit ADC and outputs an ASCII string. The device is extremely small and lightweight (29 $\times$ 45 $\times$ 9 mm and weights 35 g); it is well suitable for wearable applications.

Our previous sEMG classifier took into consideration complete bursts, which means it had to wait for the movement to complete before identifying it. This is unacceptable for an interactive device, since the control signal would be too late, so we investigated how recognition rate varies using incomplete movements.

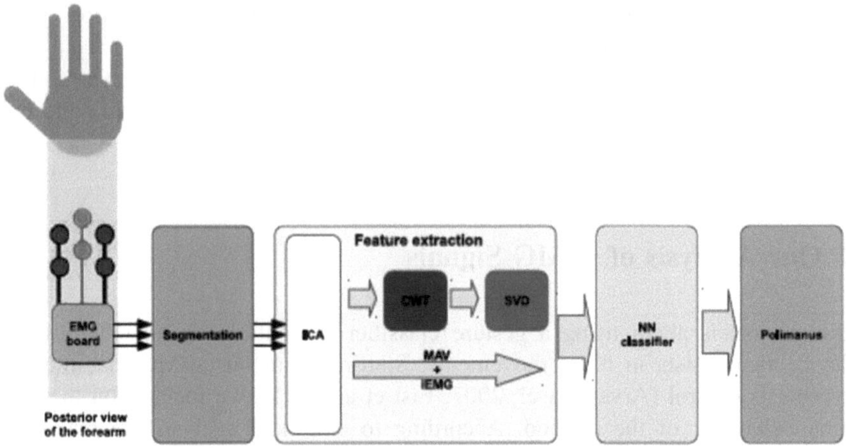

Fig. 1 System architecture

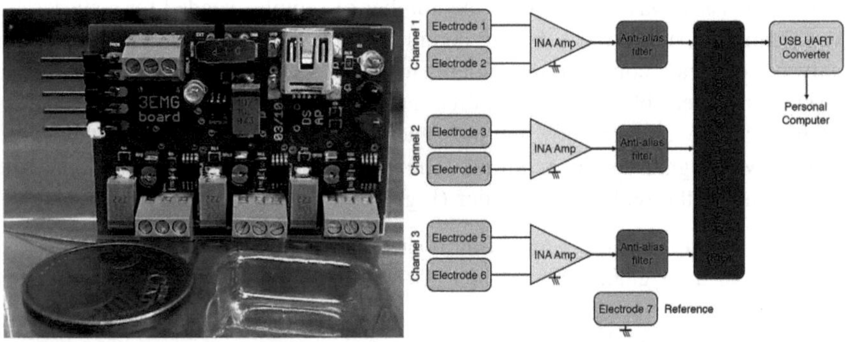

Fig. 2 **a** The Eracle board: picture compared with a 5cents coin; **b** The Eracle structure

We checked the performance of five neural networks trained on sEMG data acquired as in (Lisi et al. 2011); the set was composed by thirty bursts for seven gestures, with an average length of 200 samples each. The classification performances were computed over the testing sub-set, feeding the networks with features extracted from the initial segments of the bursts with increasing lengths.

Figure 3 displays the recognition rate over the percentage of the analyzed burst. After 50 % of the burst the recognition rate dramatically increases reaching performances close to the ones obtained analyzing a complete burst.

The test was repeated using networks trained using only half bursts. Recognition rate reached his maximum with half burst and slightly decreased for longer segments (Fig. 4). The decreasing trend near full burst is due to the fact that the network reaches the peak of his performances over the very same burst length used for his training; as the percentage of the analyzed segment moves from 50 % the

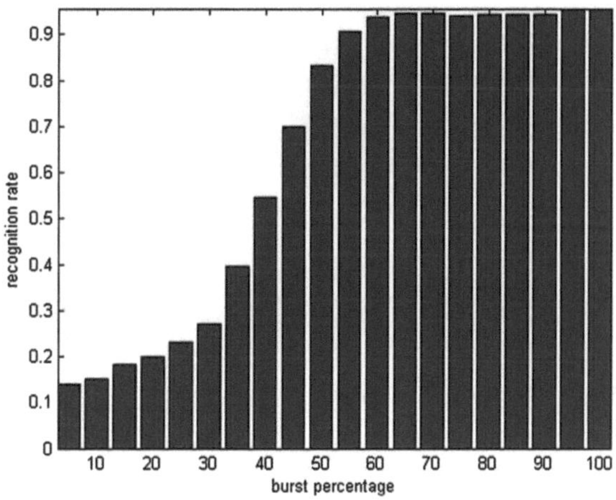

Fig. 3 Recognition rate over burst

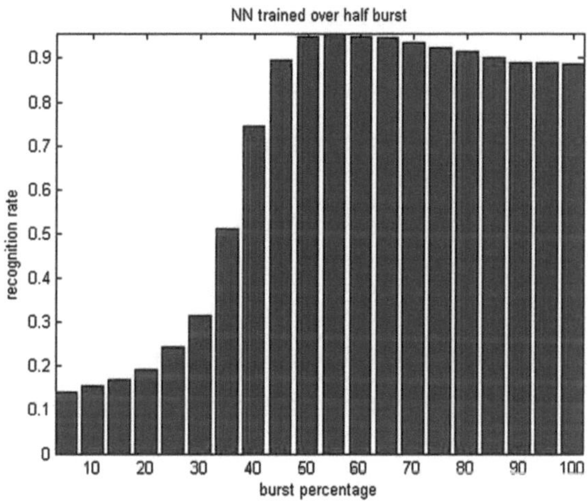

Fig. 4 Recognition rate over half burst

extracted features slightly change, thus scoring under 90 % at the end. Further tests were made training nets over segments even shorter, but no significant result was achieved.

We concluded that it is possible to obtain in an early stage a recognition rate close to the one obtained analyzing full bursts, using features extracted from the preamble and few samples right after the detection of the movement; this is what we call online classifier.

To fully develop the online classifier we selected a new reduced set for rehabilitation purposes of only 3 movements: hand opening, hand closing and precision grasp (pinch). The relevant muscles for those movements are fdp and fds that are responsible of most of the force generated for fingers and wrist flexion, the edc, responsible for fingers and wrist extension, the fpl and apb for thumb movement.

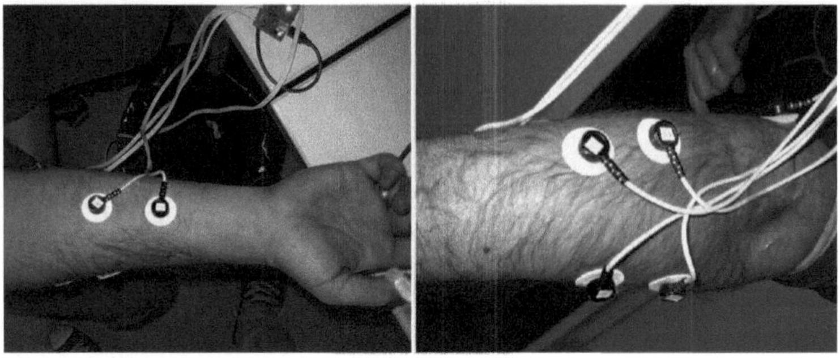

Fig. 5 Electrodes placement

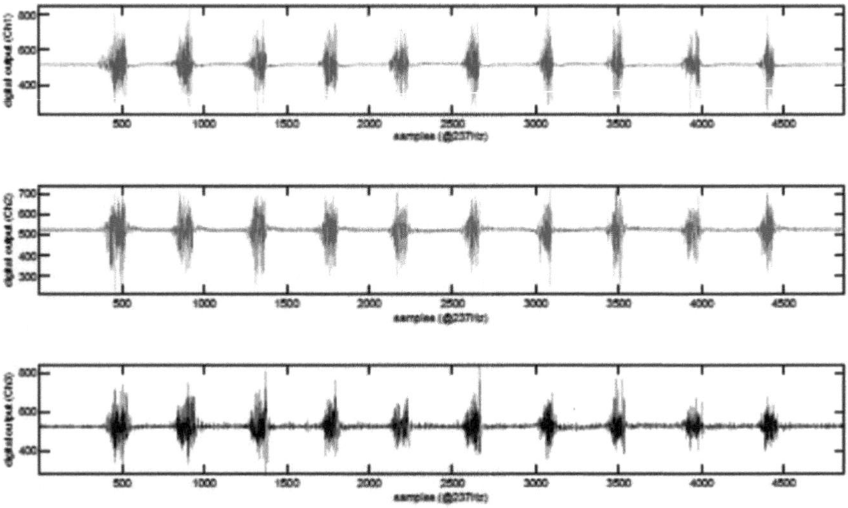

Fig. 6 The parsed signals

The choice for electrodes was intentionally limited to the ones commercially available for electro-stimulation, that are easily available at stores and whose signal keeps an acceptable signal-to-noise ratio even if used multiple times. We opted for 32 mm circular electrodes to reduce the surface and so the crosstalk.

The two electrodes of the first channel were placed in the volar side of the forearm along the fdp and fds, to highlight the muscle activity that leads to hand closing and wrist flexion. The second channel was placed over the edc, to acquire the signal of finger and wrist extension. The third channel could not be placed over the fpl and the apb because these muscles are too small and deep to generate a measurable signal; wee placed it in the internal dorsal part of the forearm (Fig. 5).

The function of Eracle's common reference is to detect the noise from the body (to subtract from the other channels); so its electrode was placed on the elbow, which is far from any involved muscle, and so records noise only.

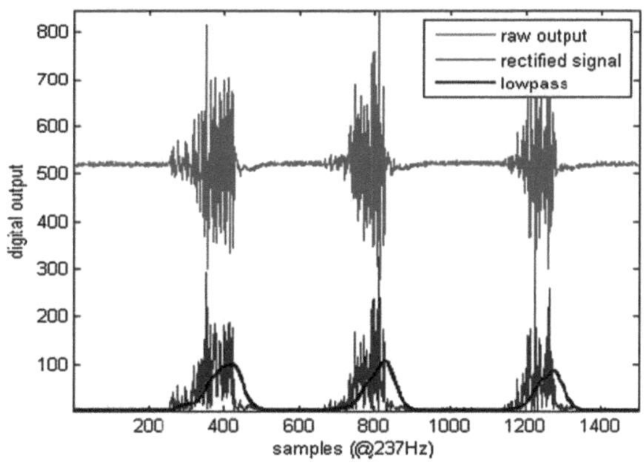

Fig. 7 The result of segmentation over 3 bursts of hand closing on channel 1

We shortly illustrate the main steps of the sEMG classifier.

1. Parsing—The signal is acquired from the board using Matlab's Serial Port Interface and converted from ASCII string to a N $\times$ 3 matrix (Fig. 6), where N is the number of acquired samples; the values are unsigned integer representing the 10 bit encoding of the signal. The input buffer is set to contain up to 1 s of samples.
2. Segmentation—Before identifying a movement we must detect it and define his boundaries. This is done subtracting the signal mean, rectifying the signal, filtering it with a second-order low-pass Butterworth filter (cut-off frequency at 2 Hz). In this way we can determine the beginning of a movement (burst's head) using a fixed threshold and checking his derivative. We consider a movement ended (burst's tail) when the signal or his derivative drops under a fixed value (empirically found). A burst is considered as open while activity in any of the channels is detected, and closed when activity does not satisfy the parameters anymore. See Fig. 7.
3. Independent component analysis (ICA)—We used the FastiICA package with Hyvarinen's fixed-point algorithm ICA allows extracting N independent source signals from at least N samples containing linear mixtures using multivariate statistical analysis. Given enough channels we could theoretically eliminate cross-talk separating the activity of every single muscle. The number of muscles however is much larger than the number of channels, so we couldn't associate a predominant signal to every channel but instead we used ICA for de-noising: we rebuilt the signal with the most significant contributions, applying an adaptive threshold to the matrix of weights. Since the FastICA is a fixed-point algorithm the weighting matrix is stored and used as initial value during further ICA analyses of the same burst, and is reset only after the closing of the burst.
4. Features extraction—The temporal features considered are the mean absolute value (MAV) and his integral (iEMG). They are closely related to signal energy and different gestures generate very different activities on different channels

caused by different patterns in recruitments of MU. For example hand closing generates a strong signal on the channels placed on the volar side, while fingers hyper-extension generates more energy in the dorsal channels. Only using these features we obtained a classification with 80 % accuracy. To improve the performance we considered also the Continuous Wavelet Transform (CWT), which is able to retain the temporal localization of the shifting frequency features. We chosen the Daubechies wavelet family, and empirically set the parameters.

5. Dimensionality reduction—The CWT for an N-samples signal generates an M $\times$ N matrix, where M is the number of scaling coefficients. For an average burst of 200 elements this means 5 $\times$ 200 because of the empirical choice to make the scale to vary between 1 and 5. The dimensionality reduction of the matrix is achieved by singular value decomposition (SVD). Therefore the neural network classifier receives in input a feature vector composed by seven elements: MAV, iEMG and the five singular values.
6. Neural network classification—Among all the techniques available we used ANN because of their ease in the setup process. We defined a feed-forward network with one hidden layer of thirty-five neurons, and tan-sigmoid transfer function. Data was partitioned using 75 % of the data for the training, 15 % of the samples for validation and the remaining 10 % for external testing. As learning algorithm Levenberg-Marquardt was selected, with early stopping.

The modules are automatically called during system execution. A Graphic User Interface was created to guide the user through the acquisition protocol and to automate the training. When the acquisition phase is complete, the interface stores the raw data of each repetition in a text file properly tagged, that is used for training. Offline classification, using the entire batch, is used during the training phase.

On the contrary, the online classifier is used to recognize the movement during the use of the system. During online recognition the EMG board is periodically polled for new samples, the new chunk is appended to the buffer and the updated signal is processed. If a burst is detected during the segmentation, and is at least 120 samples long, then the classifier is called and the resulting command is forwarded to the exoskeleton; if the burst has less than 120 samples only ICA is performed to compute the mixing matrix for the next iterations.

Since we are making a continuous acquisition, before acquiring the next signal segment a part of the old signal may be kept. There are three cases:

- If no burst is detected, the last 100 samples are kept to fill the preamble of any potential new burst.
- If an incomplete movement was detected, the signal is flushed up to the head of the burst.
- If a complete movement was detected, the buffer is flushed to the tail of the burst.

Table 1 Time for a burst classification

Function	Time (ms)
Segmentation	11.4
Feature extraction	14.7
Classification	8.6
Total	34.7

5 Results

The online classifier was tested with to determine the performances of the overall system considering the classification rate to recognize three gestures and the user perceived delay. Tests were performed over a P4-2.4 GHz PC with 4 GB of RAM and running Matlab 7.11 for Windows.

The delay analysis has been performed executing the complete analysis using 100 segments of signals containing a burst. A complete burst classification, as in Table 1, takes an average of 35 ms, which leads to a frequency of 28 analyses per second.

To test performance of the online classifier a new acquisition set was acquired for the three hand movements, for a total of ninety movements, from one subject (26 years old male, with a height of 1.83 m and weighting 73 kg). With this data set a classifier was trained, using cross-validation with 75 % of the samples for training, 15 % for validation and 10 % for external testing. The online classifier was launched and the user was asked to perform a sequence of randomly selected movements while recording the success rate.

The classifier scored an overall recognition rate of 95 %. Hand openings/closings scored a perfect recognition rate of 100 %. Some issues were instead noticed with pinch: this movement generates a mild muscular activity, hard to detect before the fingertips touch and start pushing against each other. In a few cases this movement was mistaken for hand closing because of the relatively similar activation.

The delay recorded between the beginning of the movement and the first response from the classifier was estimated to be around 200 ms (including the delay introduced by the EMG board, the serial communication, the time needed to gather enough samples for a reliable classification and finally the analysis itself), while subsequent cycles produced a new output (confirming the first one) every 20–30 ms until movement completion.

6 Conclusions

In this work we demonstrated the feasibility of an interactive controller for a rehabilitative device based on the classification of the EMG through an early analysis of the burst. We showed how to obtain good classification performances starting the analysis on a limited number of samples from the beginning of the detected movement; this way we reduced the delay under 200 ms, an interval which is under the commonly accepted limit for a smooth interaction. Thanks to the new interactive capabilities the classifier can be integrated into a rehabilitative device, allowing an assist-on-need strategy based on the residual muscle signal. The software is available at http://code.google.com/p/polimiemganalysis.

This result can significantly improve the quality of the rehabilitative training: from tools which force the patient through a set of preprogrammed movements, promoting only joint plasticity, to devices able to detect the user's intentions, quickly reacting to assist whatever movement is trying to perform. This new capability has several implications. Forcing an active effort it helps to regain muscle tone; it allows performing exercises for the rehabilitation of the neuromuscular system; it is also suitable for highly-impaired patients, whose inability to perform any movement would not permit them to benefit from robotic rehabilitation through force-controlled devices.

The new architecture of the system was also conceived to improve his modularity, decoupling the core signal analysis from the specific implementation of the external devices. This allows to easily adapting it to new devices, and reusing the system for applications even outside the field of rehabilitation, such as prosthesis control, teleoperation, and human computer interaction.

Matlab was used because of his high performances and the availability of functions and toolboxes for every application. However better time performances could be achieved porting the code on a microcontroller.

Rehabilitative robotics promises to bring significant improvements into the quality of life of victims of impairing accidents offering high intensity training and allowing to objectively compare the effectiveness of different therapies. Significant results had been achieved, but a solid framework of both knowledge and devices is yet to be established.

References

American Heart Association: Heart disease and stroke statistics-2011 update. Circulation (2011).

Arvetti, M., Gini, G., Folgheraiter, M.: Classification of EMG signals through wavelet analysis and neural networks for controlling an active hand prosthesis, Proc IEEE ICORR 2007, 531–536 (2007).

Belluco, P., Bordegoni, M. and Cugini, U.: Eracle: Electromyography system for gesture interaction. In M. Smith and G.Salvendy, editors, Human Interface and the Management of Information. Interacting with Information, volume 6771 LNCS, 391–398. Springer (2011).

Bullock, I.M. and Dollar, A.M.: Classifying human manipulation behavior. Proc. IEEE ICORR (2011).

De Luca , C. J.: Physiology and mathematics of myoelectric signals.(6):313–325 (1979).

Dipietro, L., et al.: Customized interactive robotic treatment for stroke: EMG-triggered therapy. IEEE Trans NSRE, 13(3):325–334 (2005).

Englehart, K, and Hudgins, B.: A robust, real-time control scheme for multifunction myoelectric control. IEEE Trans BME, 50(7):848–854 (2003).

Folgheraiter, M, Gini, G.: Human-like reflex control for an artificial hand, BioSystem Journal, 76, (1–3), 65–74 (2004).

Folgheraiter, M. ,Gini, G., Perkowski, M.: Adaptive Reflex Control for an Artificial Hand, 7th Int IFAC Symposium on robot control, Syroco 2003, Wroclaw, Poland, (2003).

Gini, G., M. Arvetti, M., Somlai, I. and Folgheraiter, M.: Acquisition and analysis of EMG signals to recognize multiple hand movements for prosthetic applications, Applied Bionics and Biomechanics, N 9, 145–155 (2012).

Gray, H.: Anatomy of the Human Body. (1918)., Bartebly.com books on line.

Ho, N.S.K. et al.: An emg-driven exoskeleton hand robotic training device on chronic stroke subjects: Task training system for stroke rehabilitation. Proc IEEE ICORR (2011).

Hogan, N., Mann, R.: Myoeletric signal processing: Optimal estimation applied to electromyography IEEE Trans BME 27, 382–395 (1980).

Hudgins, B., Parker, P. and Scott, R.N.: A new strategy for multifunction myoelectric control, IEEE Trans BME, 40(1):82–94 (1993).

Lisi, G. et al.: From the classification of EMG signals to the development of a new lower arm prosthesis, IFAC World Congress, Milan, 6493–6498 (2011).

Lo, A.C., et al: Robot-assisted therapy for long-term upper-limb impairment after stroke. New England Journal of Medicine, 362(19) 1772–1783 (2010).

Marchal-Crespo, L. and Reinkensmeyer, D. J.: Review of control strategies for robotic movement training after neurologic injury. J. of NeuroEngineering and Rehabilitation, 6 (2009).

Mulas, M., Folgheraiter, M., Gini, G.: An EMG-controlled Exoskeleton for Hand Rehabilitation, Proc. IEEE ICORR, 371–374 (2005).

Naik, G.R., Kumar, D.K., and Weghorn, H.: ICA based identification of sources in sEMG. Proc ISSNIP (Intelligent Sensors, Sensor Networks and Information), 619–624 (2007).

Raez, M.B.,. Hussain, M.S., and Mohd-Yasin, F.: Techniques of EMG signal analysis: detection, processing, classification and applications. In Biol Proced Online. 2006, March 2006.

Soto Martell, J. W., Gini, G.: Robotic hands: design review and proposal of new design process, Proc. World academy of science, engineering and technology, vol20, 85–90 (2007).

Squeri, V., Basteris, A. and Sanguineti, V.: Adaptive regulation of assistance 'as needed' in robot-assisted motor skill learning and neuro-rehabilitation. Proc IEEE ICORR (2011).

Szu, H., Telfer, B. and Garcia, J.: Wavelet transforms and neural networks for compression and recognition, Neural Networks, 9:695–708 (1996).

Wolbrecht, E.T., Chan, V., Reinkensmeyer, D.J. and Bobrow, J.E.: Optimizing compliant, model-based robotic assistance to promote neurorehabilitation. IEEE Trans NSRE 16(3):286–297 (2008).

Mathematical Modeling of Human Affective Behavior Aimed to Design Robot EI-Controller

A. Rodić and K. Addi

Abstract The chapter regards to building emotion-driven behavior and social development in robots based on theory of personality from personality psychology. More precisely, the chapter concerns with modeling attributes of human emotional intelligence with aim to develop robot EI-controller capable to manage and use emotions, mange relationship with others and increase the autonomy. Brief theoretical background of personality psychology, regarding categorization of human personality types and types of temperament are presented in the chapter, too. Besides, it will be analyzed how differences amongst personality traits determine human affective and social behavior in circumstances of different physical and social environmental conditions. Based on the theory from psychology, a generic model of human emotion-driven behavior as an element of emotional intelligence is proposed. Corresponding simulator is developed in the chapter, too. Designed EI-model is tested in simulation experiments. For this purpose, a "trigger" (an emotion-causal event) is assumed. Different personality profiles, exterior and interior influencing factors are varied in simulation tests. Proposed model is validated by comparison of the simulation results and results obtained experimentally by using results of the tests of human examinees. The on-line psychological questionnaires available at the Internet were used as appropriate tests.

Keywords Affective computing · Behavioral robotics · Sociable robotics · Artificial intelligence · Emotional intelligence · Emotion-driven behavior

A. Rodić (✉)
Institute Mihailo Pupin, Belgrade, Serbia
e-mail: aleksandar.rodic@pupin.rs

K. Addi
PIMENT, University of La Réunion, Saint-Denis, France
e-mail: khalid.addi@univ-reunion.fr

A. Rodić et al. (eds.), *New Trends in Medical and Service Robots*,
Mechanisms and Machine Science 20, DOI: 10.1007/978-3-319-05431-5_10,

1 Introduction

An increasing interest in emotion can be seen in the behavioral, biological and social sciences but also more and more in advanced robotics. Research over the last two decades suggests that many phenomena, ranging from individual cognitive processing to social and collective behavior, cannot be understood without taking into account affective determinants (i.e. motives, attitudes, moods, and emotions) (http://en.wikipedia.org/wiki/Affective_science). The emerging field of affective science[1] seeks to bring together the disciplines which study the biological, psychological and social dimensions of affect (Francis et al. 2009). The fact that emotions are considered to be essential to human reasoning suggests that they might play an important role in autonomous robots as well (Busher 1973; Weng et al. 2001).

To function in a complex and unpredictable physical and social environment humans are faced with applying their physical and intellectual resources to realize multiple goals in an intelligent and flexible manner. Two distinct and complementary information processing systems—*cognition* and *emotion* enable humans achieving of these goals by operating simultaneously (Picard 1997). The cognitive system is responsible for interpreting and making sense of the world, whereas the emotion system is responsible for evaluating and judging events to assess their overall value with respect to the human (e.g. positive or negative, desirable or undesirable, hospitable or harmful, etc.) (Breazeal 2003). When operating in the proper balance, the emotion system modulates the operating parameters of the cognitive system and the body to improve the overall mental and physical performance of the human. The scientific literature documents the beneficial effect of emotion on creative problem solving, attention, perception, memory retrieval, decision-making, learning, etc. As argued by Damisio (1994), too much emotion can hinder intelligent thought and behavior, however, too little emotion is even more problematic.

Today's autonomous robots can certainly improve their ability to function in complex environments and to behave appropriately in partnership with people. Using the properties of natural intelligence as a guide, a robot's cognitive system would enable it figure out what to do, whereas the emotion system would help it to do so more flexibly in complex and uncertain environments, as well as help the robot behave in a socially acceptable and effective manner with people (Breazeal 2003).

In order to interact with others (whether it is a device, robot or another person) it is essential to have a good conceptual model of how the other operates (Norman

[1] Affective science is the scientific study of emotion or affect. This includes the study of emotion expression, emotional experience and the recognition of emotions in others. In particular the nature of feeling, mood, emotionally driven behavior, decision making, attention and self-regulation, as well as the underlying physiology and neuroscience of the emotions (http://en.wikipedia.org/wiki/Affective_science).

2001). With such a model, it is possible to explain and predict what the other is about to do, its reasons to doing it, and how to elicit a desired behavior from it. There is a very practical side to developing robots that can effectively convey and communicate their internal state to people for cooperative tasks. The work in this chapter focuses on developing emotionally-driven and sociable robots for envisioned applications where the robot interacts with a person or another robot as a partner. The field of social robots and safe Human–Robot Interaction (HRI) opens new areas of applications like: healthcare, caretaking, assistance, edutainment and entertainment.

The mathematical modeling of human emotional intelligence[2] (EI) (Kluemper 2008; Mayer and Salovey 1997; Petrides et al. 2007) should result in a final extent to achieving advanced robot functionalities such as: (i) intelligent behavior in complex, unpredictable physical and social environments (ii) perceiving (sensing and recognizing) affective behavior of others (ii) ability of expression emotions and internal emotion state to others, and (iv) to respond to humans with social adaptability and appropriateness.

The chapter is organized in the following way. In Sect. 2, a state-of-the-art in this field of study is given. Brief theoretical background from personality psychology as the platform for further research consideration is given in Sect. 3. In Sect. 4 the EI model is developed and its' structure is described. The designed model is verified by simulation tests in Sect. 5 and simulation results are analyzed to assess model properties. Experimental model validation is done in Sect. 6. The novelties and future research are given in Sect. 7. The chapter is terminated by acknowledgement and list of references.

2 State-of-the-Art

While *Developmental* or *Epigenetic robotics* (Asada et al. 2009; Lungarella et al. 2003) aims at studying the developmental mechanisms, architectures and constraints that allow lifelong and open-ended learning of new skills and new knowledge in embodied machines the *affective computing* (Francis et al. 2009; http://en.wikipedia.org/wiki/Affective_computing) studies and develop systems and devices that can recognize, interpret, process, and simulate human emotions (affects). It is an interdisciplinary field spanning computer sciences, psychology, and cognitive science.

Entertainment (toy robots) and sociable robots are typically designed to have distinctive personalities which affect how they behave towards their human user or how they act within the virtual world of games (Dautenhahn 2007). Some of the

[2] Under the term *Emotional Intelligence* it is assumed the ability to identify (perceive), assess (understand), use (express), and control (manage) emotions of oneself, others, and groups (http://en.wikipedia.org/wiki/Emotional_intelligence).

advanced recent research projects in this area resulted in building intelligent sociable robots such as: Kismet and Leonardo (Breazeal 2002), PEPE (Stoytchev and Tanawongsuwan 1998), ROMAN (Hirth 2007), iCub (Metta et al. 2005), ASORO (http://www.asoro.a-star.edu.sg/robots_mika.html), PROBO (http://probo.vub.ac.be/), MAGGIE (http://roboticslab.uc3m.es/roboticslab/robot.php?id_robot=1), FURHAT (http://www.speech.kth.se/furhat/), KASPAR (http://www.kaspar.herts.ac.uk/), etc.

The "Feelix Growing" (http://en.wikipedia.org/wiki/Feelix_Growing) is a EU funded research project that was working to design robots that are capable detect and respond to human emotional cues. The project aimed to create robots that can recognize a given emotion, such as anger or fear, in a human, and adapt its behavior to the most appropriate response after repeated interactions.

Inspired by models of natural intelligence in biological systems, the authors from Massachusetts Institute of Technology (Breazeal 2003) designed an architecture that features both—cognitive system and emotion system (ES). Both systems operated in parallel and are deeply intertwined to foster optimal functioning of the robot in its environment. The overall architecture was comprised of a distributed network of interacting agent-like processes that excite and inhibit one another by spreading activation. For modeling of the ES, a learning structure based on the Gaussian mixture model combined with a Kurtoisis-based approach for dynamically deciding the appropriate number of kernels, were applied (Breazeal 2002).

Modeling of emotions is intensively worked in the video game industry. While finite state automata are easy to develop with entertainment robots, they are rather predictable. Over long game sessions, a character's static behavioral repertoire may result in repetitive behavior that hurts believability (Saltzman 1999). Therefore, many developers of computer games and robotic toys have turned to hierarchical, probabilistic and fuzzy state machines (Schwab 2004). The advantage of these systems is that layered control supports sophisticated behaviors, and probabilistic transitions make the actual behavior of the agent nondeterministic, less predictable, and more realistic. Other game developers have turned to scripting languages which allow arbitrarily sophisticated behaviors (Millington 2006). Current psychological theories model emotion in humans as three interrelated processes: (i) physiological responses, (ii) overt behaviors, and (iii) conscious feelings that occur in response to events of potential relevance (Gluck et al. 2008). Many researchers postulate that the functional role of emotions is to determine what problems are currently important and to focus the agent's mind and actions on them [e.g. (Damasio 2000; Minsky 2007)]. Simon (1983) points out that the environment presents many challenges that cannot all be met at once and that emotions provide a way to shift our focus to priorities.

Two popular emotion models in artificial intelligence are: *multiple concerns* models and *cognitive evaluation* models. *Multiple concerns* models map emotion to competing systems detecting events of importance to an agent. Features in perception or cognition act as triggers for concerns, which in turn can trigger emotions, or behavioral modes, that change how the agent selects its behaviors.

The PEPE system (Stoytchev and Tanawongsuwan 1998) for example is a multiple concerns model based on ideas from Simon (1983) and Frijda (1986). *Cognitive evaluation* models map emotions to a hierarchy of evaluations of physical and mental conditions that can affect an agent. In (Ortony et al. 1988) it was proposed a cognitive evaluation OCC-model in which emotions consists of valenced reactions to the outcome of events. The OCC model was deliberately designed to be implementable on an artificial intelligence system.

Also, there are many machine learning techniques used for modeling emotional intelligence that can exploit past experience (Alpaydin 2004; Mitchell 1997). Two popular techniques are *case-based reasoning* and *reinforcement learning*. A case based reasoning system learns by storing specific episodes, or cases; this involves deciding what parts of a current experience to store, what lesson the experience teaches, and how to label the experience for retrieval later (Kolodner et al. 1993). Once an agent has retrieved a case from its case library, it must adapt it to solve the current problem, and then ideally update its records of its experiences based on the new outcome (Kolodner 1984). Reinforcement learning, commonly used in robotic learning and control, attempts to find a scheme for selecting actions, or policy that maximizes the agent's return on a reward function (Sutton 1998). Reinforcement learning and case-based reasoning can be combined. The LARC model (Santamaria 1997) stores cases that trace the recent history of the agent's perceptions and behaviors along with the accompanying reward function.

In Gadanho and Hallam (2001a) a non-symbolic emotion model was developed that takes the form of a recurrent artificial neural network where emotions both depend on and influence the perception of the state of the world. This emotion model was integrated in a reinforcement-learning architecture with three different roles: influencing perception, providing reinforcement value, and determining when to reevaluate decisions.

In Li et al. (2010) was proposed an improved three-level structure of affective model as "personality-emotion-mood" for intelligent and emotional virtual characters. Also, the emotion state space was presented, as well as the emotion updating functions to generate authentic and expressive emotions. In order to achieve the complexity and variety of behaviors, the authors brought forward a behavior organizing structure as the behavior tree.

The question under examination in (Gadanho and Hallam 2001b) was whether the role of emotions can be useful for a robot which adapts to its environment. For this purpose, an emotion model was developed and integrated in a reinforcement learning framework.

Francis et al. (2009) presented an artificial intelligence model inspired by the psychological results in which an emotion model triggers case-based emotional preference learning and behavioral adaptation guided by personality models.

In the chapter Kirby and Forlizzi (2010) a general affective model for social robots was developed and particular details of implementation of this model in the robot Roboceptionist.

Table 1 Personality traits of the dichotomy pair (E)–(I)

Extraversion versus introversion (E)–(I)	
Talkative and sociable	Private
Expressive	Reserved
Would rather speak than listen	Would rather listen than speak
Comfortable around people	Tire quickly in social settings
Dislike being alone	Comfortable being alone
Get energized by communicating with other people	Get energized by being alone
Think while speaking	Think before speaking

3 Theoretic Background

The platform for development mathematical model of human emotionally driven and social behavior is the Meyers-Briggs theory on personality (Myers-Briggs 1995) widely used in personality psychology. According to this theory, the personality type and temperament dominantly determine human psychological behavior.

3.1 Personality Types

Personality psychology is a branch of psychology that studies personality and its individual differences (http://en.wikipedia.org/wiki/Personality_psychology). According to the theory, "personality" is a dynamic and organized set of characteristics possessed by a person that uniquely influences individual cognitions, emotions, motivations, and behaviors in various situations. Personality also refers to the pattern of thoughts, feelings, social adjustments, and behaviors consistently exhibited over time that strongly influences one's expectations, self-perceptions, values, and attitudes. It also predicts human reactions to other people, problems, and stress (Myers 2010; Winnie and Gittinger 1973). This scientific discipline uses the Myers-Briggs Type Indicator (MBTI) assessment as a psychometric questionnaire designed to measure psychological preferences in how people perceive the world and make decisions (http://en.wikipedia.org/wiki/Myers-Briggs-Type-Indicator). The MBTI sorts psychological differences into four opposite pairs, i.e. dichotomies: Extravert-Introvert (Table 1), Sensing-iNtuitive (Table 2), Feeling-Thinking (Table 3) and Perceiving-Judging (Table 4). That results in 16 possible psychological types. None of these types are better or worse. However, Briggs and Myers theorized that individuals naturally prefer one overall combination of type differences (http://en.wikipedia.org/wiki/Personality_psychology). In the same way that writing with the left hand is hard work for a right-hander, so people tend to find using their opposite psychological preferences more difficult, even if they can become more proficient (and therefore behaviorally flexible) with practice and development. The 16 personality types are typically referred to by an abbreviation of four letters, e.g. ESTJ, INTJ, ISTP, etc.

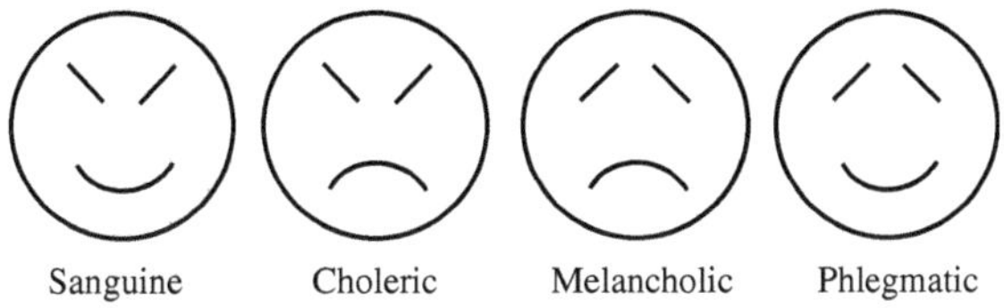

Fig. 1 Emoticon representation of four temperament types

3.2 Types of Temperaments

Under the notion "temperament" it is assumed in psychology, unlike to the term "personality", the individual kinds of the psyche traits that determine dynamics of human psychological activity (http://en.wikipedia.org/wiki/Four_temperaments). The temperament traits are expressed in an even manner in any activity nevertheless to its' content, goals and motives, remaining invariant in the later years and which, in their interconnections, characterize the type of temperament (http://en.wikipedia.org/wiki/Four_temperaments). The temperaments are (Fig. 1): *sanguine* (pleasure-seeking and sociable), *choleric* (ambitious and leader-like), *melancholic* (introverted and thoughtful), and *phlegmatic* (relaxed and quiet).

The characteristics of different temperament types are systematized in Table 5 (La Haye and 1984; http://en.wikipedia.org/wiki/Four_temperaments). A temperament type can be determined by filling corresponding questionnaires (tests) available at the Internet (http://neoxenos.org/wp-content/blogs.dir/1/files/temperaments/temperament_test.htm).

4 Modeling of Emotional Intelligence

While the artificial intelligence (AI) copes with tasks such as pattern recognition, spatial reasoning, context reasoning, decision making, etc., the emotional intelligence (EI) is responsible in humans for self awareness, self management, awareness of others and relationship management (Kluemper 2008; Mayer and Salovey 1997; Petrides et al. 2007). According to the theory of personality (considered in Sect. 3), individual emotional conditions primarily depend on three factors (Myers 2010): (i) personality type (ii) personality character, and (ii) type of temperament. These factors are determined by the genetic code of an individual and it is acquired by birth. Besides, the behavior of individuals is strongly influenced by additional exterior and interior factors (Fig. 2) such as: (i) "exterior world" (ii) "interior stimuli" as well as (iii) "social factors". The personality character, as an important factor, will be disregarded in this research being it is related mostly to certain pathologic conditions and that is not of our interest.

Under the term "exterior world" our physical and social environment (that includes trigger-events, -situations, -acts or relationships with other persons) are

Table 2 Personality traits of the dichotomy pair (S)–(N)

Sensing versus intuition (S)–(N)	
Spend most of the time focusing on what can be touched, seen or experienced	Spend most of the time focusing on what can be imagined
More interested in practical matters than ideas	More interested in ideas than practical matters
Down-to-earth	Head in the clouds
More observant than imaginative	More imaginative than observant
Focus on the past or the present	Focus on the future
Notice the details, but might miss the bigger picture	See the bigger picture, but might miss details
Trust experience	Trust instinct

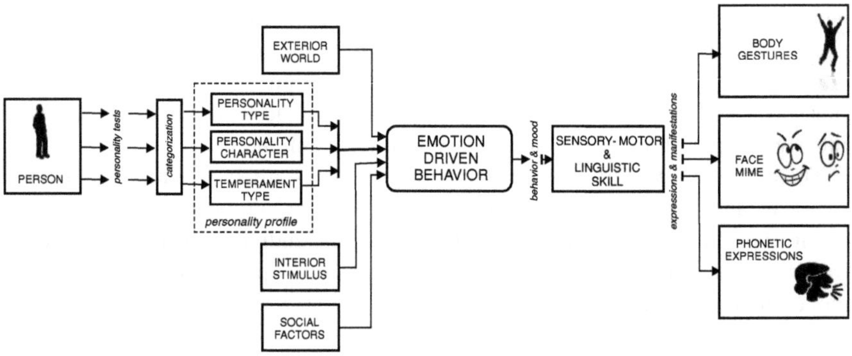

Fig. 2 High-level model description: trigger/stimuli—personality profile—behavior—actions

assumed. The "interior stimuli" mainly concerns with our physical and psychological conditions (regarding to body and psyche) such us senses of fatigue, pain, disease, etc. Under the same term, the feelings like love, depression, anger, hatred, fear, satisfaction etc., are assumed, too. The "social factors" regard to the conditions that influence some features of individual behavior. The "social factors" includes: family and school education, influence of companions, religion and affiliation to the social groups e.g. political parties, civil communities, clubs, fans, etc. Bearing in mind the previous facts, a psychological (affective) behavior of an individual is determined by plenty of different exterior and interior factors.

To derive a generic model of human psychological behavior the following assumptions are assumed. The considered biological system can be approximated by a deterministic, dynamic, non-linear, multi-input–multi-output (MIMO) system of arbitrary complexity. The input and output variables of the emotion-driven behavior (EDB) model are hardly measurable but they can be quantified by using corresponding psychological questionnaires (http://www.16personalities.com/free-personality-test; http://neoxenos.org/wp-content/blogs.dir/1/files/temperaments/temperament_test.htm).

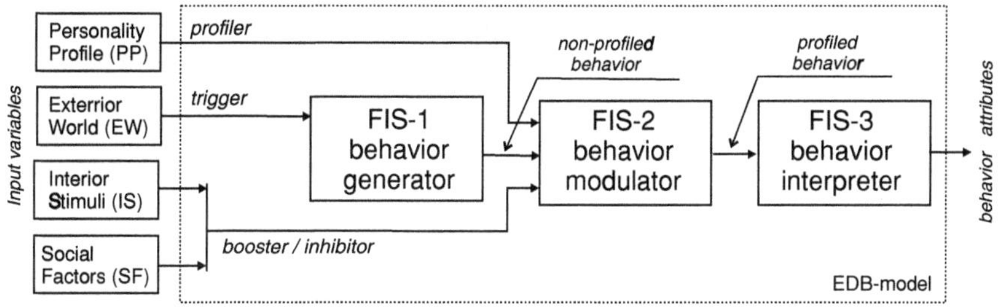

Fig. 3 Structure of the three-stage EDB-model with fuzzy blocks: behavior generator, behavior modulator and behavior interpreter

The variables of interest required for modeling EDB (Fig. 3) include qualitative information regarding personality profile, physical and social environment, emotional and health conditions, social factors, etc. They are quite heterogeneous and rather linguistic and descriptive than measurable and numerical. Generally observed, humans use to behave (in psychological sense) in a fuzzy manner. That means, people use their sensory-motor skills, symbolic body and facile gestures as well linguistic forms to express their psychological state—behavior attributes, mood, etc. Due to a fuzzy nature of human behavior, the modeling approach to be proposed in this chapter consequently belongs to the knowledge-based type. It assumes utilization of the fuzzy inference system i.e. fuzzy logic structure. Accordingly, the appropriate structure of the EDB model can be represented by a three-stage block structure (Fig. 3). It consists of three fuzzy inference systems FIS-1 to FIS-3 aligned in the cascade with aim to propagate individual behavior attributes towards the output of the model. Achieved behavior attributes depends on information entered to the model by the input variables such as: "personality profile" (PP), "exterior world" (EW), "interior stimuli" (IS) and "social factors" (SF).

A biological mechanism of human affective behavior produces the emotive reactions based on three excitation signals (information carriers): (i) "trigger" of behavior (that arouses different psychological reactions) (ii) "profiler" (that shapes event-driven behavior to fit the personality profile of the individual), and (iii) behavior "booster" or "inhibitor" (that increases or decreases the expressiveness of the individual affective manifestations).

The trigger of psychological behavior (mood) is the "exterior world" according to the Fig. 3. The EW represents our physical and social environment (type of event, situation, inter-personal relationship and interaction or acts). The initiated emotional state is then gained by influence of some "interior stimuli" and "social factors". According to the Fig. 3, the trigger variables are led to the input of the FIS-1 block named "behavior generator". This block produces at its' output the "non-profiled" behavior (mood). It can be also called the "non-personalized" (being it does not reflect an individual affective behavior but one estimated by an experience based on emotional behavior of a large sample of individuals). For example, a sad and a frightening event (situation) certainly cause with majority persons corresponding feeling of sadness as well fear as the normal psychological reactions to be expected. But, the expressiveness of feelings differs from person to person depending on their personality profiles (personality type and temperament), interior stimuli and social factors. Because of that, the individual traits (personality type and temperament) represent so called the "behavior profiler[3]" while the "interior stimuli" and "social factors" represent the "behavior booster" or "behavior inhibitor" depending if it increases or decreases energy of emotions. Both, the behavior "profiler" and the "booster" (or "inhibitor") shape the "non-profiled" behavior making of it one that is "profiled" and called also "personalized" since its' behavior attributes are individually-specific. The fuzzy block FIS-2 (Fig. 3) is called "behavior modulator[4]" because the adjustment (modulation) of the non-profiled behavior is achieving in this block.

Fuzzy model blocks FIS-1 to FIS-3 (Fig. 3) are assumed to be of Mamdani type. The input and output vectors are of the arbitrary number depending on how complex (general) model wish to be developed. Being the considered biological system is non-linear, the corresponding input and output membership functions (MFs) of the FIS-1 to FIS-3 blocks are assumed to be the Gauss curve or the Sigmoidal function. The number of fuzzy rules in the corresponding rules data-bases can vary depending on how refined behavior properties intend to fit by our model. If one requests from the model to provide high resolution (distinction) between the similar psychological states then it is required larger number of rules in the corresponding data-base. The proposed model architecture (Fig. 3) with fuzzy blocks aligned in a cascade enables easy monitoring of the intermediate model states (behavior attributes that correspond to the non-personalized or personalized states) generated at the particular FIS blocks. Also, such modular structure enables easier analysis of the separated or synergetic influence of the "interior stimuli" and "social factors" upon the individual affective behavior.

The attributes that characterize event (situation, act or relationship with others) can be numerous and different regarding types. The list of the basic event types assumed for the model derivation in this study is given in Table 6. The actual number of possible types is certainly much larger than the presented ones given in Table 6. The larger number of the trigger variables introduced in the model, the more complex and complete the model is. Anyway to the number of input/output variables, the global model structure is invariant regardless to the model complexity. The trigger-events considered in the chapter represent in a general case

---

[3] The "profiler" variable is a set of information regarding to the personality profile. It enables modulation of the event-driven behavior (information carrier generated at the FIS-1 output). Behavior profiling is achieved by instrumenting knowledge-based structure in FIS-2 in a way determined by the information transmitted by the variable "profiler".

[4] Behavior modulation is process of changing properties (qualitatively and quantitatively) of the event-driven behavior attributes, called "carrier of information", by using profiling variables which contain individual-specific information regarding personality profile.

Table 3 Personality traits of the dichotomy pair (F)–(T)

Feeling versus thinking (F)–(T)	
Listen to the heart	Listen to the head
Kind	Tough
Closer to "bleeding heart" than "ice in the veins"	Closer to "ice in the veins" than "bleeding heart"
Sensitive to criticism	Insensitive to criticism
Emotional reaction to conflicts	Rational reaction to conflicts
Want to be seen as warm, sensitive and sincere	Want to be seen as rational, calm and just
Compassion above truth	Truth above compassion

combination of several basic event types listed in Table 6. For example, a birthday anniversary represents a combination of the cheerful, funny, perhaps surprising and socially-driven event types. Single-event types are rather rare in a real life.

The model blocks "behavior generator" and "behavior modulator" produce at the output ports corresponding emotional states (mood) such as for example happy, sad, anger, shame, disgusted, etc. The generated psychological states are characterized by combination of different emotions (feelings). Such emotions can be classified in the five categories according to the dominant feeling such as: joy, sadness, anger, fear and confusion. The list of the existing human emotions is rather numerous. The power of emotions (their expressiveness) can be formally quantified in the range 0–100 %. Within this range it is possible to make further additional gradation from minimum to maximum like for example: not at all, somewhat, moderate, significant and completely. Such fine resolution of emotion intensities is suitable for implementation with fuzzy models.

The fuzzy block FIS-3 represents the "behavior interpreter". The input vector to this block consists of variables that transmit information about the generated behavior attributes of individual. The output vector of the FIS-3 consists of the variables that carries on information about the emotive reactions (expressions and manifestations) caused by the psychological state generated by model. The psychological reactions regard to the sensory-motor, emotionally driven response of the individual including variety of body gestures, facile and phonetic expressions (speech, voice, etc.). The scale of psychological reactions varies from low intensity to a very expressive. Regarding body gestures it is assumed the emotion-driven manifestations to be accomplished by head (wobble), arms (swinging) or entire body (twisting, bending, etc.). Face mime includes expressions of smile, fear, anger, hatred, confusion, etc. Phonetic expressions include accordingly speech, lough, clamor, etc.

5 Model Simulation

In order to get better insight into the EI-model properties the corresponding simulator is developed. For the purpose of simulation tests, a case study (emotion-causal event) from real-life is assumed.

Case study
At the dinner table, someone told a funny joke. While laughing, you have suddenly burped loudly.

The chosen case study can be experienced in a different way by persons of different personality type and subjected to influence of different exterior and interior factors. In that sense, the following tasks (examples) are tested by the simulator.

Task imposed
It is required to simulate emotionally driven behavior of a person who reacts to the test-scenario assumed. The generic model proposed in this chapter is used and the following input conditions are introduced:

T.1 Personality type: (Extrovert = 60 %, Sensing = 57 %, Thinking = 78 %, Perceiving = 69 %); Type of temperament: (Phlegmatic = 60 %); Interior stimuli: (emotional condition—*not expressed*); Social factor: (family education—*liberal*);

T.2 Personality type: (Introvert = 60 %, iNtuitive = 57 %, Feeling = 78 %, Judging = 69 %); Type of temperament: (Melancholic = 60 %); Interior stimuli: (emotional condition—completely *moody*); Social factor: (family education—*strict*);

T.3 Compare the emotional reactions of two competitive persons considered in the tasks T.1 and T.2. Which person is more affective in a psychological sense?

The test-event used in simulation combines properties of several complementary basic event types (see Table 6). The quantification (scoring) of the test-event properties are given in Fig. 4. The attributes are expressed in percentages. The quantification scheme was obtained by interview accomplished with 10 independent human examinees. They are requested to score this test-event according to their personal feeling (opinion). The tests are quite subjective but the final score are objective obtained by taking a statistical average of the declared individual results reported by examinees. Results of scoring are shown by a slider-graph in Fig. 4.

In the similar way, the indicators "interior stimuli" and "social factors" are quantified, too. With aim of simplicity, the emotive condition (the antagonist pair cheerful—moody) and family education (the antagonist pair liberal—strict) are considered only as the characteristic representatives of IS and SF. The number of potential IS and SF factors are more numerous and they are not considered in this example.

The structural information regarding to the fuzzy model blocks FIS-1 to FIS-3 (Fig. 3) is given in Tables 7, 8, and 9. The Gaussian curve and the Sigmoidal

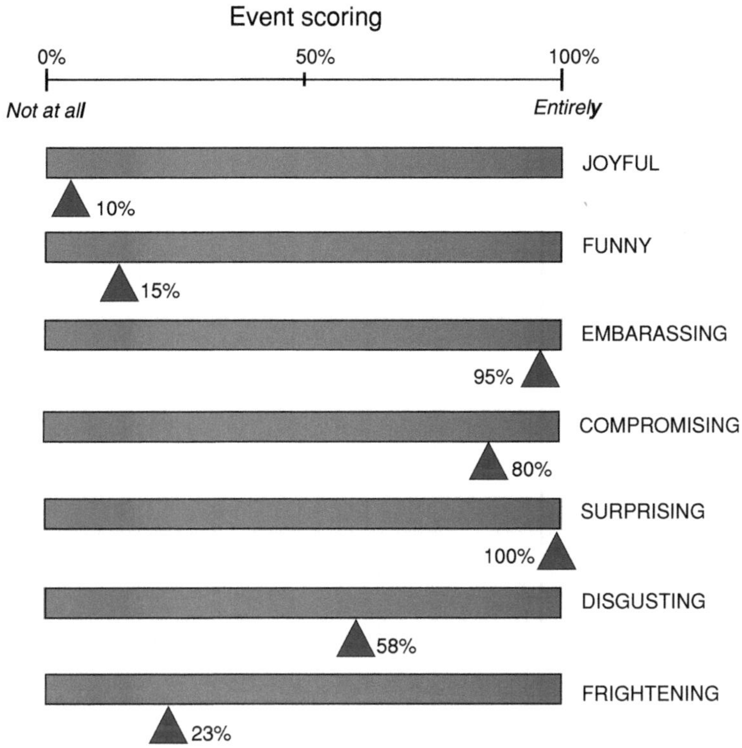

Fig. 4 Quantification of test-event attributes taking into account the basic event properties only

Table 4 Personality traits of the dichotomy pair (P)–(J)

Perceiving versus judging (P)–(J)	
Focus on options	Focus on schedules
Do not mind unpredictability	Cannot stand unpredictability
Playful about work	Very serious about work
Dislike long-term plans	Make long-term plans
Not that worried about order	Orderly
Indecisive	Inflexible
Dislike rules	Like rules

function defined by (1) and (2) are used in the model as the appropriate membership functions that fit well a non-linear nature of human emotions.

$$G(c,\sigma) = e^{-\frac{(x-c)^2}{2\sigma^2}} \tag{1}$$

$$S(\alpha,c) = \frac{1}{1+e^{-(x-c)}} \tag{2}$$

Table 5 Overview of type temperaments and corresponding behavior attributes

Temperament traits	Temperament type			
	Sanguine	Choleric	Phlegmatic	Melancholic
Sensitivity	Reduced	Reduced	Reduced	Increased
Activity	High	High	High	Low
Reactivity	High	High	Low	Low
Correlation between activity and reactivity	Balanced	Reactivity overcomes activity	Balanced (but activity overcomes reactivity)	Low level of correlation
Emotional sensitivity	Increased (to the positive events)	Increased	Reduced	Increased (to the negative events, depressive)
Tempo of reactions (psychological rate)	Accelerated	Accelerated	Slow	Slow
Worry	Reduced	Reduced	Reduced	Increased
Extraversion/Introversion	Extraverted	Extraverted	Introverted	Introverted
Communicativeness	Increased (talkative)	Increased (talkative)	Reduced (mum)	Reduced (mum)
Rigidity/Flexibility	Flexible	Rigid	Rigid	Rigid
Resistance	High	High	High	Low

Table 6 Basic types of events used in this study for model derivation

Cheerful	Funny	Humane	Interesting
Boring	Embarrassing	Compromising	Provoking
Confusing	Surprising	Irritating	Frustrating
Frightening	Disgusting	Demoralizing	Encouraging
Depressing	Sexually-driven	Socially-driven	Religious

Table 7 Structure parameters of the FIS-1 model block

FIS-1				
	Membership functions			
Input variables	Joyful	Some G(15, 0)	Very G(15, 50)	Entirely G(15, 100)
	Funny	Some G(15, 0)	Very G(15, 50)	Entirely G(15, 100)
	Embarrassing	Some G(15, 0)	Very G(15, 50)	Entirely G(15, 100)
	Compromising	Some G(15, 0)	Very G(15, 50)	Entirely G(15, 100)
	Surprising	Some G(15, 0)	Very G(15, 50)	Entirely G(15, 100)
	Disgusting	Some G(15, 0)	Very G(15, 50)	Entirely G(15, 100)
	Frightening	Some G(15, 0)	Very G(15, 50)	Entirely G(15, 100)
Output variables	Unpleasant	Some G(15, 0)	Very G(15, 50)	Entirely G(15, 100)
	Guilty	Some G(15, 0)	Very G(15, 50)	Entirely G(15, 100)
	Shame	Some G(15, 0)	Very G(15, 50)	Entirely G(15, 100)
	Afraid	Some G(15, 0)	Very G(15, 50)	Entirely G(15, 100)
	Excited	Some G(15, 0)	Very G(15, 50)	Entirely G(15, 100)
	Disgusted	Some G(15, 0)	Very G(15, 50)	Entirely G(15, 100)
	Worried	Some G(15, 0)	Very G(15, 50)	Entirely G(15, 100)

FIS-1 model—Mamdani type, 7 inputs, 7 outputs, 29 rules, defuzzification method—centroid

Fuzzy rules in fuzzy blocks FIS-1 and FIS-3 are designed based on life-experience or can be determined experimentally by testing of the examinees. Design of the fuzzy rules in the FIS-2 block requires specific knowledge from psychology regarding theory of personality. In this study, the basic knowledge regarding personality preferences and behavior traits of different temperament types, systematized in Tables 2, 3, 4, 5, and 6 and adapted in form of fuzzy rules, are used. The finite number of fuzzy rules is used to describe a psychological behavior in the test-example. As more rules are introduced in the data-base the more accurate and comprehensive model is.

The simulation results obtained with regards to the imposed tasks T.1–T.3 are presented in the graph and compared by use of a 2D column graph presentation. Affective behavior of an ESTP (extravert-sensing-thinking-perceiving) phlegmatic person faced with experiencing the test-event (task T.1) is shown in Fig. 5. Also, the behavior of an INFJ (introvert-intuitive-feeling-judging) melancholic

Table 8 Structure parameters of the FIS-2 model block

FIS-2						
	Membership functions					
Input variables	Non-profiled behavior	Not at all G(8, 0)	Some G(8, 25)	Moderate G(8, 50)	Very G(8, 75)	Completely G(8, 100)
	Extravert	Low S(-0.15, 50)	Null G(4, 50)		High S(0.15, 50)	
	Introvert	Low S(−0.15, 50)	Null G(4, 50)		High S(0.15, 50)	
	Sensing	Low S(-0.15, 50)	Null G(4, 50)		High S(0.15, 50)	
	Intuitive	Low S(-0.15, 50)	Null G(4, 50)		High S(0.15, 50)	
	Feeling	Low S(-0.15, 50)	Null G(4, 50)		High S(0.15, 50)	
	Thinking	Low S(-0.15, 50)	Null G(4, 50)		High S(0.15, 50)	
	Perceiving	Low S(-0.15, 50)	Null G(4, 50)		High S(0.15, 50)	
	Judging	Low S(-0.15, 50)	Null G(4, 50)		High S(0.15, 50)	
	Sanguine	Weak G(6.6, 0)	Moderate G(6.6, 15)		Strong S(0.15, 22.5)	
	Choleric	Weak G(6.6, 0)	Moderate G(6.6, 15)		Strong S(0.15, 22.5)	
	Melancholic	Weak G(6.6, 0)	Moderate G(6.6, 15)		Strong S(0.15, 22.5)	
	Phlegmatic	Weak G(6.6, 0)	Moderate G(6.6, 15)		Strong S(0.15, 22.5)	
	Moody	Cheerful S(-0.15, 35)	Neutral G(4.15, 50)		Moody S(0.15, 35)	
	Strict	Liberal S(-0.15, 35)	Neutral G(4.15, 50)		Strict S(0.15, 35)	
Output variables	Profiled behavior	Not at all G(8, 0)	Some G(8, 25)	Moderate G(8, 50)	Very G(8, 75)	Completely G(8, 100)

FIS-2 model—Mamdani type, 15 inputs, 7 outputs, 50 rules, defuzzification method—centroid

Table 9 Structure parameters of the FIS-3 model block

FIS-3						
	Membership functions					
Input variables	Extravert	Low	Null	High		
	Introvert	Low	Null	High		
	Unpleasant	Some	Very	Entirely		
	Guilty	Some	Very	Entirely		
	Shame	Some	Very	Entirely		
	Afraid	Some	Very	Entirely		
	Excited	Some	Very	Entirely		
	Disgusted	Some	Very	Entirely		
	Worried	Some	Very	Entirely		
	IS-emotive condition	Cheerful	Neutral	Moody		
	SF-family education	Liberal	Neutral	Strict		
Output variables	Face smiled	Not at all	Somewhat	Very	Radiant	
	Face gloomy	Not at all	Somewhat	Very		
	Face fear	Not at all	Somewhat	Very		
	Face sad	Not at all	Somewhat	Very	Cloudy	
	Astonished	Not at all	Somewhat	Very		
	Face anxious	Not at all	Somewhat	Very		
	Overwrought	Not at all	Somewhat	Very		
	Voice	Silent	Quiet	Audible	Loud	Noisy
	Body gesture	Static	Slow	Active	Dynamic	

FIS-3 model—Mamdani type, 11 inputs, 9 outputs, 31 rules, defuzzification method—centroid

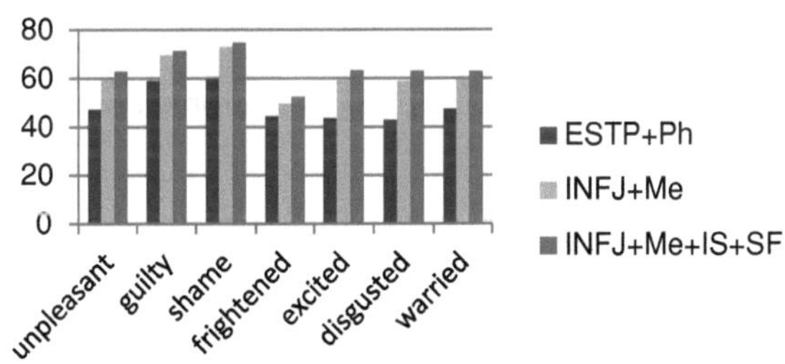

Fig. 5 Simulation results of modeling human emotion-driven behavior. Model sensitivity to different personality profiles and exterior/interior factors imposed

person in the same circumstances is presented in the same graph (task T.2). Besides, behavior of the INFJ person with entirely negative emotional state (moody = 100 %) and with completely strict family education (task T.3) is shown in Fig. 5, too. The obtained affective behavior attributes are compared in the graph. The results presented on the graph in Fig. 5 prove that the generic fuzzy model is sensitive to variation of personality profile parameters, interior stimuli and social factors.

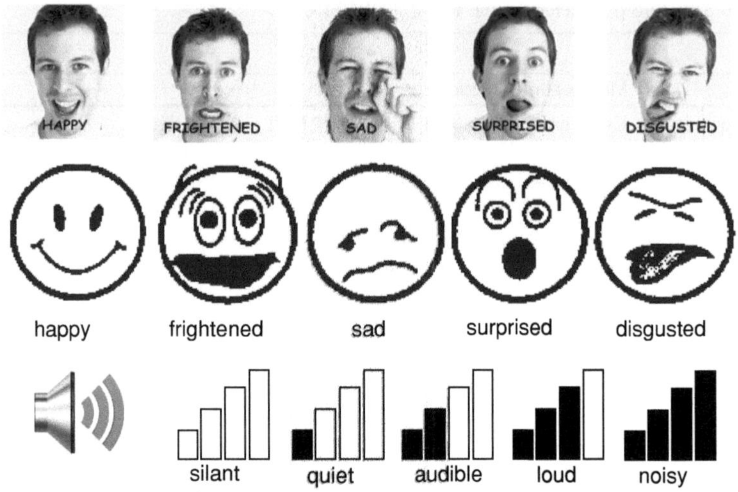

Fig. 6 Expression examples of different affective reactions. Facile expressions, graphic emoticons and audio features characteristic for different emotional states

In order to track the changes of emotional behavior attributes produced by the model simulator a customized graphical user interface (GUI) was developed. The GUI emulates the emotional reactions (affective manifestations) as the output of the FIS-3 block. Basic five emotional expressions are presented in Fig. 6 by face mimes and symbolic emoticons. Besides, the scale of phonetic levels (in the range from minimum to maximum) characteristic for some affective reactions is shown in Fig. 6, too. Developed interface enable us to get a better insight into the model properties through a multimodal interpretation of behavior attributes.

6 Model Validation

Model validation was done experimentally with human examines by use on-line tests. Several persons of different gender and age were requested to fill out the personality test available at the Internet (http://www.16personalities.com/free-personality-test). The same examinees were asked to do the test for identification of temperament type, too (http://neoxenos.org/wp-content/blogs.dir/1/files/temperaments/temperament_test.htm). The scoring of personality traits of the examinees was performed and the results are displayed in the Table 10. The same examinees were asked to fill out the questionnaire regarding to their hypothetic

Table 10 Results of personality tests

Examinee	E/I Percentage	N/S	T/F	J/P	Sang.	Chol.	Meln.	Phlg.
A.R	I-36	N-16	T-02	J-16	10.0	50.0	22.5	17.5
J.R	E-01	S-10	F-08	J-24	17.5	15.0	40.0	27.5
S.S	E-02	N-14	T-02	J-22	07.5	15.0	42.5	35.0
A.Ć	E-01	S-08	F-02	J-35	02.5	07.5	30.0	60.0
I.Sv	E-25	N-22	F-02	J-24	12.5	65.0	17.5	05.0
I.St	I-36	N-02	T-44	P-16	05.0	22.5	45.0	27.5
M.T	E-36	N-28	F-34	J-10	22.5	40.0	20.0	17.5
B.M	I-14	N-16	T-02	J-16	15.0	10.0	30.0	45.0
S.P	I-22	N-12	F-02	J-24	02.5	07.5	60.0	30.0

Quantification of the personality preferences and temperament types performed with the subjected group of the examinees by using web-questionnaires

Table 11 Results of the questionnaire

A.R	J.R	S.S	A.Ć	I.Sv	I.St	M.T	B.M	S.P
B	C	B	A	B	C	B	A	C

Responses of examinees to the same trigger-event depending on their dominant personality traits

affective reactions as response to the trigger-event described in the Sect. 5. The following answers were offered in the questionnaire:

A. I would feel as nothing was happened and that everything is normal
B. I would kindly smile and apologize because of the occasional inattention
C. I would feel myself extremely unpleasantly and embarrassingly keep silent
D. I would repeat the same to demonstrate that it's a natural deed to make anybody ashamed
E. I would feel the guilty, leave the place and no return back
F. None of the offered answers…

The answers of the examinees are given in Table 11.

Model validation was done by comparing experimentally acquired affective reactions of the examinees and simulation results of the affective behavior model developed in the chapter for the same input conditions (personality profiles, trigger-event and reactions). The validation tests proved that the generic human emotion-driven model has satisfactory congruence with the biological model.

7 Conclusion

The chapter concerns with development of artificial EI attributes through synthesis of new generic model of human emotion-driven behavior. The model developed in the chapter is aimed to building cognitive robot interface (EI-controller). The purpose of the artificial EI in robots is to increase their autonomy through building advance cognitive features such as: emotion understanding, self-management, managing relationship with others, etc. The novelties given in the chapter regards to the modeling approach of human affective behavior based on the theory from personality psychology. Unlike to the methods commonly used in the "developmental" or "epigenetic" robotics that allow lifelong, incremental learning of new affective behavior and social skills, the approach presented in this chapter is based on utilization of the structured and systematized knowledge about human emotional behavior. A three-stage fuzzy logic model architecture proved that the model proposed fits well a non-linear nature of human affective behavior. The future researches are planned to extend the present model by introducing new behavior attributes as well as to make more detailed experimental verification.

Acknowledgments The research in the chapter is funded by the Serbian Ministry of Science under the grants TR-35003 and III-44008. It is partially supported by the SNSF IP project IZ74Z0_137361/1 as well by the Serbia-Portugal "COLBAR" research project under the grant 451-03-02338/2012-14/12. The authors express thanks to the scientists from the Department of Experimental Psychology, Faculty of Human Sciences, University of Belgrade for the useful suggestions.

References

Affective science: http://en.wikipedia.org/wiki/Affective_science.

Affective computing. http://en.wikipedia.org/wiki/Affective_computing.

Alpaydin, E.: *Introduction to machine learning*. Cambridge, MA: The MIT Press. (2004).

Asada, M., Hosoda, K., Kuniyoshi, Y., Ishiguro, H., Inui, T., Yoshikawa, Y., Ogino, M. and Yoshida, C.: Cognitive developmental robotics: a survey. IEEE Transactions on Autonomous Mental Development, Vol.1, No.1, pp.12–34, (2009).

ASORO sociable robot. http://www.asoro.a-star.edu.sg/robots_mika.html.

Breazeal, C.: Function Meets Style: Insights from Emotion Theory Applied to HRI. *IEEE Transactions in Systems, Man, and Cybernetics, Part C*, 34(2), 187–194. (2003).

Breazeal, C.: Designing sociable robots. MIT Press. Cambridge. (2002).

Busher, H.J.: Human Intelligence its Nature and Assessment, Harfer Torbchbooks, NewYork, (1973).

Damasio, A.,: Descartes Error: Emotion, Reason, and the Human Brain. G.P Putnam's sons, New York. (1994).

Damasio, A.: A second chance for emotion. In R. D. Lane & L. Nadel (Eds.), *Cognitive neuroscience of emotion* (pp. 12–23). New York: Oxford University Press. (2000).

Dautenhahn, K.: Socially intelligent robots: dimensions of human - robot interaction, Philosophical Transactions of the Royal Society B: Biological Sciences, 362(1480), pp. 679–704. (2007).

Developmental robotics: http://en.wikipedia.org/wiki/Developmental_robotics.
Emotional intelligence: http://en.wikipedia.org/wiki/Emotional_intelligence.
Francis, A.G., Mehta, M.J., Ram, A.: Handbook of Research on Synthetic Emotion and Sociable Robotics: New Applications in Affective Computing and Artificial Intelligence. Ed. J. Vallverdú, D. Casacuberta. Chapter XX: Emotional Memory and Adaptive Personalities. Informatlon science reference, Hershey-NewYork, pp. 391–412 (2009).
Frijda, N.: *The emotions.* New York: Cambridge University Press. (1986).
FURHAT sociable robot. http://www.speech.kth.se/furhat/.
Gadanho, S. C. and Hallam, J.: Robot learning driven by emotions. In: Journal of Adaptive Behavior. Vol. 9, Issue 1, pp. 42–64, MIT Press Cambridge, MA, USA (2001a)
Gadanho, S. C. and Hallam, J.: Emotion-triggered Learning in Autonomous Robot Control. In: Cybernetics and Systems. (2001b).
Gluck, M., Mercado, E. and Myers, C.: *Learning and memory: From brain to behavior.* New York: Worth Publishers. (2008).
Hirth, J., Schmitz, N., Berns, K.: Emotional Architecture for the Humanoid Robot Head {ROMAN}. Proceedings of the IEEE International Conference on Robotics and Automation (ICRA) - 2150–2155, Rome, Italy (2007).
KASPAR sociable robot. http://www.kaspar.herts.ac.uk/.
Kirby, R., Forlizzi, J., Simmonsa, R.: Affective social robots. Robotics and Autonomous Systems. ELSEVIER, Vol. 58, pp. 322–332 (2010).
Kluemper, D.H.: Trait emotional intelligence: The impact of core-self evaluations and social desirability. Personality and Individual Differences, 44(6), 1402–1412, (2008).
Kolodner, J.L.: *Case-based reasoning.* San Francisco, CA: Morgan Kaufmann. (1993).
Kolodner, J.L.: *Retrieval and organization strategies in conceptual memory: A computer model.* Northvale, NJ: Lawrence Erlbaum Associates. (1984).
La Haye, T.: Your Temperament: Discover Its Potential. Tyndale Publishing. (1984).
Li, L., Liu, G., Zhang, M., Pan, Z., Song, E.: BAAP: a behavioral animation authoring platform for emotion driven 3D virtual characters. In: Proceedings of ICEC'10 Proceedings of the 9th international conference on Entertainment computing, pp. 350–357, Springer-Verlag-Berlin, Heidelberg (2010).
Lungarella, M., Metta, G., Pfeifer, R. and Sandini, G.: Developmental robotics: a survey. Connection Science, 15:151–190, (2003).
Mayer, J.D. and Salovey, P.: What is emotional intelligence? In: P. Salovey & D. Sluyter (Eds.), Emotional development and emotional intelligence: Implications for educators, pp. 3–31, New York: Basic Books, (1997).
MAGGIE sociable robot. http://roboticslab.uc3m.es/roboticslab/robot.php?id_robot=1.
MBTI: http://en.wikipedia.org/wiki/Myers-Briggs-Type-Indicator.
Metta, G., et al.: The RobotCub project—an open framework for research in embodied cognition, Humanoids Workshop, IEEE—RAS International Conference on Humanoid Robots. (2005).
Millington, I. (2006). *Artificial intelligence for games.* San Francisco, CA: Morgan Kaufmann.
Minsky, M.: *The emotion machine: Commonsense thinking, artificial intelligence, and the future of the human mind.* New York: Simon & Schuster. (2007).
Mitchell, T.: *Machine learning.* McGraw Hill. (1997).
Myers, D. G. Psychology (9th ed.). New York: Worth Publishers. (2010).
Myers-Briggs, I. and Myers, P.: Gifts Differing: Understanding Personality Type. Mountain View, CA: Davies-Black Publishing. (1995).
Norman, D.: How might humans interact with robots. Keynote address to the DARPA/NSF Workshop on Human-Robot Interaction, San Luis Obispo, CA. (2001).
On-line personality test: http://www.16personalities.com/free-personality-test.
On-line temperament test: http://neoxenos.org/wp-content/blogs.dir/1/files/temperaments/temperament_test.htm.
Ortony, A., Clore, G.L., & Collins, A.: *The cognitive structure of emotions.* Cambridge University Press. (1988).
PROBO sociable robot. http://probo.vub.ac.be/.

Project "Feelix Growing". http://en.wikipedia.org/wiki/Feelix_Growing.
Personality psychology: http://en.wikipedia.org/wiki/Personality_psychology.
Petrides, K.V., Pita, R., Kokkinaki, F.: The location of trait emotional intelligence in personality factor space. British Journal of Psychology, 98, 273–289, (2007).
Picard, R. Affective computation. MIT Press, Cambridge, MA. (1997).
Saltzman, M.: (Ed.) *Game design: Secrets of the sages.* Indianapolis, IN: Brady Publishing. (1999).
Santamaria, J.C.: Learning adaptive reactive agents. Unpublished doctoral dissertation. Georgia Institute of Technology, Atlanta, GA. (1997).
Schwab, B.: *AI game engine programming.* Hingham, Massachusetts: Charles River Media. (2004).
Simon, H.A.: *Reason in human affairs.* Stanford, CA: Stanford University Press. (1983).
Stoytchev, A., Tanawongsuwan, R.: PEPE—PErsonal PEt. In *Video Proceedings of the AAAI-98 Mobile Robot Exhibition*, Madison, WI. (1998).
Sutton, R.S., & Barto, A.G.: *Reinforcement learning: an introduction.* Cambridge, MA: MIT Press. (1998).
Temperament types: http://en.wikipedia.org/wiki/Four_temperaments.
Weng, J., McClelland, Pentland, A., Sporns, O., Stockman, I., Sur, M., and E. Thelen: Autonomous mental development by robots and animals. Science, vol. 291, pp. 599–600, (2001).
Winnie, J.F. and Gittinger, J.W.: An introduction to the personality assessment system. Journal of Clinical Psychology, Monograph Supplement, 38, 1=68 (1973).

Robot Skill Acquisition by Demonstration and Explorative Learning

Bojan Nemec and Ales Ude

Abstract The chapter presents a survey of methods used at Humanoid and Cognitive Robotics Lab for the robot skill acquisition and self-improvement of the learned skill. Initial demonstration are parameterized as Dynamic Movement Primitives and stored into a data base of actions. Whenever needed, the robot retrieves previous learned skill from the data-base and generalizes it to a new situation. If the generalization itself cannot generate an appropriate action for the given situation, the robot refines its skill by means of the reinforcement learning. In order to speed up the learning process, the algorithm searches first in the constrained manifold of demonstrated movements. For final tuning, it explores also the full dimensional space of a parameterized policy. The approach is validated with illustrative examples, taken from everyday life.

Keywords Learning by demonstration · Reinforcement learning · Skill acquisition

1 Introduction

Autonomy is one of the most important issues in contemporary robotics. In order to become fully autonomous, a robots has to be able to generalize to new actions from previously shown or learned examples. Generally, this is a hard problem, since the search space the robot has to explore is potentially huge (Schaal 1999).

B. Nemec (✉) · A. Ude
Humanoid and Cognitive Robotics Lab, Department for Automatics, Biocybernetics and Robotics, Jozef Stefan Institute, Jamova 39, 1000 Ljubljana, Slovenia
e-mail: bojan.nemec@ijs.si

A. Ude
e-mail: ales.ude@ijs.si

A. Rodić et al. (eds.), *New Trends in Medical and Service Robots*,
Mechanisms and Machine Science 20, DOI: 10.1007/978-3-319-05431-5_11,

The size of the search space depends on the number of degrees of freedom of the robot, representation of the motion and on the objects involved in the action. Furthermore, external objects can affect the search space indirectly. To overcome problems arising from high-dimensional and continuous perception-action spaces, it is necessary to guide the search process. One of the most successful paradigms that can be used for this purpose is imitation or robot programming by demonstration (Schaal 1999; Dillmann 2004). When observing either good or bad examples, one can reduce the search for a possible solution, by either starting the search from the observed good solution (local optima), or conversely, by eliminating from the search space what is known as a bad solution (Billard and Calinon 2007). Imitation is also familiar to everybody from daily experience, where a teacher demonstrates a movement and immediately the student is capable of approximately repeating it (Schaal et al. 2004). In order to successfully accomplish the task imposed by the demonstration, the subject (student) has to adapt it according to it's physical capabilities and constraints. Thus, imitation does not mean simple copy of the demonstrated motions. Moreover, it is important that the subject is capable of generalization of example trajectories to new situations that were not observed during training. In general, this requires a data-base containing example movements well distributed across the search space. In the case of the sparse data-base, where some example trajectories are missing, generalisation to a new situation might fail or does not result in skill reproduction within the required precision. In such a case, it is important that the agent itself finds the missing example trajectories by means of reinforcement learning.

The goal of the chapter is to propose a unified approach for the skill learning and generalisation to a new situation as it arises. As the underlaying motion representation we apply Dynamic Movement Primitives. Our approach can be summarised in the following steps:

- acquisition of the demonstrated skill and storing them into an example motion data-base
- parametrisation of the motion using the Dynamic Movement Primitives framework
- statistical generalisation of the available training data to new situations as they arise
- retrieve missing training data by means of Reinforcement learning
- adding of newly learned movement to the example motion data-base

Each step is described more in detail in the rest of the chapter.

2 Motion Acquisition

Robot programming by demonstration requires the acquisition of example trajectories, which can be captured in various ways. Motion capture techniques based on optical or magnetic tracking devices were applied successfully to replicate

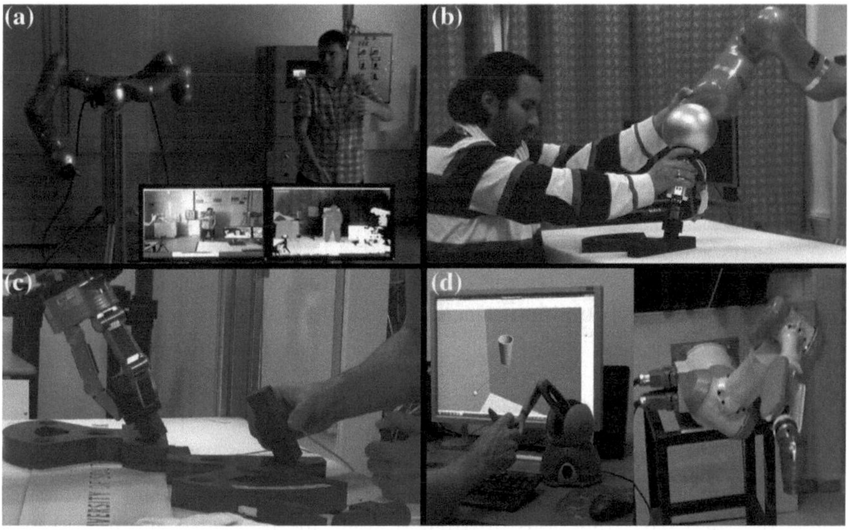

Fig. 1 Different methods of guidance for learning: **a** using RGBD camera **b** using kinesthetic guidance **c** using magnetic tracker **d** using haptic device

complex movements on humanoid robots such as dancing, which would be difficult to program manually (Ude et al. 2004). Computer vision techniques that aim to capture human motion without special markers are slowly getting matured (Moeslund 2006), but the application of specialized tracking devices is still preferred inmost of the recent works in order to avoid the pitfalls of computer vision approaches (Fig. 1a). Alternatively, a robot can be physically guided through the desired trajectory, which is recorded proprioceptively (Fig. 1b). This method requires that the robot is back-drivable (Peters and Schaal 2008) or can compensate for the influences of external forces (Albu-Schäffer et al. 2007). The advantage of kinesthetic guiding is that the movements are recorded directly on the learning robot and do not need to be first transferred from a system with different kinematics and dynamics. Another motion demonstration method which involves also the possibility to deal with environment forces is direct guiding using magnetic sensor (Fig. 1c) or using haptic device (Fig. 1d).

3 Motion Parametrisation

Our approach relies on a parameterized policy using Dynamic Movement Primitives (Ijspeert et al. 2013). Within this framework, every degree of freedom is described by its own dynamic system, but with a common phase to synchronize them. For point-to-point movements (also referred to as discrete movements), given either in joint or in task space, the trajectory of each robot degree of freedom y is described by the following system of nonlinear differential equations

$$\tau\dot{z} = \alpha_z(\beta_z(g - y) - z) + f(x), \tag{1}$$

$$\tau\dot{y} = z, \tag{2}$$

$$\tau\dot{x} = -\alpha_x x, \tag{3}$$

where x is the phase variable and z is an auxiliary variable. α_x, α_z, β_z and τ should be defined in such a way that the system converges to the unique equilibrium point $(z, y, x) = (0, g, 0)$. The nonlinear term f contains free parameters that are used to modify the dynamics of the second-order differential equation system to approximate any smooth point-to-point trajectory from the initial position y_0 to the final configuration g

$$f(x) = \frac{\sum_{i=1}^{N} w_i \Psi_i(x)}{\sum_{i=1}^{N} \Psi_i(x)} x, \; \Psi_i(x) = \exp\left(-h_i(x - c_i)^2\right), \tag{4}$$

with the given initial velocity and final velocity equal to zero. Here c_i are the centers of radial basis functions distributed along the trajectory and $h_i > 0$ their widths. Weights w_i are estimated in such a way that the DMP encodes the desired trajectory. N denotes the number of gaussian kernel functions used in nonlinear term $f(x)$. Generally, higher N means more precise description of the parameterized policy. In the equations above, α_x, α_z, and β_z are constant. They are set so that the underlying second order linear dynamic system is critically damped (Schaal et al. 2007).

A trajectory represented by the Dynamic Movement Primitives is parameterized with the initial velocity and position, the final goal position g, trajectory duration τ and a set of weights w_i associated with radial basis functions. All parameters except weights w_i can be obtained directly from the demonstrated trajectory. Here, we will show how to calculate weights w_i using regression. We assume that from human demonstration or kinesthetic guiding we obtain K trajectory data points $\{y_d(t_j), \dot{y}_d(t_j), \ddot{y}_d(t_j),\ t_j \in [0, T]\}$. By replacing the system of two first order Eqs. (1, 2) with one equation of the second order we obtain

$$f(t_j) = \tau^2\ddot{y}(t_j) + \tau\alpha_z\dot{y}(t_j) - \alpha_z\beta_z(g - y(t_j)), \tag{5}$$

where $f(t_j)$ is the value of the nonlinear function $f(x)$ (Eq. 4) in time t_j. Writing

$$\mathbf{w} = \begin{bmatrix} w_1 \\ \vdots \\ w_N \end{bmatrix}, \quad \mathbf{f} = \begin{bmatrix} f(t_0) \\ \vdots \\ f(t_K) \end{bmatrix}, \tag{6}$$

we obtain the following system of linear equations

$$\mathbf{A}\mathbf{w} = \mathbf{f}, \tag{7}$$

where the $(K \times N)$ system matrix $\mathbf{A}$ is given by

$$\mathbf{A} = \begin{bmatrix} \frac{\psi_1(x(t_0))x(t_0)}{\sum_{j=1}^{N}\psi_j(x(t_0))} & \dots & \frac{\psi_N(x(t_0))x(t_0)}{\sum_{j=1}^{N}\psi_j(x(t_0))} \\ \vdots & \vdots & \vdots \\ \frac{\psi_1(x(t_K))x(t_K)}{\sum_{j=1}^{N}\psi_j(x(t_K))} & \dots & \frac{\psi_N(x(t_K))x(t_K)}{\sum_{j=1}^{N}\psi_j(x(t_K))} \end{bmatrix}.$$

Set of weights that solve set of linear Eq. (7) in least square sense is then calculated using

$$\mathbf{w} = \mathbf{A}^{+}\mathbf{f}, \tag{8}$$

where $\mathbf{A}^{+}$ denotes the Moore-Penrose pseudo-inverse of the system matrix $\mathbf{A}$.

4 Motion Generalisation

In this section we show how to generalize previously learned policies to a new situation. Lets assume that we have a set of example trajectories together with the parameters characterizing the task

$$\mathscr{Z} = \{y_{\mathrm{d}}^{k}(t_{k,j}), \dot{y}_{\mathrm{d}}^{k}(t_{k,j}), \ddot{y}_{\mathrm{d}}^{k}(t_{k,j}); \mathbf{q}_k | k = 1, \ldots, M, j = 1, \ldots, T_k\}, \tag{9}$$

where $y_d^k(t_j)$, $\dot{y}_d^k(t_j)$, $\ddot{y}_d^k(t_j)$ are the measured positions, velocities, and accelerations on trajectory k, M is the number of examples, and T_k the number of sampling points on each trajectory. Indexing of the degrees of freedom is omitted from Eq. (9) for clarity. $\mathbf{q}_k \in \mathbb{R}^n$ are the parameters describing the task in a given example situation. The trajectories can be specified either in joint or task space. The issue is how to generate a DMP specifying a movement for every new query point $\mathbf{q}$, which in general will not be one of the example queries $\mathbf{q}_k$.

To generalize the example movements to new situations, we need to learn a function

$$\mathbf{G}(\mathbf{q}; \mathscr{Z}) \mapsto [\mathbf{w}^T, \tau, g]^T = \theta. \tag{10}$$

In general, the functional relationship between $\mathbf{q}$ and set of parameters θ describing the policy π given in a set of examples $\mathscr{Z}$ is unknown. Note that $\mathbf{G}(\mathbf{q}; \mathscr{Z})$ becomes a function only by constraining the generalized trajectories to be as similar as possible to the example trajectories. For example, there are many different ways of how to throw the ball into the basket. The relationship between the basket positions (query point $\mathbf{q}$) and DMP parameters describing the robot motion becomes a function only by requiring that the generalized movements are similar to the example movements (see Fig. 2a). In most cases it is difficult to find

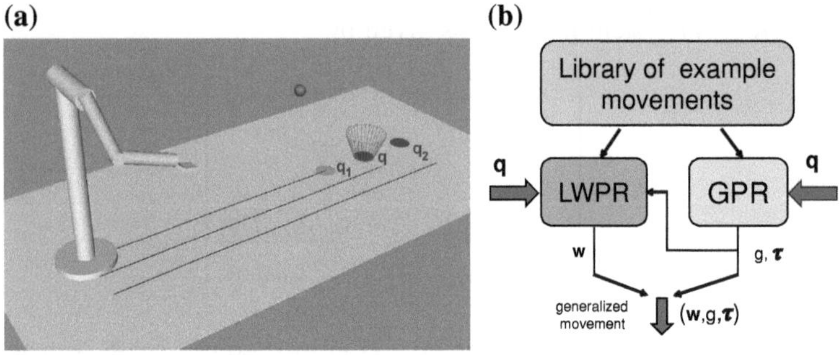

Fig. 2 **a** Generalisation of the ball throwing: Given two robot trajectories associated with the throw to the position described with q_1 and q_2, respectively, the generalisation procedure predicts the robot trajectory that results in the throw to the position q. **b** Generalisation of example trajectories using different statistical methods: LWPR: Locally Weighted Projected Regression, GPR: Gaussian Process regression

a global model that provides a good approximation for the function $\mathbf{G}(\mathbf{q}; \mathscr{X})$. We therefore avoid global model identification and rather apply regression techniques to generalize the movements. Due to significantly different sizes of data sets involved in the calculation of parameters $\mathbf{w}$ on the one hand, and g and τ on the other hand, different methods can be utilized to estimate them. In particular, in (Ude et al. 2010) we applied locally weighted regression for the estimation of the shape parameters and Gaussian process regression (Rasmussen and Williams 2006) to estimate g and τ, as it is schematically show in the Fig. 2b. More details about this work can be found in (Ude et al. 2010). The important point is to realize that a functional relationship between the query points $\mathbf{q}$ and DMP can be learned from example movements. The accuracy of the generalized motion depends on the nature of the problem and the number and density of the query points. If there are only few example query points, we might not reach the desired performance and we have to refine the generated movement by means of reinforcement learning.

5 Policy Learning

During the policy learning, we can generally not rely on the environment models, because they are either too complex either not available. Widely accepted technique to deal with model-free learning is Reinforcement Learning (RL) (Sutton et al. 1998). The general goal of the policy learning can be described as an optimization process, where the goal is to determine policy parameters $\mathbf{q} \in \mathbb{R}^n$, such that they maximize the expected return of the state value cost function

$$J(\theta) = E\left[\sum_{k=0}^{H} a_k r_k(\theta)\right]. \tag{11}$$

E denotes the expectation value, k is the time step, a_k are time-step dependent weighting factors, H is the horizon, which in case of discrete DMPs is equal to the number of sampling steps along the trajectory, and r_k is the reward received at each time step. $\mathbf{q}$ are the parameters describing the selected movement representation, e.g. DMPs. There are numerous methods how to optimize the above cost function. In continuation we will focus on policy gradient methods and direct policy improvement methods, which are widely accepted in robotics and sensory-motor learning.

5.1 Learning in Unconstrained Parameter Space

Policy gradient methods follow the steepest descent of the expected return in an episodic task, where the general parameter update rule can be written as

$$\theta_{m+1} = \theta_m + \alpha_m \nabla_\theta J(\theta). \tag{12}$$

Parameter α_m denotes the learning rate. The convergence to at least a local minimum can be guaranteed providing that the gradient estimate is unbiased and that the learning rate fulfills $\sum_{m=0}^{\infty} \alpha_m > 0$ and $\sum_{m=0}^{\infty} \alpha_m^2 = \text{const}$ (Peters and Schaal 2008). Note that one of the most important advantages of policy gradient methods over traditional reinforcement learning techniques (like Q-learning or SARSA) is that the update step can be controlled with the learning rate parameter. This becomes extremely important in learning actions of physical agents, e.g. robots. A drastic change of policy parameters can result in unpredicted motion, which can be hazardous both for the robot and for its environment. Moreover, as it was demonstrated in Schaal (1999), a drastic change can make the initialization of the policy based on imitation learning useless, as the initial parameters may vanish after a single update step.

Policy gradient methods require a good estimator for the policy gradient $\nabla_\theta J(\theta)$. If a deterministic model of the system was available, we could directly compute this gradient by

$$\nabla J = \frac{\partial \sum_{k=0}^{H} a_k r_k}{\partial \theta}. \tag{13}$$

Such a model is normally not available, therefore the main problem is how to estimate the policy gradient. A number of policy gradient estimation methods were proposed, for example finite gradient methods (Peters and Schaal 2008), likelihood ratio methods (Williams 1992), natural policy gradients (Kakade 2002), to name just a few. The main problem is high dimensionality of parameters to be learned. For example, a typical control policy encoded by DMPs might require 30–50 parameters for each joint, which makes the search space huge. Recently, new stochastic methods PI^2 and PoWER, which combine the well-developed methods from statistical learning and empirical inference with classical reinforcement learning (RL) algorithms, were proposed (Theodorou et al. 2010; Kober and Peters

2009). Such algorithms can scale to significantly more complex learning systems and minimize the number of tuning parameters. Although the parameter update rule has similar form as given in Eq. (12), PI^2 and PoWER are probabilistic policy improvement algorithms, not gradient algorithms. Unlike the policy gradient methods, they do not require the tuning of the learning rate α_m because they compute the optimal parameter update. The general form of a parameter update algorithm can be given as

$$\theta_{m+1} = \theta_m + \Upsilon(\pi, \Theta, \mathbf{r}), \tag{14}$$

where π, Θ and $\mathbf{r}$ denote set of all trajectories, parameters and rewards obtained during the exploration, respectively, and Υ denotes the learning algorithm, e.g. PI^2 (Theodorou et al. 2010) or PoWER (Kober and Peters 2008). In order to reduce the parameter and reward sets and to speed up the learning, importance sampling techniques are commonly used (Sutton et al. 1998). Initial parameters θ_0 can be obtained either by the parametrisation of the demonstration either by the statistical generalisation. In most cases a stochastic exploration rule is applied for RL, where the exploration parameters θ_l in each roll-out are selected according to $\theta_l = \theta_m + \varepsilon_l, \varepsilon_l \sim \mathcal{N}(0, \sigma^2)$. Noise variance σ^2 remains the only tuning parameters in policy improvement RL algorithms.

5.2 Learning in Constrained Parameter Space

In the previous section we presented how to improve policy given the initial policy described with the initial parameters θ_0. In this section, we will show how to speed up learning of new policies combining the methods of statistical generalisation and RL. Let us assume, that we have only few demonstration trajectories and using the statistical generalisation only we can not derive the policy, that will accomplish the given task with the required accuracy. Lets further assume that $\mathbf{G}(\mathbf{q}; \mathscr{Z})$ is an exact (ideal) function and $\hat{\mathbf{G}}(\mathbf{q}; \mathscr{Z})$ its approximation and that the relationship $\theta = \mathbf{G}(\mathbf{q}; \mathscr{Z}) = \hat{\mathbf{G}}(\mathbf{q} + \Delta\mathbf{q}; \mathscr{Z})$ exists. The idea is to learn a new query $\hat{\mathbf{q}} = \mathbf{q} + \Delta\mathbf{q}$ that fulfils the task instead of learning of the full set of parameters θ. Doing so, the learning problem defined in Eq. (11) can be converted into

$$\hat{J}(\hat{\mathbf{q}}) = E\left[\sum_{k=0}^{H} a_k \hat{r}_k(\hat{\mathbf{q}})\right], \quad \hat{r}_k(\hat{\mathbf{q}}) = r_k(\hat{\mathbf{G}}(\hat{\mathbf{q}}; \mathscr{Z})), \tag{15}$$

and the update step (12) becomes

$$\hat{\mathbf{q}}_{m+1} = \hat{\mathbf{q}}_m + \alpha_m \nabla_{\hat{\mathbf{q}}} \hat{J}(\hat{\mathbf{q}}), \tag{16}$$

where the dimensionality of $\hat{\mathbf{q}}$ is much lower than the dimensionality of θ. Because of this, we can successfully apply also simple optimisation methods (like finite gradients), which normally can't scale with high dimensional problems. We can

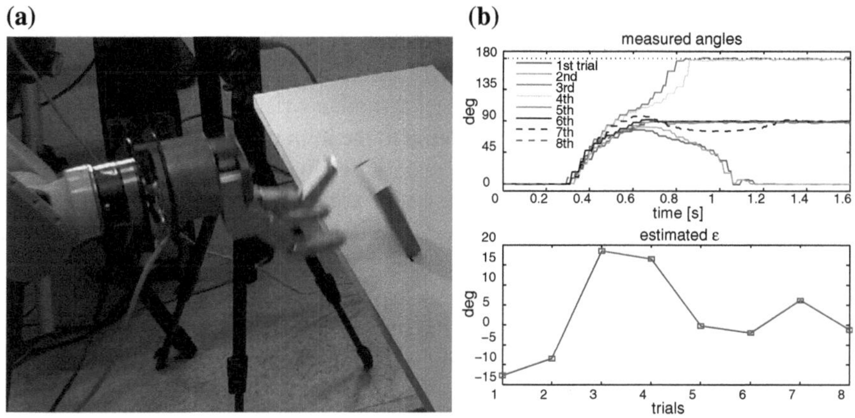

Fig. 3 **a** Learning of the matchbox flip-up with a robot. **b** Results of 8 trials of learning, where the *upper* and the *lower* graph show the estimated angle and the estimated error respectively. In this case the robot has learned the policy in 5 trials

even further simplify learning rule if we introduce error vector ε, which denotes the difference between the desired query $\mathbf{q}_0$ and the actually obtained query $\mathbf{q}_a = \mathbf{q}_0 + \Delta\mathbf{q} = \hat{\mathbf{G}}^{-1}(\mathbf{G}(\hat{\mathbf{q}};\mathscr{X});\mathscr{X})|_{\hat{\mathbf{q}}=\mathbf{q}_0}$,

$$\varepsilon = \mathbf{q}_0 - \mathbf{q}_a. \tag{17}$$

Defining the final reward as $r = \varepsilon^T\varepsilon$ and computing $\nabla_{\mathbf{q}}\hat{J}$ for this case yields

$$\nabla_{\mathbf{q}}\hat{J} = -2\frac{\partial \mathbf{q}_a}{\partial \mathbf{q}}\varepsilon \approx -\mathbf{K}\varepsilon, \tag{18}$$

where the matrix $\mathbf{K}$ is an approximation for the partial derivative $\frac{\partial \mathbf{q}_a}{\partial \mathbf{q}}$ around the desired query point. Note that in the case of the ideal generalization, i.e. $\mathbf{G} = \hat{\mathbf{G}}$, this matrix is an identity matrix. In practice, the matrix $\mathbf{K}$ can be approximated using numerical derivatives of the generalization function. Taking into account that we have to minimize the cost, we obtain the following error-based learning algorithm (Nemec et al. 2013; Wolpert et al. 2011)

$$\hat{\mathbf{q}}_{m+1} = \hat{\mathbf{q}}_m + \mathbf{K}\varepsilon. \tag{19}$$

If enough demonstration trajectories are available around the desired query point, the gain matrix $\mathbf{K}$ can be directly estimated from the example trajectories database, thus eliminating exploration. Alternatively, due to the low dimensionality of the problem, we can apply also line search optimisation algorithm to determine the optimal query update $\Delta\hat{\mathbf{q}}$.

We will demonstrate the usage of this policy learning method in constrained parameter space on a challenging task, where the robot has to flip-up the matchbox to stand upright on the narrower side (Fig. 3a). The flip-up is a very challenging task even for humans, in most cases we can succeed to do it only occasionally. For this reason, we recorded two unsuccessful attempts. In the first attempt the matchbox flipped back and in the second it flipped over. Every example trajectory $\mathscr{X}$ was generated by mapping the recorded Cartesian human wrist motion to the robot wrist motion and the human middle finger motion to the joint motion of the middle finger of the robot hand. The reward is given upon how close the matchbox came to the upright position by measuring the angle with a camera. When it flips forward, the reward is assigned upon the angular velocity in upright position, which is estimated from the angle measured 0.05 s after the matchbox has reached the upright position. The results of learning using the parameters update given by the Eq. (19) are shown in Fig. 3b. Due to noise introduced by the real hardware into the system, the error oscillates around 0 until it reaches steady state 0, typically in 5 trials.

6 Combined Learning in Constrained and Unconstrained Parameter Space

In this section we will consider the case, where the learning only in constrained domain can not find the policy with the required performance, i.e. we can not find such $\Delta\mathbf{q}$ that fulfills the equation $\mathbf{G}(\mathbf{q}; \mathscr{X}) = \hat{\mathbf{G}}(\mathbf{q} + \Delta\mathbf{q}; \mathscr{X})$. In such a case, we have two possibilities. (a) To proceed with learning in full parameter space using algorithm given with the Eq. (14) after finding the best possible approximation of the query $\mathbf{q}$ using the algorithm (19) (b) Combine learning in both constrained and unconstrained parameter space (Nemec et al. 2012). In the latter case we assume the process model described as $\theta = \hat{\mathbf{G}}(\hat{\mathbf{q}}; \mathscr{X}) + \Delta\theta$. Our goal is to learn such $\hat{\mathbf{q}}$ and $\Delta\theta$, which will maximize the reward r. For that, we define an extended parameter set in the form

$$\theta^* = [\hat{\mathbf{q}}, \Delta\theta]^T \tag{20}$$

and estimate the extended parameter set using Eq. (14) and the stochastic exploration policy

$$\theta_i^* = \theta_m^* + \varepsilon_i, \quad \varepsilon_i \sim [\mathcal{N}(0, \sigma_1^2), \mathcal{N}(0, \sigma_2^2)], \tag{21}$$

where different exploration noise σ_1^2 and σ_2^2 is used for the search in the constrained and full parameter space, respectively. The noise variance σ^2 is highly dependent on the process parameters θ^*. Generally, higher values of σ^2 speed up the learning and lower values of σ^2 lead to more accurate results. As shown in the previous section, learning in constrained domain characterized by $\mathbf{q}$ benefits from faster search because the search space is considerably smaller with the proper choice of the constrained configuration space. Thus, with proper choice of σ^2 the search in constrained space dominates over the search in unconstrained parameter space. Physical units of $\mathbf{q}$ are also considerably different from the policy parameters $\Delta\theta$,

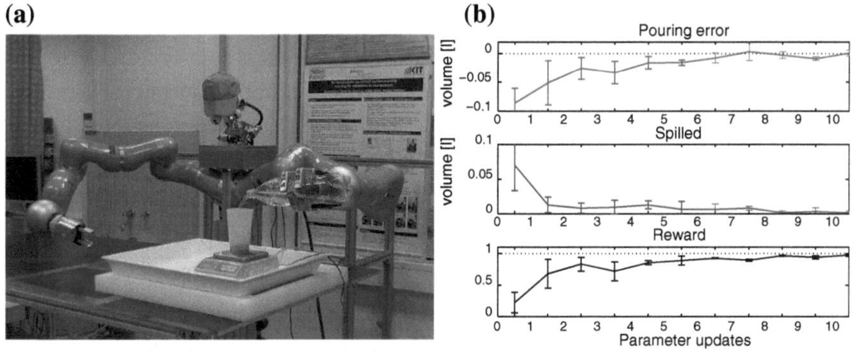

Fig. 4 **a** Learning of the pouring. **b** Results of 10 parameters updates using combined learning. *Vertical bars* denote standard deviation of 5 experiments. The robot quickly learns the policy that pours the required quantity of liquid without spilling

therefore we propose to use one noise variance for the query estimation and a different one for the general movement parameters. Noise variation is difficult to guess if we start learning from scratch. However, in our system we have a number of training trajectories available, hence the appropriate σ^2 can be calculated as $\sigma^2 = \max_{i,j}\{\|\theta_i - \theta_j\|\}s$, where s is a suitably chosen constant, which defines the span of parameter exploration.

Combined learning will be demonstrated in learning of a barman skill, where the task of the robot is to pour the same quantity of liquid into a glass from bottles containing different volumes of liquid (Nemec et al. 2012). Using the kinesthetic guiding, we provided two demonstration of pouring movements, which poured 0.2 l of liquid into the glass from a bottle containing 0.3 and 1.0 l of liquid, respectively. Demonstration trajectories were captured in joint coordinates. The quantity of liquid in the glass was measured with a precision scale after the execution of the pouring movement. No vision sensors were used to detect either the glass position or the level of liquid in the glass. Learning in joint coordinates induces additional nonlinearities in the system and, consequently, the generalization in joint coordinates with only two example trajectories caused that the robot was spilling the liquid during the execution of the pouring movement. It was therefore necessary to apply the combined learning in order to learn a pouring policy without spilling. The reward function was $r = 1 - 5\|v_d - v_m\| - 5v_s$, where v_d is the desired volume of the liquid in the glass, v_m is the measured poured volume and v_s is the volume of the spilled liquid. The demonstrated trajectories describing the motion of each of 7 joints were encoded as DMPs with 30 Gaussian kernel functions. Thus, the total number of θ^* parameters (including query $\mathbf{q}$, kernel weights $\mathbf{w}$ and the duration τ) was 212. Figure 4 shows the mean value of the pouring error, spilled volume, and the reward from 5 learning experiments with 10 parameters updates, where we learned to pour from a bottle containing 0.5 l of liquid. Note that each parameter update requires three additional roll-outs, therefore we have four roll-outs per parameter update.

7 Conclusions

In the chapter we presented unified approach to the robot sensorimotor learning, generalisation and self-improvement of the learned skill. We demonstrated how to capture demonstration policies and store them a data base of actions. As the underlying representation of parameterized policies we used DMPs and showed how to obtain the corresponding parameters using regression technique. Whenever the robots encounter new situation, it explores the database of the example policies and generate the required policy using the statistical generalisation. If the newly generated policy does not meet the required precision, it has to be refined by means of RL. We considered three cases: (1) learning in full (unconstrained) parameter set describing the policy, (2) learning in constrained parameter set characterised by a query imposed by the statistical generalisation (3) combined learning in constrained and unconstrained parameter set. Newly learned policy is then added to the policies data-base. In such a way, robot has to learn new policies only when necessary. The described framework inherits life-long learning, which can successfully solve the problem arising from changing environments and robot triteness. Our approach was validated with illustrative examples taken from everyday problems a service robot might encounter during the autonomous operation.

References

S. Schaal, "Is imitation learning the route to humanoid robots?" *Trends in Cognitive Sciences*, vol. 3, no. 6, pp. 233–242, 1999.

R. Dillmann, "Teaching and learning of robot tasks via observation of human performance," *Robotics and Autonomous Systems*, vol. 47, no. 2-3, pp. 109–116, 2004.

A. Billard and S. Calinon, "Force control," in *Robot Programming by Demonstration*, B. Siciliano and O. Khatib, Eds. 1em plus 0.5em minus 0.4em Berlin, Heidelberg: Springer, 2007, pp. 1371–1394.

S. Schaal, A. Ijspeert, and A. Billard, *Computational approaches to motor learning by imitation.* 1em plus 0.5em minus 0.4em oxford university press, 2004, no. 1431, pp. 199–218.

A. Ude, C. G. Atkeson, and M. Riley, "Programming full-body movements for humanoid robots by observation," *Robotics and Autonomous Systems*, vol. 47, no. 2-3, pp. 93–108, 2004.

A. Moeslund, T. B. Hilton and V. Krüger, "A survey of advances in vision-based human motion capture and analysis," *Comput. Vis. Image Understanding*, vol. 104, no. 2, p. 90GÇô126, 2006.

J. Peters and S. Schaal, "Reinforcement learning of motor skills with policy gradients," *Neural Networks*, vol. 21, pp. 682–697, 2008.

A. Albu-Schäffer, C. Ott, and G. Hirzinger, "A unified passivity based control framework for position, torque and impedance control of flexible joint robots," *Int. J. Robot. Res.*, vol. 26, no. 1, p. 2339, 2007.

A. J. Ijspeert, J. Nakanishi, H. Hoffmann, P. Pastor, and S. Schaal, "Dynamical movement primitives: Learning attractor models for motor behaviors," *Neural Computation*, vol. 25, no. 2, pp. 328–373, 2013.

S. Schaal, P. Mohajerian, and A. Ijspeert, "Dynamics systems vs. optimal control – a unifying view," *Progress in Brain Research*, vol. 165, no. 6, pp. 425–445, 2007.

A. Ude, A. Gams, T. Asfour, and J. Morimoto, "Task-specific generalization of discrete and periodic dynamic movement primitives," *IEEE Trans. Robotics*, vol. 26, no. 5, pp. 800–815, 2010.

C. E. Rasmussen and C. Williams, *Gaussian Processes for Machine Learning.* 1em plus 0.5em minus 0.4em Cambridge, MA: MIT Press, 2006.

R. Sutton and A. Barto, *Reinforcement Learning: An Introduction.* 1em plus 0.5em minus 0.4em Cambridge, MA: MIT Press, 1998.

R. J. Williams, "Simple statistical gradient-following algorithms for connectionist reinforcement learning," *Machine Learning*, vol. 8, no. 23, 1992.

S. A. Kakade, "Natural policy gradient," *Advances in neural information processing systems*, vol. 14, pp. 1531–1538, 2002.

E. A.Theodorou, J. Buchli, and S. Schaal, "A generalized path integral control approach to reinforcement learning," *Journal of Machine Learning Research*, no. 11, pp. 3137–3181, 2010.

J. Kober and J. Peters, "Learning motor primitives for robotics," in *Proc. IEEE Int. Conf. Robotics and Automation*, Kobe, Japan, 2009, pp. 2112–2118.

J. Kober, J. Peters, "Policy search for motor primitives in robotics," *Neural Information Processing Systems (NIPS)*, 2008.

B. Nemec, R. Vuga, and A. Ude, "Efficient sensorimotor learning from multiple demonstrations," *Advanced Robotics*, vol. 27, no. 13, pp. 1023–1031, 2013.

D. M. Wolpert, J. Diedrichsen, and J. R. Flanagan, "Principles of sensorimotor learning." *Nature reviews. Neuroscience*, vol. 12, no. 12, pp. 739–51, Dec. 2011.

B. Nemec, D. Forte, R. Vuga, M. Tamošiūnaitė, F. Wörgötter, and A. Ude, "Applying statistical generalization to determine search direction for reinforcement learning of movement primitives," in *2012 12th IEEE-RAS International Conference on Humanoid Robots*, Osaka, Japan, 2012.

[illegible]

Two Faces of Human–Robot Interaction: Field and Service Robots

Rodrigo Ventura

Abstract This chapter reports on recent research and development done at Institute for Systems and Robotics (ISR) on Human-Robot Interaction (HRI), encompassing two different perspectives. On the one hand, we have conducted research on field robots tele-operated by remote human operators, targeting Urban Search And Rescue scenarios. Here, research is focused on the challenge of conveying the operator with an effective situation awareness of the robot surroundings. Situation awareness is here understood as "the perception of the elements in the environment within a volume of time and space, the comprehension of their meaning, and the projection of their status in the near future" (Drury et al. 2003). Our approach is based on decoupling operation of the robot perception from the motion command: an Head-Mounted Display displays in stereo a video stream from the cameras onboard the robot, while the gaze of these cameras is controlled by the operator head, and the robot motion is commanded from a gamepad held by the operator. On the other hand, we have addressed the challenge of service robots designed to perform tasks requested by users. Humans interact with these robots, firstly to request a task, and secondly during task execution. The main research challenge is to have these robots to be aware of their own limitations, and ask humans for help to overcome those limitations. We are currently addressing the challenge of developing robust localization and navigation methods targeting office environments.

Keywords Human-robot interaction · Urban search and rescue · Service robots · Head-mounted display · Immersive teleoperation · Interactive mapping · Fast-marching methods

R. Ventura (✉)
Institute for Systems and Robotics, Instituto Superior Técnico, Lisbon, Portugal
e-mail: rodrigo.ventura@isr.ist.utl.pt

A. Rodić et al. (eds.), *New Trends in Medical and Service Robots*,
Mechanisms and Machine Science 20, DOI: 10.1007/978-3-319-05431-5_12,

1 Introduction

Human-Robot Interaction (HRI) is a field of study focused on the reciprocal action (interaction), including communication (verbal and non-verbal), between humans and robots [see (Fong et al. 2003; Goodrich and Schultz 2007) for reviews]. This interaction can take various forms, depending on the modality (visual, speech, etc.), on the proximity between humans and robots (collocated or remote), and on many other dimensions [see (Yanco and Drury 2002; Yanco et al. 2004) for a thorough taxonomy of the design space of HRI].

In this chapter we present recent research conducted in Institute for Systems and Robotics[1] (Instituto Superior Técnico, Lisbon) on two distinct application areas: field and service robotics. The former concerns the use of mobile robots on unstructured environments. In particular, we target Urban Search And Rescue (USAR) scenarios. In this case, the interaction is primarily concentrated on the teleoperation of the robot by a remote human operator, where the operator has total control over the robot operation. The latter area encompasses mobile robots that perform services requested by humans, where we focus on office environments. HRI happens in two situations: first, the operation of requesting a task—remotely, e.g., using the web, or locally, e.g., speech commands to the robot, and second, interaction with humans during task execution, e.g., requesting a human to open a door. The rest of this chapter is structured as two major sections, Sects. 2 and 3, covering each one of these areas of research. We wrap up the chapter with some concluding remarks on the Sect. 4.

2 Field Robotics

Field robotics concerns the use of sturdy robots in unstructured environments. By unstructured environments we mean environments for which there is no a priori map and the ground is not necessarily horizontal. A major application area where these environments can be found is Urban Search And Rescue (USAR). After a major disaster (natural or human made) affecting a urban region, victims are often found trapped inside buildings partially collapsed (and close to collapse). In many cases, these buildings pose a serious threat to human teams, and therefore, the use of teleoperated robots become a much safer option. In particular, robots can be sent in cases where human teams are unable to go due to imminent danger of collapse.

Since 2003 that ISR has been involved in the design, construction, and use of tracked wheel robots for USAR scenarios: RAPOSA, which was developed from scratch in a joint project lead by a spin-off (IdMind), and RAPOSA-NG, built upon

[1] http://www.isr.ist.utl.pt

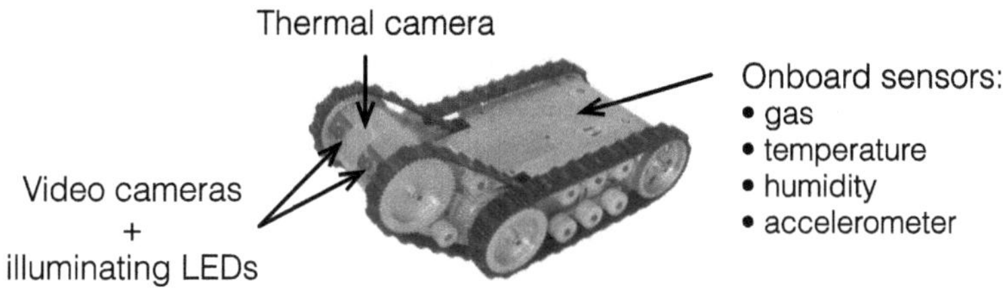

Fig. 1 Photo of the RAPOSA platform with the location of its sensors indicated

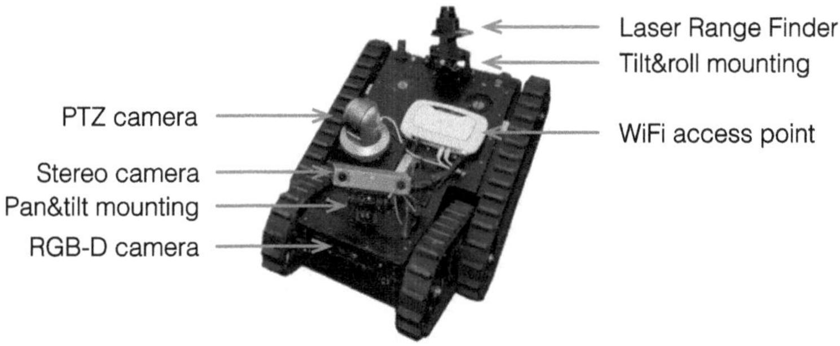

Fig. 2 Photo of RAPOSA-NG platform with the onboard equipment indicated

a commercial, barebones, and significantly improved version of RAPOSA (made by IdMind). In the following two sections these two platforms are briefly presented, followed by an overview of the conducted research on HRI issues with these platforms. Both robots have track wheel fors traction and feature two separate bodies: the main body where most of the equipment resides (batteries, motors, etc.), and an frontal arm actuated by a motor (Figs. 1 and 2). Both bodies have tracks, thus maximizing the area of traction with the gound.

2.1 RAPOSA

The first prototype was developed jointly with the IST spin-off company IdMind and the Lisbon firefighters brigade (RSBL) during the 2003–2005 period. This prototype, called RAPOSA (Fig. 1), is a tracked wheel platform whose specifications were driven by a set of requirements for USAR missions, including the capability of climbing standard-size stairs and moving along standard-size pipes, remote voice communication with victims, having environmental sensors (relevant gases, humidity, and temperature) and thermal camera. This robot is physically similar to other robots developed around the same time, notably the iRobot Packbot (Yamauchi 2004), however it is distinctive by an innovative aspect: there is a tether cable carrying power and an embedded wireless Access Point (AP), that can be remotely attached and detached from the body without direct human intervention (Marques et al. 2007, 2006). The remote operator commands the robot to move towards the cable, using a rear camera, inside behind the cable attachment outlet of the robot. The cable is physically attached to the robot by a motorized locker mechanism that grips the cable end. The RAPOSA is equipped with a broad range of sensors: two frontal video cameras, one frontal thermal camera, one rear camera (for cable attaching), and various environmental sensors. The communication with the base station, from which the remote operator commands the robot, is based on digital wireless communications (WiFi), either directly to the base station or using the AP at the cable end.

After the development and construction of the platform, it have been intensively used for research. Besides the work on HRI, that will be described in Sect. 2.3, we have also focused on autonomous behaviors. Since USAR operations are often always conducted under a strict chain of command, the use of semi-autonomy is usually preferred over fully autonomous ones. The concept of adjustable autonomy stems from the observation that the level of autonomy is something that is decided and set by the human operator (Goodrich et al. 2001; Murphy and Rogers 1996). Under this umbrella we have addressed two autonomous behaviors: stair climbing and cable docking. We have developed a successful stair climbing method, combining visual servoing for approaching the stairs, and the use of the onboard accelerometers in closed loop to climb the stairs while keeping the robot movement orientation orthogonal with the stair edges (Ferraz and Ventura 2009). Autonomous cable docking is achieved using visual servoing techniques using the camera images captured by the rear camera (Ferreira and Ventura 2009).

2.2 RAPOSA-NG

Following the success of RAPOSA, the IdMind company developed a commercial version of RAPOSA, improving it in various ways. Notably, the rigid chassis of RAPOSA, which eventually ends up being plastically deformed by frequent shocks, was replaced by semi-flexible structure, capable of absorbing non-elastically shocks, while significantly lighter than the original RAPOSA.

ISR acquired a barebones version of this robot, called RAPOSA-NG, and equipped it with a different set of sensors, following lessons learnt from previous research with RAPOSA (see Fig. 2). In particular, it is equipped with:

- a stereo camera unit (PointGrey Bumblebee2) on a pan-and-tilt motorized mounting;
- a Laser-Range Finder (LRF) sensor on a tilt-and-roll motorized mounting;
- an pan-tilt-and-zoom (PTZ) IP camera;
- an Inertial Measurement Unit (IMU).

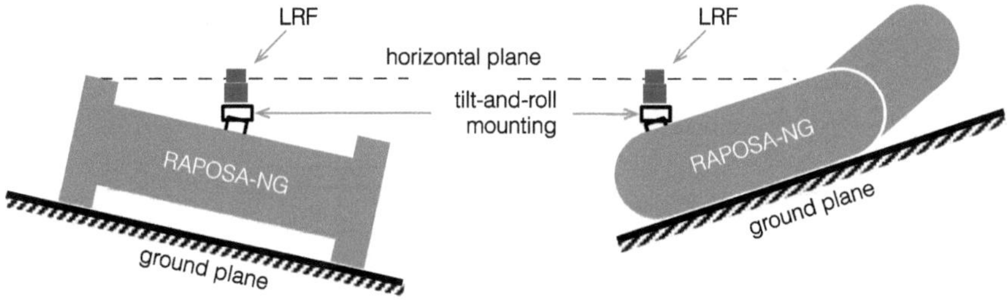

Fig. 3 Tilt-and-roll mounting for stabilizing the LRF

This equipment was chosen not only to fit better our research interests, but also to aim at the RoboCup Robot Rescue competition (see Sect. 2.5).

The stereo camera is primarily used jointly with an Head-Mounted Display (HMD) wear by the operator: the stereo images are displayed on the HMD, thus providing depth perception to the operator, while the stereo camera attitude is controlled by the head tracker built-in the HMD (see Fig. 4). This system will be explained in detail in Sect. 2.3.

The LRF is being used in one of the following two modes: 2D and 3D mapping. In 2D mapping we assume that the environment is made of vertical walls. However, since we cannot assume horizontal ground, we use a tilt-and-roll motorized mounting to automatically compensate for the robot attitude, such that the LRF scanning plane remains horizontal, as depicted in Fig. 3. An internal IMU measures the attitude of the robot body and controls the mounting servos such that the LRF scanning plane remains horizontal.

The IP camera is used for detail inspection: its GUI allows the operator to orient the camera towards a target area and zoom in into a small area of the environment. This is particularly relevant for remote inspection tasks in USAR. The IMU is used both to provide the remote operator with reading of the attitude of the robot, and for automatic localization and mapping of the robot.

2.3 HRI for Teleoperation

One of the challenges of using tele-operated robots in USAR scenario is to provide the remote operators with an effective situation awareness of the robot surroundings. We have been addressing this challenge by using a stereo camera pair on the robot together with an HMD equipped with an head tracker, wear by the remote operator: the stereo camera pair streams stereo imagery to the remote operator HMD, while the HMD head tracker controls the motion of the camera. With this arrangement we achieve several goals. Firstly, since the video stream is composed of stereo images, the remote operator experiences depth perception of the environment (also known as stereopsis). This allows improved perception of

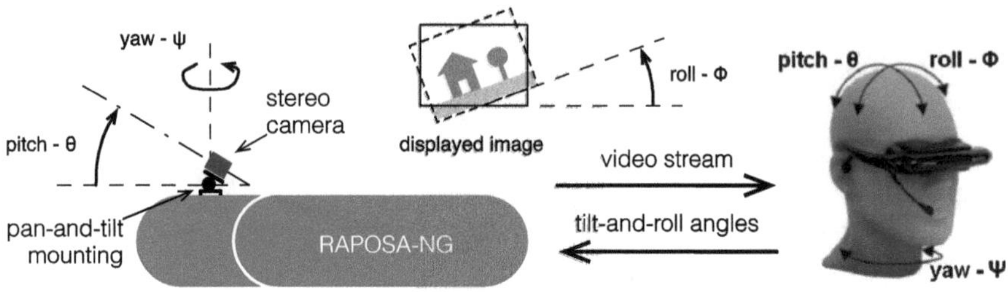

Fig. 4 Teleoperation using HMD and pan-and-tilt camera mounting

distances, than using monocular images. And secondly, by controlling the gaze of the cameras using the HMD head tracker, we allow the remote operator to control the camera orientation with his head. This frees his hands for other tasks, namely to command the robot motion using a gamepad interface.

We evaluated this architecture in both RAPOSA and RAPOSA-NG. Since the RAPOSA frontal cameras are fixed on the frontal body, we chose to orient the cameras in the following way: adjust the frontal body arm for the tilt movement, and change the heading of the robot (using the tracks) for the pan movement. We evaluated this system in a controlled user study (Martins and Ventura 2009), over a set of tasks involving RAPOSA. The results show the benefit of both stereopsis and HMD, however, they also show that controlling the heading of the robot using the HMD head tracker degrades task performance. One possible reason for this negative result lies on the fact that humans move the head and the walking direction independently. In other words, whenever the remote operator turns his head, he does not expect the moving direction of the robot to change.

Driven by this result, we decided to install the stereo camera on RAPOSA-NG using a motorized pan-and-tilt mounting. This allows the camera orientation can be changed independently than the robot heading. The HMD pitch and yaw angles control the mounting tilt and pan angles, while the roll angle rotates the images with respect to the center (see Fig. 4). Additionally, we introduced the concept of virtual pan-and-tilt: we emulate a (small) change of pan/tilt angles by re-projecting the camera image to a different optical axis (but same focal point) and cropping the result. Figure 5 illustrates the physical and reprojected optical axis. This reduces the effective field of view as seen by the operator, however, the field of view of the stereo cameras is quite large.[2] We combine the physical and the virtual pan-and-tilt so that we are able to provide fast pan/tilt image movements, up to certain limits. We evaluated this system on RAPOSA-NG in another user study (Reis and Ventura 2012), which has shown the benefits of the system.

[2] Pointgrey Bumblebee2 with an horizontal field-of-view of 97°.

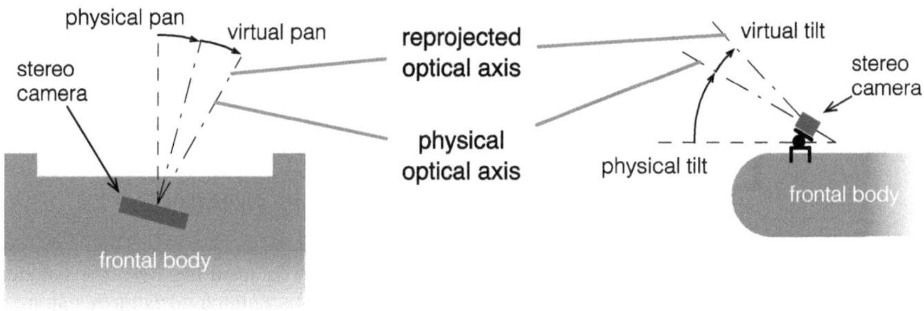

Fig. 5 The physical and reprojected optical axis in the virtual pan-and-tilt of the stereo camera

2.4 Interactive Mapping

Most methods of 2D or 3D mapping rely on matching a sequence of sensor data scans to find the best fit among scans. Having this, sensor data is registered into a map. The most commonly used method is the Iterative Closest Point (ICP) (Besl and McKay 1992), followed by a large variety of variants. However, most scan matching methods are prone to local minima. When this happens, misalignment of scan data occurs and the map turns out showing severe distortions. We have addressed this problem taking a semi-automatic approach according to which a human user corrects these misalignments. The method is based on a graphical user interface that allows the user to interact with individual scans. Any scan can be individually translated and rotated. The innovation we have introduced lies in a technique to assist moving scans in the interface. In particular, scans can be moved along the directions of higher ambiguity (Vieira and Ventura 2012a, b, 2013). For instance, when moving scans of a straight corridor, as shown in Fig. 6, movement tends to be constrained along the corridor, while transmitting a feeling of being "stuck" on the orthogonal direction. This results from moving the selected point cloud D, with respect to M, such that a virtual force F_m caused by a mouse drag movement is balanced by a reaction force F_r given by the gradient of the ICP cost function. This effect resembles the so called "magnetic" effect in most vector drawing programs.

This methods was applied to the adjustment of both 2D scans taken from a LRF and 3D scans acquired by a RGB-D sensor. Figure 7 shows an example of a set of 2D point clouds from a segment of an office floor, (a) before alignment, (b) after running ICP, and (c) after interactive mapping. The local minima phenomena that results from ICP alone is clearly visible in the deformation of the resulting map in (b), while the involvement of a human is capable of effectively correct those deformations, as shown in (c). However, we have to acknowledge the fact that humans have prior knowledge about typical office floors, while ICP alone has not. But in fact that is the strength of having the human-in-the-loop in tasks that machines are uncapable of performing alone.

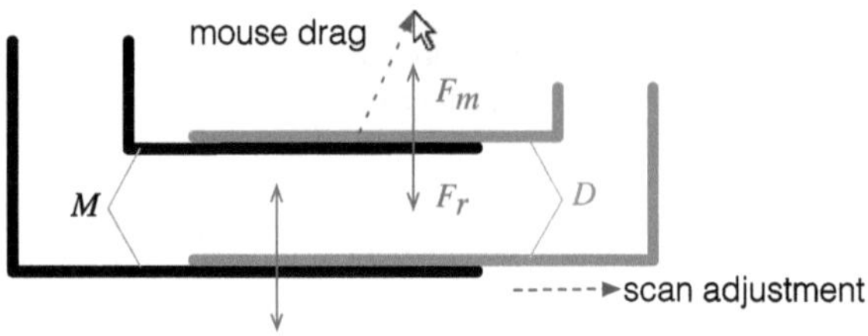

Fig. 6 Interactive adjustment of a pointcloud D with respect to M resulting from the balance between a mouse force F_m and a reaction force F_r. As a result, the pointcloud D moves along a direction parallel to the corridor

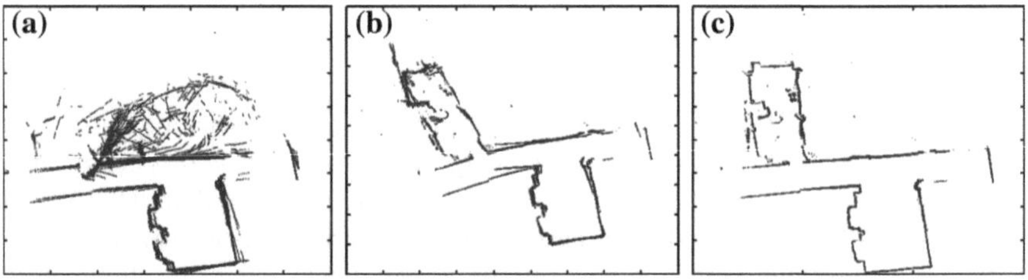

Fig. 7 Results of interactive mapping applied to 2D scans from a LRF. **a** The original raw data, **b** after running ICP, **c** after interactive mapping

2.5 Scientific Competitions as Benchmark

Evaluation and benchmarking is a fundamental part of any development cycle in science and engineering. Benchmarking aims at evaluating, with respect to an established common ground, alternative approaches to a given problem. However, many evaluation setups are *ad-hoc*, designed to specifically show in a controlled lab environment the benefits of a specific solution. In recent years, a broad range of competitions have been proposed in the area of computer science to foster benchmarking on independently controlled conditions. Examples of these competitions include semantic robot vision (Helmer et al. 2009), planning (Long and Fox 2003), and chatterbots (Mauldin 1994). In the robotics area, RoboCup has emerged as one of the most prominent scientific event comprising a broad range of competitions (Kitano et al. 1997), being robotic soccer the first one. The first competition was held in Nagoya in 1997, and since then the range of competitions has grown to include USAR—leagues Rescue Robot and Rescue Simulation (Kitano and Tadokoro 2001)—as well as service robots for home—league @Home (van der Zant and Wisspeintner 2007). All these competitions, not only allow benchmarking over a common scenario, but perhaps more importantly fosters and motivate research and development of more advanced and robust solutions. It should also be mentioned the remarkable effect of these competitions on the dissemination of science and technology to the society.

The ISR has been actively involved in RoboCup since 1998, initially in the robotic soccer leagues, and latter in the Rescue Robot one. We have participated with the RAPOSA-NG platform in the GermanOpen in 2012 (Magdeburg, Germany) and in RoboCup in 2013 (Eindhoven, Netherlands). The RoboCup Rescue Robot league evaluates the performance of USAR robots in an abridged version of the NIST standard scenario (Jacoff et al. 2003). It comprises finding simulated victims, within a limited timeframe (typically 15–20 minutes), in either a fully autonomous robot situation or a teleoperated one. When in teleoperation, the remote operator is sitting on a booth without any direct visual contact with the scenario.

These competition has pushed our development efforts along three main lines. First, in the direction of a more effective HRI, namely the stereo teleoperation with the HMD, as described in Sect. 2.2. This has proven extremely useful in competition, in particular understanding the situation of the robot in the challenging scenarios put by the NIST scenario. Second, the competition pressure demands for a real focus on the robustness of the robot. For instance, simple solutions such as remotely being able to perform an hardware reset of the onboard computer allowed us to overcome severe onboard computer hang-ups. And third, to explore the best configuration of the suite of sensors. For instance, besides the stereo cameras, we also choose to equip RAPOSA-NG with a PTZ camera for examining details that were hard to spot using the stereo camera, and with a LRF on a tilt-and-roll mounting for 2D mapping.

3 Service Robotics

Traditionally, service robots are seen as autonomous robots that perform tasks for users. The robot design is such that it is in principle capable of completing the requested task autonomously. Thus, the set of tasks is limited by the robot capabilities. For instance, if a robot has no arms, it will never be able to pick up objects by itself.

In recent years a different approach to service robots have been pursued, based on the concept of symbiotic human-robot interaction (Coradeschi and Saffiotti 2006; Rosenthal et al. 2010), according to which capability limitations of robots are coped with the help of humans. This approach has been actively pursued by the group of Manuela Veloso at CMU using the robot platform CoBot (Veloso et al. 2012). This platform is designed to navigate autonomously in office environments and to interact naturally with people. This platform is based on an omnidirectional drive base and is equipped with a suite of sensors for navigation and interaction. Research on CoBot has included a broad variety of topics, such as Kinect-based localization (Biswas and Veloso 2011), symbiotic planning (Haigh and Veloso 1998; Rosenthal et al. 2011), remote task scheduling (Ventura et al.2013), interaction with users (Rosenthal and Veloso 2010), and telepresence (Coltin et al. 2011).

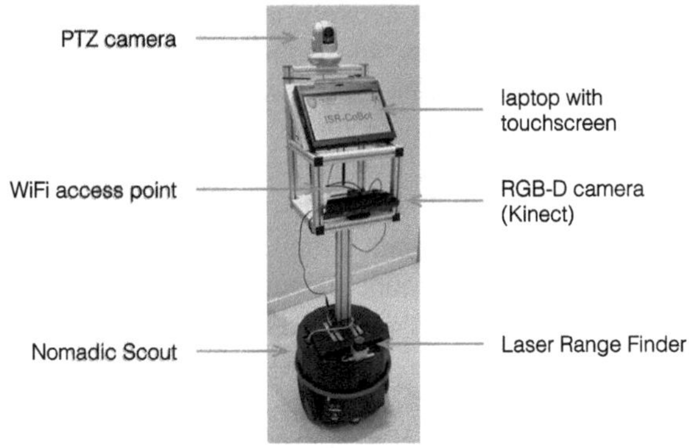

Fig. 8 ISR-CoBot platform with the onboard equipment indicated

Following a collaboration with CMU on CoBot, we have started developing a platform following the same design principles of CoBot. The platform is called ISR-CoBot, shown in Fig. 8, being currently based on a Nomadic Scout platform customized by IdMind. On top of it a pedestral supports the main equipment onboard: a laptop with touchscreen for user interface, a PTZ camera for telepresence, a Kinect sensor, and a wireless access point.

ISR-CoBot is a differential drive platform, however we are currently working on migrating to a omnidirectional base. The main advantage is that the kinematics of an omnidirectional platform is the capability of deviation from obstacles without changing the robot heading. This is a consequence of its non-holonomy (Pin and Killough 1994).

3.1 Localization

Most localization algorithms for indoor environments match range sensor measurements with a 2D map, relying on the presence of vertical walls. We have been working on a localization method that does not depend on vertical walls, but rather matches the map with the shape of the ground. To do so, we estimate the shape of the visible part of the ground using a RGB-D camera, extract its edges, and match those with the map (Vaz and Ventura 2013).

RGB-D cameras provide point clouds defined in 3D space, relative to the camera reference frame. After an initial calibration, the geometric parameters of the ground plane are estimated. This allows the classification of the points from a given point cloud among two classes: ground and non-ground. Then, the concave hull of the ground points is computed, yielding a polygon delimiting these points. The edges of this polygon are then filtered, in order to ignore the edges corresponding to the edges of the sensor field of view. The remaining ones are then matched against a map of the environment.

3.2 Motion Planning and Guidance

For navigation we use a standard occupancy grid map (Elfes 1989), obtained from off-the-shelf SLAM software.[3] This map is used both for motion planning, using Fast Marching Method (FMM) (Sethian 1999), and localization, using off-the-shelf software.[4]

Motion planning is based on a FMM approach (Sethian 1999). Unlike other methods based on explicit path planning, e.g., RRT (LaValle and Kuffner 2001), followed by path tracking, we adopt here a potential field approach. Given a map constraining the workspace of the robot, together with a feasible goal point, a (scalar) potential field $u(x)$, for $x \in R^2$, is constructed such that, given a current robot location $x(t)$, the path towards the goal results from solving the ordinary differential equation $\dot{x}(t) = -\nabla u(x)$. In other words, given an arbitrary current location of the robot x, the robot should follow a gradient descent of the field $u(x)$. Using potential fields for motion planning was proposed in the 80's (Borenstein and Koren 1989) but they were found to be prone to local minima (Koren and Borenstein 1991). This problem can be solved by the use of harmonic potential fields (Kim and Khosla 1992), however, it does not guarantee absence of local minima at the frontier. Thus, we decided to employ a more recent approach, FMM, which provides: (1) local minima free path to goal across the gradient, (2) allows the specification of a spatial cost function, that introduces a soft clearance to the environment obstacles, and (3) does not require explicit path planning and trajectory tracking.

The FMM is based on the Level Set theory, that is, the representation of hypersurfaces as the solution of an equation $u(x) = C$. The solution of the Eikonal equation

$$\begin{aligned} |\nabla u(x)| &= F(x) \\ u(\Gamma) &= 0 \end{aligned} \tag{1}$$

where $x \in \Omega$ is a domain, Γ the initial hypersurface, and $F(x)$ is a cost function, yields a field $u(x)$ (Sethian 1999). The level sets of this field define hypersurfaces $u(x) = C$ of points that can be reached with a minimal cost of C. The path that minimizes the integral of the cost along the trajectory can be shown to correspond to the solution of $\dot{x}(t) = -\nabla u(x)$ with the initial condition of $x(0)$ set to the initial position and the initial condition $u(\Gamma) = 0$ set at the goal.[5] Intuitively it corresponds to the propagation of a wave front, starting from the initial hypersurface, and propagating with speed $1/F(x)$. FMM is a numerically efficient method to solve the Eikonal equation for a domain discretized as a grid.

---

[3] GMapping (http://wiki.ros.org/gmapping, retrieved 16 October 2013).

[4] AMCL (http://wiki.ros.org/amcl, retrieved 16 October 2013).

[5] Γ corresponds to the boundary of an arbitrarily small ball around the goal.

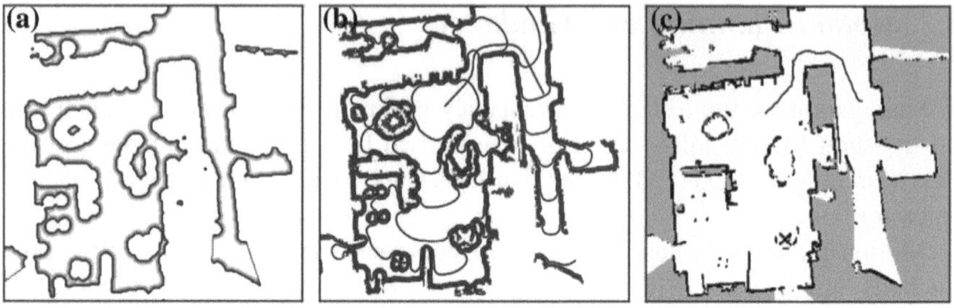

Fig. 9 Motion planning using FMM: **a** the cost function $F(x)$ (*darker* means a higher cost), **b** the solution field $u(x)$ (*level curves*) together with the gradient descent $\dot{x}(t) = -\nabla u(x)$ solution (from the *right* to the *left*), and **c** the real path traveled by the robot

Since FMM employs a grid discretization of space, it can be directly applied to the occupancy grid map, where domain Ω corresponds to the free space in the map. As cost function we use

$$F(x) = \frac{1}{\min\{D(x), D_{\max}\}} \tag{2}$$

where $D(x)$ is the distance to the nearest occupied cell in the map and $D_{\max}$ is a threshold to clip the cost function. This cost function induces a slower wave propagation near the obstacles, and thus making the optimal path to display some clearance from them. The clipping at $D_{\max}$ prevents the robot to navigate in the middle of free areas, regardless of their size. The $D(x)$ function can be directly obtained using an Euclidean Distance Transform (EDT) algorthm, taking the occupied cells as the boundary. Figure 9 illustrates the results of this approach: the cost function $F(x)$ for the given map is shown in (a), from which, given a goal location, a field $u(x)$, shown in (b) is obtained (the goal corresponds to the minimum value of the field), and in (c) the real path taken by the robot is shown.

Using FMM on a previously constructed map does not account for unmapped or moving obstacles. Thus, the field $v(x)$ used to control the robot in real-time results from combining the field $u(x)$ obtained from FMM with a repulsive potential field $r(x)$ of obstacles sensed by the LRF. This repulsive field is obtained from running EDT on a small window around the robot, such that the value of $r(x)$ corresponds to the minimum distance between any obstacle and point x. The fields are combined using

$$v(x) = u(x) + \frac{\lambda}{r(x)} \tag{3}$$

where λ is a parameters specifying the strength of the repulsive field (higher values of λ tend to increase the clearance from perceived obstacles).

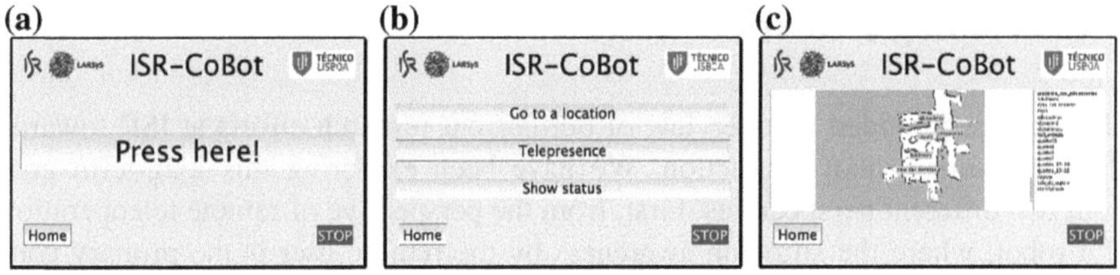

Fig. 10 Three screenshots of the onboard GUI: the welcome screen on (**a**), from which the main menu on (**b**) follows, and the destination location screen on (**c**)

The method described above have proven to be very effective, even in cluttered environments full of people crowded around the robot. We have demoed the robot in a public event—the European Researcher's Night (September 27th, 2013, in the Pavilion of Knowledge science museum, Lisbon)—where people from all ages crowded around ISR-CoBot. We have also tested the robot in an hospital environment, in the context of our participation in the FP7 European project MOnarCH (Sequeira 2013).

3.3 Interaction with Users

Currently the interaction with users is limited to setting goal locations on a displayed map of the environment, with minimal voice feedback. We decided at this stage not to use voice as input channel, since speech recognition on a mobile robot with background noise is still an open challenge (many systems are available, but they still lack the robustness needed for an engaging interaction). Therefore, even though the robot provides voice feedback of its actions in the form of canned sentences, the input is limited to the onboard touchscreen.

Screenshots of the graphical user interface can be found in Fig. 10. After a welcoming message, the user is invited to choose among three possibilities:

1. select, from either a map or a list (Fig. 10c), a location for the robot to autonomously navigate to: the shown map was previously manually labeled with relevant locations (we do not allow users to set arbitrary locations in the map, for safety reasons);
2. choose to engage in telepresence, that is, a QR-code is shown containing a URI to the Skype contact of ISR-CoBot; once called, a remote user establishes voice and visual contact with whoever is nearby the robot; and
3. display a status panel showing the current robot location and other relevant information (namely battery levels).

We demoed this interface in the aforementioned European Researcher's Night and observed that most people used appropriately the interface without any prior instruction or training.

4 Concluding Remarks

This chapter provided an overview of our current research efforts at ISR towards effective human-robot interaction. We have been exploring this long-term goal from two different perspectives. First, from the perspective of remote teleoperation of a robot, where the situation awareness by the remote user is the primary concern. In this respect, we have been using technologies and methods that aim at providing a natural interface to the operator. And second, from the perspective of autonomous service robots, which are required to robustly navigate in a structured environment, being capable of reacting appropriately to unknown obstacles, and interacting in a natural way with people.

In the future we will continue to pursue these goals. In what concerns teleoperated robots, we intend to explore augmented reality techniques to superimpose in the camera images relevant information from the map being constructed. On the service robots, we will pursue engaging interaction under the principle of symbiotic autonomy.

Acknowledgments Most of the results here presented were only possible due to the hard work of many students and grantees supervised by the author, namely Jorge Ferraz, Fausto Ferreira, Henrique Martins, João José Reis, Pedro Vieira, Miguel Vaz, Filipe Jesus, and João Mendes.

This work was partially funded by FCT [PEst-OE/EEI/LA0009/2013], [PTDC/EIA-CCO/113257/2009], and EU Project MOnarCH.

References

Besl, P.J., McKay, N.D.: A method for registration of 3-D shapes. IEEE Transactions on Pattern Analysis Machine Intelligence **14**(2), 239–256 (1992)

Biswas, J., Veloso, M.: Depth camera based localization and navigation for indoor mobile robots. In: RGB-D Workshop (RSS-2011) (2011)

Borenstein, J., Koren, Y.: Real-time obstacle avoidance for fast mobile robots. IEEE Transactions on Systems, Man and Cybernetics **19**(5), 1179–1187 (1989)

Coltin, B., Biswas, J., Pomerleau, D., Veloso, M.: Effective semi-autonomous telepresence. In: Proceedings of the RoboCup Symposium. Istanbul, Turkey (2011)

Coradeschi, S., Saffiotti, A.: Symbiotic robotic systems: Humans, robots, and smart environments. IEEE Intelligent Systems **21**(3), 82–84 (2006)

Drury, J., Scholtz, J., Yanco, H.: Awareness in human-robot interactions. In: IEEE International Conference on Systems, Man and Cybernetics, vol. 1, pp. 912–918 (2003)

Elfes, A.: Using occupancy grids for mobile robot perception and navigation. IEEE Computer **22**(6), 46–57 (1989)

Ferraz, J., Ventura, R.: Robust autonomous stair climbing by a tracked robot using accelerometer sensors. In: Mobile Robotics: Solutions and Challenges (CLAWAR-2009), pp. 415–422. World Scientific (2009)

Ferreira, F., Ventura, R.: Autonomous docking of a tracked wheels robot to its tether cable using a vision-based algorithm. In: Workshop on Robotics for Disaster Response, IEEE International Conference on Robotics and Automation (ICRA-09). Kobe, Japan (2009)

Fong, T., Nourbakhsh, I., Dautenhahn, K.: A survey of socially interactive robots. Robotics and autonomous systems **42**(3), 143–166 (2003)

Goodrich, M.A., Schultz, A.C.: Human-robot interaction: A survey. Foundations and Trends in Human-Computer Interaction **1**(3), 203–275 (2007)
Goodrich, M.A., Olsen, D.R., Crandall, J.W., Palmer, T.J.: Experiments in adjustable autonomy. In: Proceedings of IJCAI Workshop on Autonomy, Delegation and Control: Interacting with Intelligent Agents, pp. 1624–1629 (2001)
Haigh, K.Z., Veloso, M.M.: Interleaving planning and robot execution for asynchronous user requests. Autonomous Robots **5**(1), 79–95 (1998)
Helmer, S., Meger, D., Viswanathan, P., McCann, S., Dockrey, M., Fazli, P., Southey, T., Muja, M., Joya, M., Little, J., Lowe, D., Mackworth, A.: Semantic robot vision challenge: Current state and future directions. arXiv preprint arXiv:0908.2656 (2009)
Jacoff, A., Messina, E., Weiss, B.A., Tadokoro, S., Nakagawa, Y.: Test arenas and performance metrics for urban search and rescue robots. In: Proceedings of IEEE/RSJ International Conference on Intelligent Robots and Systems (IROS-2003), vol. 4, pp. 3396–3403 (2003)
Kim, J., Khosla, P.: Real-time obstacle avoidance using harmonic potential functions. IEEE Transactions on Robotics and Automation **8**(3), 338–349 (1992)
Kitano, H., Tadokoro, S.: RoboCup rescue: A grand challenge for multiagent and intelligent systems. AI Magazine **22**(1), 39–52 (2001)
Kitano, H., Asada, M., Kuniyoshi, Y., Noda, I., Osawa, E.: RoboCup: The robot world cup initiative. In: Proceedings of the First International Conference on Autonomous Agents (Agents'97), pp. 340–347. ACM Press, New York (1997)
Koren, Y., Borenstein, J.: Potential field methods and their inherent limitations for mobile robot navigation. In: Proceedings of the IEEE International Conference on Robotics and Automation (ICRA-91), pp. 1398–1404 (1991)
LaValle, S., Kuffner Jr, J.: Randomized kinodynamic planning. The International Journal of Robotics Research **20**(5), 378–400 (2001)
Long, D., Fox, M.: The 3rd international planning competition: Results and analysis. Journal of Artificial Intellligence Research (JAIR) **20**, 1–59 (2003)
Marques, C., Cristovão, J., Lima, P., Frazão, J., Ribeiro, M.I., Ventura, R.: RAPOSA: Semi-autonomous robot for rescue operations. In: Proceedings of IROS2006 — IEEE/RSJ International Conference on Intelligent Robots and Systems (2006)
Marques, C., Cristovão, J., Alvito, P., Lima, P., Frazão, J., Ribeiro, M.I., Ventura, R.: A search and rescue robot with tele-operated tether docking system. Industrial Robot **34**(4), 332–338 (2007)
Martins, H., Ventura, R.: Immersive 3-d teleoperation of a search and rescue robot using a head-mounted display. In: Proceedings of 14th IEEE International Conference on Emerging Technologies and Factory Automation (ETFA-2009) (2009)
Mauldin, M.L.: Chatterbots, tinymuds, and the turing test: Entering the loebner prize competition. In: Proceedings of AAAI-94, pp. 16–21 (1994)
Murphy, R.R., Rogers, E.: Cooperative assistance for remote robot supervision. Presence **5**(2), 224–240 (1996)
Pin, F.G., Killough, S.M.: A new family of omnidirectional and holonomic wheeled platforms for mobile robots. IEEE Transactions on Robotics and Automation **10**(4), 480–489 (1994)
Reis, J.J., Ventura, R.: Immersive robot teleoperation using an hybrid virtual and real stereo camera attitude control. In: Proceedings of Portuguese Conference on Pattern Recognition (RecPad) (2012)
Rosenthal, S., Veloso, M.: Using symbiotic relationships with humans to help robots overcome limitations. In: Proceedings of the AAMAS'10 Workshop on Collaborative Human/AI Control for Interactive Experiences. Toronto, Canada (2010)
Rosenthal, S., Biswas, J., Veloso, M.: An effective personal mobile robot agent through symbiotic human-robot interaction. In: Proceedings of the 9th International Conference on Autonomous Agents and Multiagent Systems, vol. 1, pp. 915–922. International Foundation for Autonomous Agents and Multiagent Systems (2010)
Rosenthal, S., Veloso, M., Dey, A.: Task behavior and interaction planning for a mobile service robot that occasionally requires help. In: Proceedings of the AAAI Workshop on Automated Action Planning for Autonomous Mobile Robots. San Francisco, CA (2011)

Sequeira, J., Lima, P., Saffiotti, A., Gonzalez-Pacheco, V., Salichs, M.A.: MOnarCH: Multi-robot cognitive systems operating in hospitals. In: ICRA 2013 Workshop on Many Robot Systems (2013)

Sethian, J.A.: Fast marching methods. SIAM review **41**(2), 199–235 (1999)

van der Zant, T., Wisspeintner, T.: Robotic Soccer, chap. RoboCup@Home: Creating and Benchmarking Tomorrows Service Robot Applications, pp. 521–528. Itech Education and Publishing (2007)

Vaz, M., Ventura, R.: Ground-plane based indoor mobile robot localization using RGB-D sensor. In: Proceedings of Portuguese Conference on Pattern Recognition (RecPad) (2013)

Veloso, M., Biswas, J., Coltin, B., Rosenthal, S., Brandao, S.D., Kollar, T., Meri cli, C., Samadi, M., Ventura, R.: CoBots: Collaborative robots servicing multi-floor buildings. In: IEEE/RSJ International Conference on Intelligent Robots and Systems (IROS-12). Vila Moura, Portugal (2012)

Ventura, R., Coltin, B., Veloso, M.: Web-based remote assistance to overcome robot perceptual limitations. In: AAAI Conference on Artificial Intelligence (AAAI-13), Workshop on Intelligent Robot Systems. AAAI, Bellevue, WA (2013)

Vieira, P., Ventura, R.: Interactive 3D scan-matching using RGB-D data. In: IEEE International Conference on Emerging Technologies and Factory Automation (ETFA'12). Kraków, Poland (2012a)

Vieira, P., Ventura, R.: Interactive mapping in 3D using RGB-D data. In: IEEE International Symposium on Safety Security and Rescue Robotics (SSRR'12). College Station, TX (2012b)

Vieira, P., Ventura, R.: Interactive mapping using range sensor data under localization uncertainty. Journal of Automation, Mobile Robotics & Intelligent Systems **6**(1), 47–53 (2013)

Yamauchi, B.M.: PackBot: a versatile platform for military robotics. Proceedings of SPIE **5422**, 228–237 (2004)

Yanco, H.A., Drury, J.L., Scholtz, J.: Beyond usability evaluation: analysis of human-robot interaction at a major robotics competition. Human-Computer Interaction **19**(1), 117–149 (2004)

Yanco, H.A., Drury, J.L.: A taxonomy for human-robot interaction. In: Proceedings of the AAAI Fall Symposium on Human-Robot Interaction, pp. 111–119 (2002)

Advanced Gesture and Pose Recognition Algorithms Using Computational Intelligence and Microsoft KINECT Sensor

D. Katić, P. Radulović, S. Spasojević, Ž. Đurović and A. Rodić

Abstract This research work suggests one kind of approach in developing a natural human–robot interface that will be used for control of four wheels differentially steered mobile robot. The designed system is capable of extracting, understanding and learning a sequence of full body gestures and poses, that were previously captured in standard RGB and IC DEPTH videos. The starting set of robot commands in first study case, includes the following 4 postures: START, WAIT A MINUTE, STOP and SLOW DOWN, while in the second study case 5 gestures were realized: START, TURN RIGHT, TURN LEFT, SPEED UP and SLOW, while command STOP is realized as pose. The special feature of proposed classifier system is fact that human user is always in visual domain of camera but without fixation for defined position or orientation. Two different kinds of classifiers were implemented: first, support vector machine (SVM) classifier and second, based on multiple interconnected FUZZY Logic systems. The research showed satisfactory results in small classification error, simple human operator training and user comfort.

Keywords Gesture recognition · Pose recognition · Computational intelligence · Robot vision · Human–robot interface

D. Katić (✉) · S. Spasojević · A. Rodić
Mihailo Pupin Institute, University of Belgrade, Belgrade, Serbia
e-mail: dusko.katic@pupin.rs

S. Spasojević
e-mail: sofija.spasojevic@pupin.rs

A. Rodić
e-mail: aleksandar.rodic@pupin.rs

P. Radulović · Ž. Đurović
Department of Electrical Engineering, University of Belgrade, Belgrade, Serbia
e-mail: rpetar@t-com.me

Ž. Đurović
e-mail: zdjurovic@etf.rs

A. Rodić et al. (eds.), *New Trends in Medical and Service Robots*,
Mechanisms and Machine Science 20, DOI: 10.1007/978-3-319-05431-5_13,

1 Introduction

Remote robot control or robot teleoperation is especially important in some robotics applications as mobile manipulation and medical applications (surgery, rehabilitation). In the last few years, thanks to rapid development of new computer vision technologies and capture motion systems, various optical based human movements systems for remote robot control have widespread use in man's daily activities. Optical motion capture systems are based on installation on several calibrated cameras which record images using active or passive markers attached to the human operator's body (special gloves or exoskeleton) (Hanai et al. 2009; http://www.vicon.com/System/TSeries) or by recording image of the body or body parts. There are also different approaches for remote robot control, based on hand gesture detection and recognition (Ghobadi et al. 2008; Raheja et al. 2010). There is a wide range of activities that the robot can execute on set gesture commands, where most of the activities related to the gestures demonstrated robot control (Iba et al. 1999; Waldherr et al. 2000).

In the last years, markerless optical motion capture systems are becoming very popular because of the comfort for human operator of not carrying any special device (http://www.ipisoft.com/products.php; Kean et al. 2011). These systems only need a group of cameras installed in the environment and an initial calibration process where the limbs of the human operator are related to the bones of a skeleton in the images of cameras. Israel company PrimeSense, which is in collaboration with Microsoft rolled out a Kinect, a new optical system that is extremely facilitate image segmentation and recognition of some specific objects that are in the camera's field of vision. A new method of determining the depth maps are based on infrared light sensors mounted on the device in addition to the standard RGB camera. The great advantage of Kinect is that it has a built-in algorithm of detection of the human skeleton and the ability to read and store 3D coordinates of typical joints of the human figure. These 3D positions of the joints are input to the gesture recognition algorithm. This led to the development of a large number of applications that use these software packages to simply obtain joint position of users in a Cartesian coordinate system related to the center of the camera. Upon receipt of such information, it can be used further for the design of intelligent systems in the purpose of the classification of poses and movements made by the user and their interpretation.

The aim of designing a system that will be described in this chapter, is the control of differentially driven mobile robot on four wheels using a natural user interface. This interface based on KINECT sensor allows the user or operator that movements of their body sets are transferred to the robot to execute the command. Kinect sensor was used to remotely command a different type of robots, specially in domain of industrial robots (Vasilijević et al. 2012). Also, there are research works based on KINECT gesture recognition techniques in area of control of mobile robots, using different learning and classifying algorithms (Hsu et al. 2013; Pourmehr et al. 2013). Hence, as second aim of research, it is necessary to design appropriate classifier that decides which gesture is recognized. There are several different approaches to the design of classifiers and techniques that can be used for this purpose. Some of them are linear classifier (if the classes are linearly separable), quadratic classifier (classes are nonlinear separable), classification using neural networks and fuzzy logic. In this chapter, for the design of the classifier, a two computational intelligence paradigms were selected. First method based on *support vector machines* (SVM) is used. SVM are mathematical models based on supervised learning, which consist of integrated training algorithms and analysis of input data and the testing of new data. The second method is based on a network of connected *fuzzy logic classifiers* that receive as input 3D joint positions of interest, and provide as output a sequence of commands that is observed in the image. As an end result, we have an algorithm that with high percentage of success recognize the predefined gestures that are executed in an arbitrary long recording images of Kinect camera.

2 Basic Features of Kinect Device

Kinect is the new generation device developed by Microsoft that unites the technology of generating and processing audio and visual signals. It was originally designed for commercial use in combination with an Xbox 360 console or Windows operating system (http://www.microsoft.com/en-us/kinectforwindows/). Kinect have algorithms for detecting human skeleton, movements and motion at a distance of approximately 0.6–4 m and storing of 3D coordinates of points in space. Kinect system consists of variable-resolution RGB camera, 3D depth sensor (infrared projector combined with a monochrome CMOS sensor—the camera sensitive to IR rays sent by the projector i.e. depth camera) and broadband microphone, and it has a corresponding user interface. Kinect can achieve up to 30 frames per second.

Due to wide range of raw and processed signals that Kinect can send as outputs through a USB connection, developers and researchers have come up with the idea that the Kinect could be used also for the scientific research and development. For this purpose, Microsoft has provided a software development tool Kinect for Windows SDK, which contains of functions and procedures for communication and generating output signals from Kinect. However, this software tool in addition to the many significant possibilities has some limitations that are established by the policy of Microsoft. Therefore, some new software packages have been developed in order to enable more direct access and more effective communication with Kinect, such as OpenNI software tool, used in this research (http://www.openni.org/). Complex depth sensing combined with RGB sensing will become a trend in robotics and Human-computer interaction (HCI) in general.

The optical subsystem consists of sensors for determining the depth image and a standard RGB camera VGA resolution (640 × 480), although the hardware is capable of a higher quality picture in a small number of frames per second.

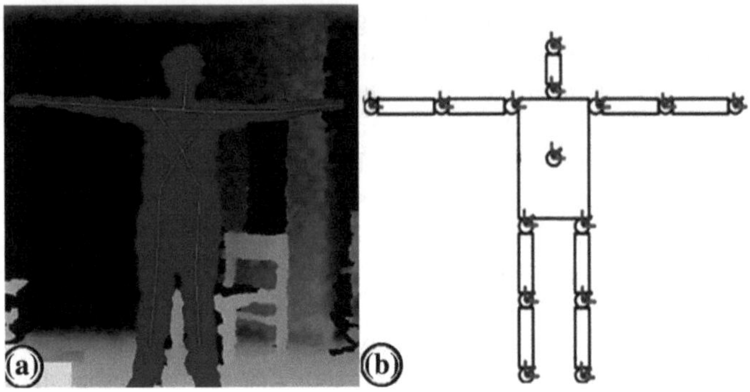

Fig. 1 Skeleton tracking (**a**) and joints of interest (**b**) given by KINECT

Determination of the depth image is made of structured light technology, which requires a projector IR (infrared light) and CMOS sensors infrared radiation. The procedure can be summarized as follows: projector emits known pattern (pattern) infrared light to objects in the visual field of the camera, the sensor detects the scene and observed changes in the patterns that depend on the distance to the area of objects and sends them to the CPU, which then process gray scale image which corresponds to the distance of objects from the camera.

Using *Microsoft's Kinect SDK* or *OpenNI* software libraries, it is possible to recognize and track more people at the same time. Six people can identify and locate, and skeleton track is only possible for two users. Figure 1 shows the 3D position of joints which can be obtained with these program me.

3 System for Gesture Recognition-Based Remote Robot Control

Current research in gesture-based interfaces typically relies on computer vision for observing and classifying the human gestures (Burger et al. 2012; Mitra and Acharya 2007; Yang et al. 2007), and numerous researchers have investigated using visually identified gestures for commanding robots, including point-to-object operations. Vision-based approaches have the advantage of avoiding human-worn equipment, with best results in controlled indoor environments, often requiring constant camera–human spatial relationships and consistent lighting.

The proposed system is designed for recognizing full body gestures using Microsoft Kinect for Windows platform (Fig. 2).

The problem of recognizing gestures in order to form a natural user interface is more specific compared to the standard classification problem. First, unlike most of the problems in pattern recognition, this is equally important not to reject

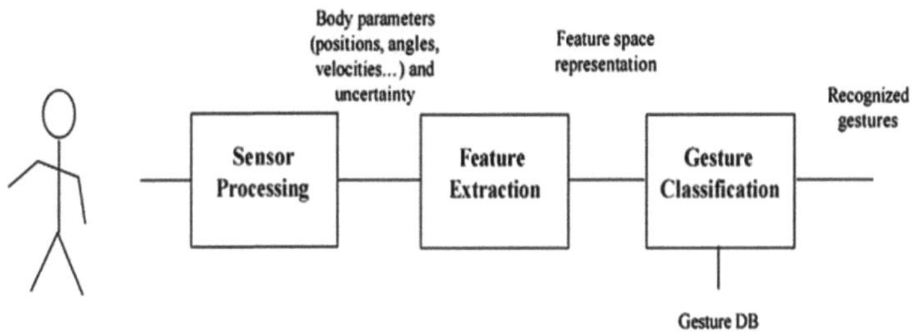

Fig. 2 Gesture recognition procedure

gesture commands and how to recognize the command itself. This area is infinitely large, and must be determined by imposing restrictions in defining properly executed movement. These limits represents variations, that a user can enter into the performance of a gesture (that it is correctly classified), and thus reduce users' freedom when using the system. Compromise between comfort from the user's side and the number of events in the undefined area of movement which will be recognized as commands is a crucial issue in the design of any modern gesture recognizing system. Another peculiarity of this problem is the choice of the classes that we want to use. While most of the other application classes get some measurements on the results of which we can not influence, this is one of the tasks of the designer to define a set of gestures that the system will recognize. This raises the question of freedom of choice in order to give commands, based on two conditions: motion must be sufficiently different from each other to make it easier to classify, but must be sufficiently simple and easy to perform in order for the system to be more comfortable for the user.

3.1 Support Vector Machines (SVM) Classifier

Support vector machines (SVMs) are a relatively new classification method. They are considered as state of the art classifiers because they deliver high performance in real-world applications. First approaches that utilized SVMs for object recognition applied the basic method that deals with a two-class classification problem. In the context of object recognition, a binary tree strategy (Guo et al. 2001; Pontil and Verri 1998) was proposed to solve the multiclass problem. While this approach provides a simple and powerful classification framework, it cannot capture correlations between the different classes since it breaks a multi-class problem into multiple independent binary problems (Crammer and Singer 2001). In addition, the result is not independent of how the candidate objects are paired. In this chapter, we used a binary approach based on the design of the SVM classifier for one versus other classes.

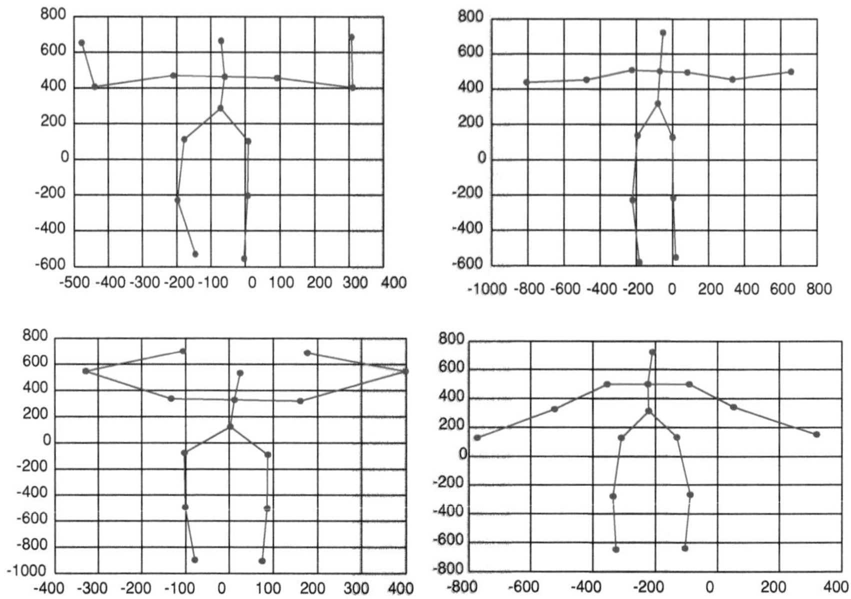

Fig. 3 Postures for recognition

3.1.1 Implementation of the Algorithm

The task of the algorithm is to recognize four static gestures that have been captured by the Kinect device. The first algorithmic step is the forming of input data, i.e. gesture acquisition. Process of gesture acquisition is based on skeleton tracking and collecting of 3D joints positions using Kinect. Some functions from OpenNI software package (Lin and Lee 1996) designed for work with 3D sensors were used in order of collecting information from Kinect. During skeleton tracking, 3D coordinates of 15 joints (Fig. 1) of the human skeleton for each frame are stored. Postures for recognition are shown in Fig. 3.

Based on the 3D coordinates of skeleton joints, feature vectors were formed and used for training of SVM. Given the choice of poses for recognition (Fig. 3) only elbow and hand joints are important, because other joints are negligible moved during recording. In order to represent results of classification in 2D space, two-dimensional feature vectors are formed. The first feature is the difference of x-coordinate values of the position of the left elbow and left hand, while the second feature relates to the ratio of distance between the left and right hand and distance between the left and right elbow. Training set consists of 100 patterns for each of the four classes, where each pattern is described with a two-dimensional feature vector. One person recorded gestures for training set, while the another person was involved in the formation of testing set. The training process is done using RBF kernel function.

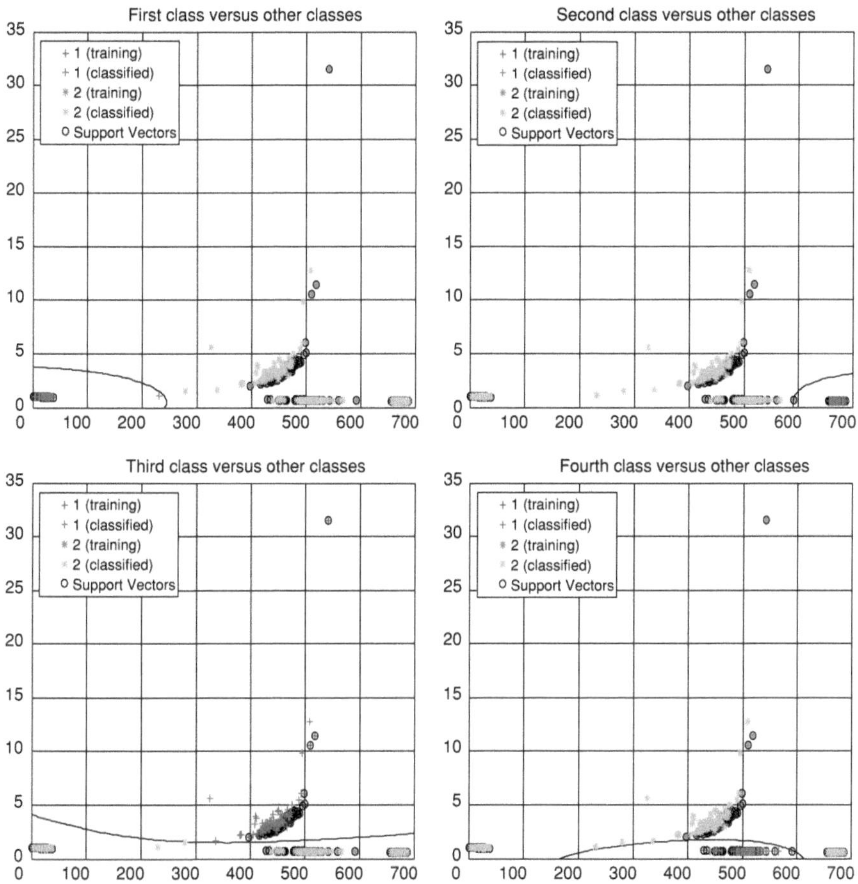

Fig. 4 Classification in 2D space

Classification is based on principle one class versus all. The result of classification process is information about affiliation of testing patterns to some class. The visual results of classification in 2D space are given on the Fig. 4.

The results of the classification are presented through matrix of success in Table 1. The reason of using RBF kernel function is its robustness and possible application in the case of non-linearly separable classes.

Testing set consists of 100 new shapes for each class. Only three shapes were wrong classified between first and third class. The accuracy of the system is 99.25 %.

Table 1 Matrix of successes of classification

	Posture 1	Posture 2	Posture 3	Posture 4
Posture 1	99	0	2	0
Posture 2	0	100	0	0
Posture 3	1	0	98	0
Posture 4	0	0	0	100

3.2 Fuzzy Classifiers

The purpose of the classifier is obtained by forming human–robot interface to facilitate control of differentially driven mobile robot, using recognition of a set of robot commands. Initial set, which was implemented at this stage of research, involves the following six commands: START, STOP, TURN RIGHT, TURN LEFT, SPEED UP and SLOW DOWN, while the STOP command from the needs of safe and reliable identification is realized as a pose, and the rest in the form of defined gestures. In Figs. 5, 6, 7, 8, 9 and 10 mentioned commands are defined. The special peculiarity of this classification system is that the user is in the camera field of view, but is not fixed to a particular position or orientation, and particular attention must be oriented to the choice of the features. The features must be such, that they do not change their properties with the change of a user position in the camera coordinate system. In accordance with these requirements, chosen features used to classify gestures are angles and relative distances, obtained from the joint position for specified commands.

Every angle is defined by three joints (e.g. 1, 2, 3), obtained from their positions, by first subtracting from each joint coordinates of angle top, forming vectors A and B as in Fig. 11 and then apply the expression (1):

$$\alpha_{123} = \arccos\left(\frac{\vec{A}\cdot\vec{B}}{|\vec{A}||\vec{B}|}\right) \tag{1}$$

It is important to notice, that in the classification of certain gestures, much more correct results are obtained, by calculating the angle between projections of vectors A and B on a plane. The relative distance between two joints is calculated as the ratio of the Euclidean distance of the two joints and the estimated height of person whose skeleton is observed. Take for example the command, TURN RIGHT. As indicated in Fig. 11 to define this movement, we need four values: α_1, angle that is defined by joints 5, 9 and 12 (top of the joint 9), α_2 angle defining the joints 12, 9 and 2 (top of the joint 9), d_1 distance between joints 5 and 12 and, d_2 distance between joints 8 and 13. The first three values are used to define the movement, while the distance between the left hand and the hip is used primarily for the protection of incorrect classification of a properly executed movement.

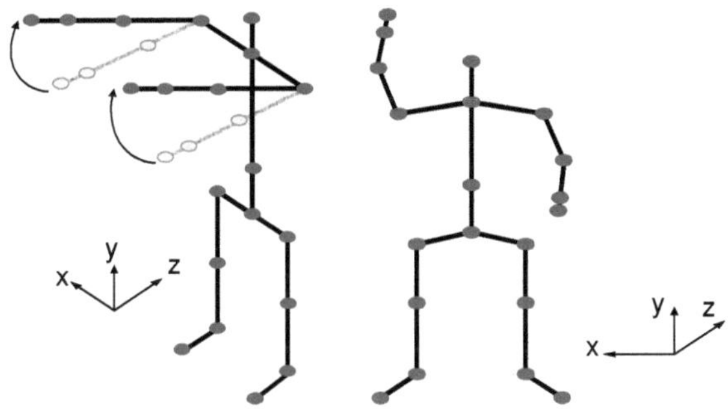

Fig. 5 Commands: START and STOP

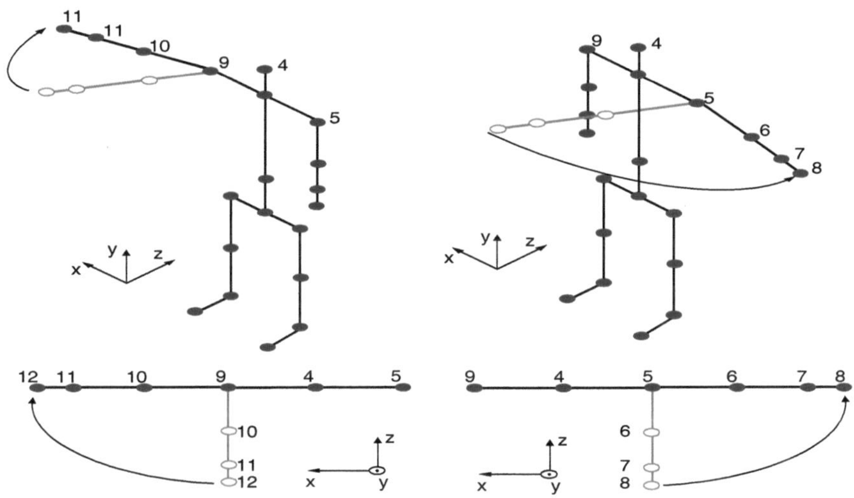

Fig. 6 Commands: TURN RIGHT and TURN LEFT

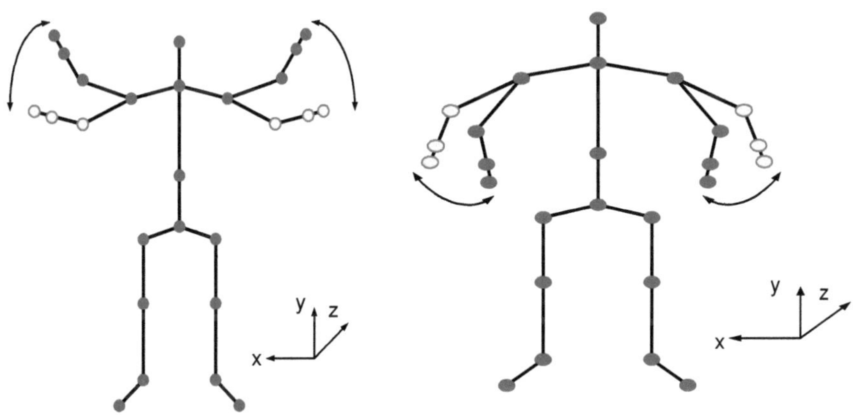

Fig. 7 Commands: SPEED UP and SLOW DOWN

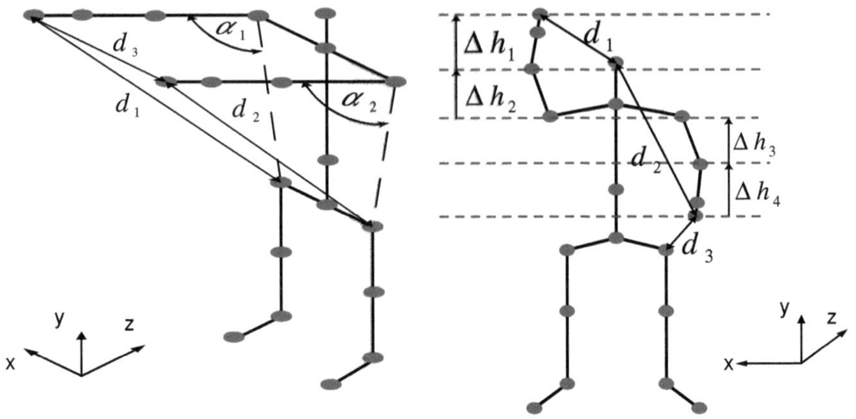

Fig. 8 Features necessary to recognize START and STOP

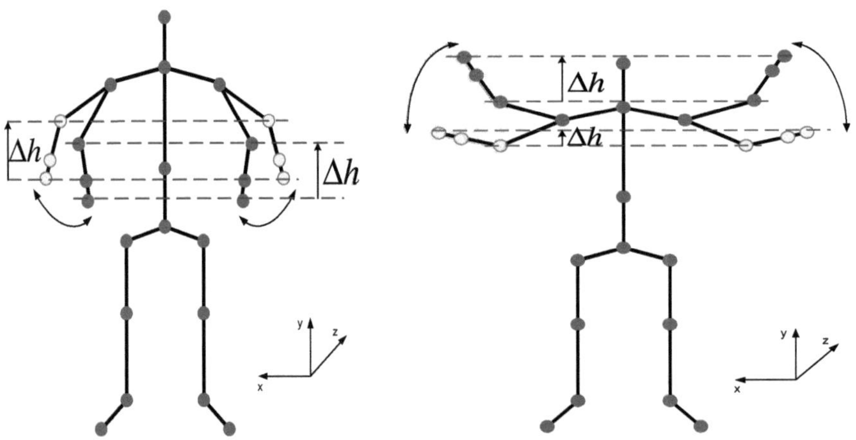

Fig. 9 Features necessary to recognize SLOW DOWN and SPEED UP

Let us explain in more detail the general algorithm for gesture recognition (Fig. 12), which uses previous four values to classify gesture TURN RIGHT (as example). First, it is necessary to define the position of the body that corresponds the beginning of the execution of the command. In this case, it would be the position of the body in which the left hand is relaxed, the left hand is on the left hip (small d_2), while the right hand is extended $\left(d_{1poc}^{+} > d_1 > d_{1poc}\right)$. The angles α_1 and α_2 are close to the 90° angle. So, each time a new frame that is passed to the processing algorithm, in case that in some of a previous moment, it was not identified start of the executing one of the commands, algorithm should to examine whether the current arrangement of the joints correspond to a defined initial position.

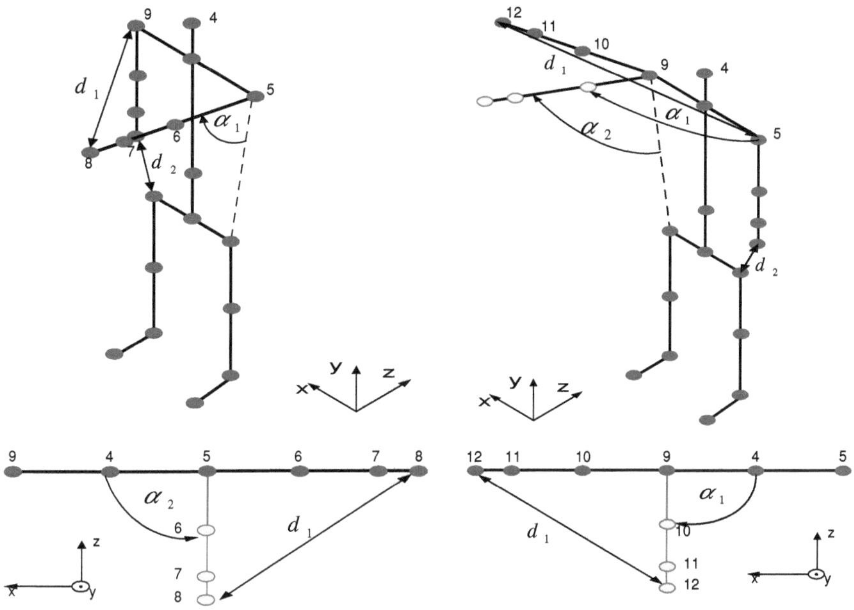

Fig. 10 Features necessary to recognize TURN RIGHT and TURN LEFT

Fig. 11 Calculation of angle α

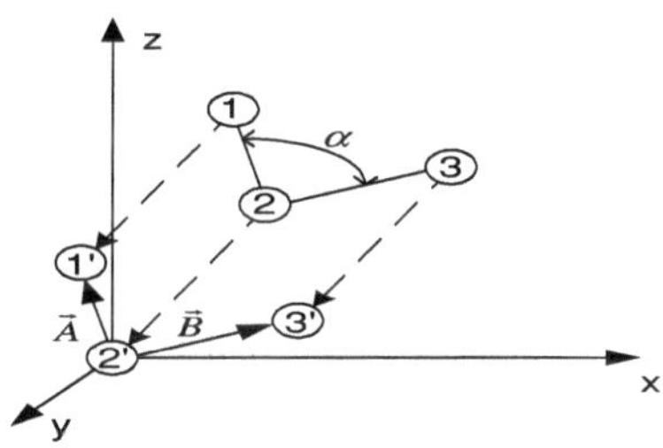

In the second phase of identification, observation of the following frames and tracking of changes in the position of the joints are realized. In the case of command TURN RIGHT, it is expect that the distance d_2 is still small, the angle α_2 still has a value close to the 90° angle, and the values of the α_1 and d_1 are constantly increasing, with some expected speed. The second phase of classification is to be repeated as long as its conditions are satisfied and the body has not been in a position corresponding to the end of the execution of a gesture. In this case it would be moment when the angle α_1 is close to 90° angle and the d_1 has reached a predefined value. Then we can say that the gesture is executed correctly and identified and after that return to the start of the algorithm in anticipation of the execution of the next gesture.

The whole classification process is based on a comparison of the current feature values with some of their values that are determined by previous analyzes of a

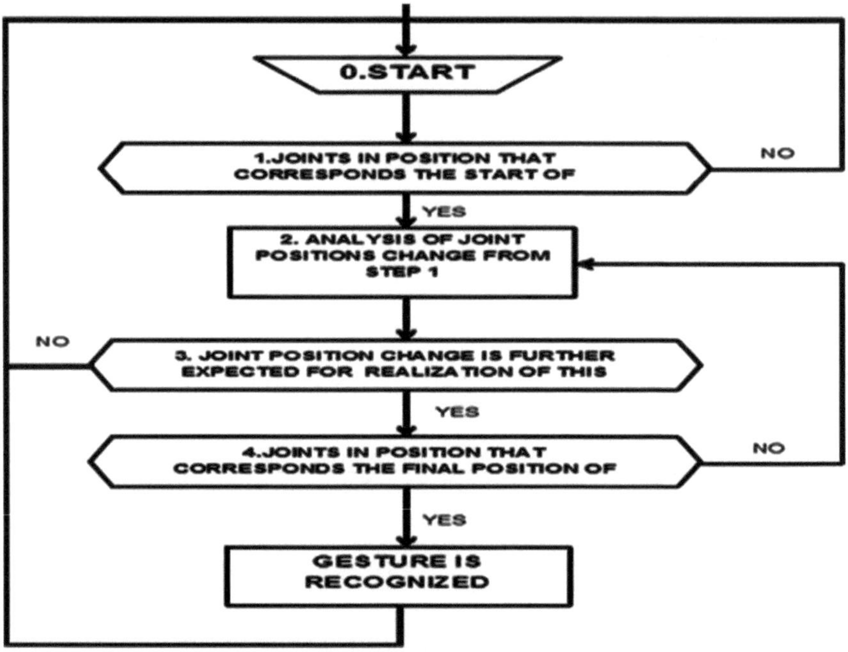

Fig. 12 General algorithm for recognition of movement

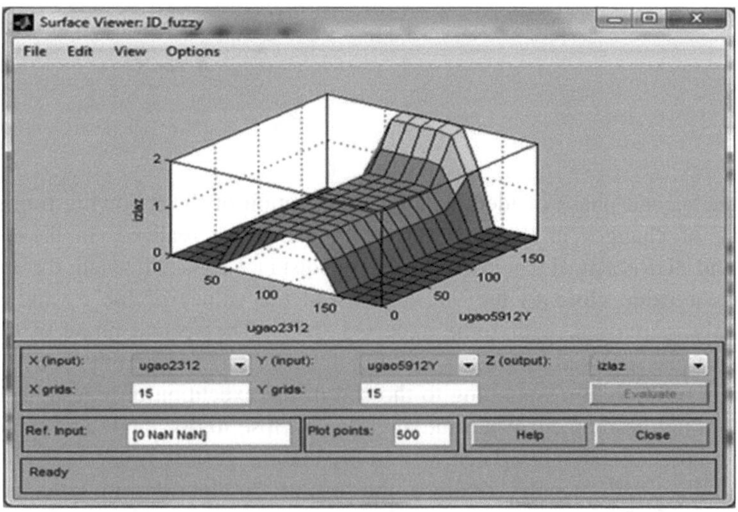

Fig. 13 Surface of fuzzy system that perform the third step in the algorithm for recognition the command TURN RIGHT

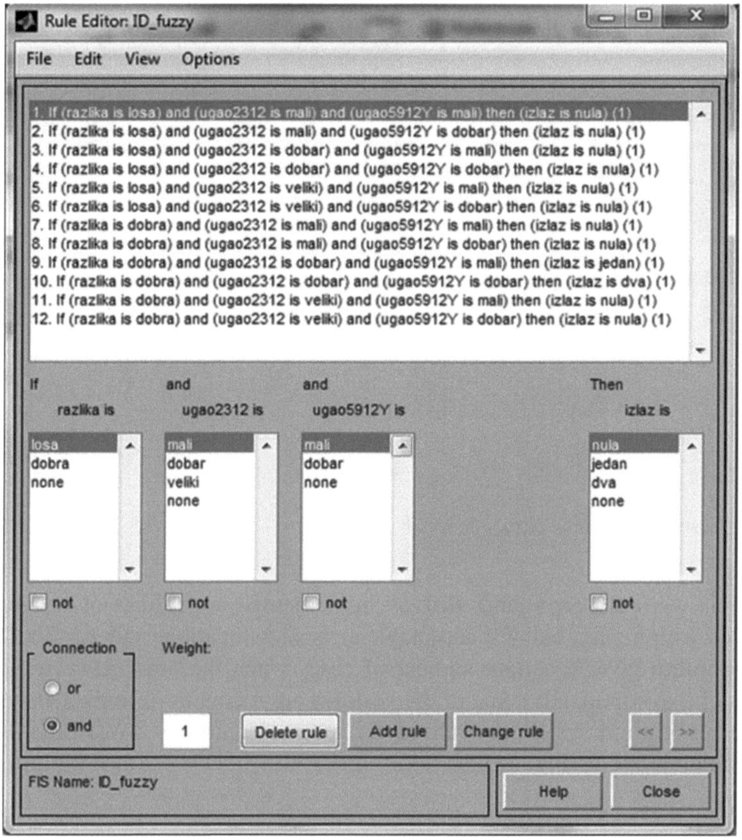

Fig. 14 Decision rules for third step in the algorithm for recognition the command TURN RIGHT

large number of images for specific command. That is the reason why this system is the right candidate for the implementation of fuzzy expert algorithm. Because of the need for the various stages of classification response, we get YES/NO form when designing the system based on Sugeno type fuzzy classifier (Lin and Lee 1996). Illustrated in Fig. 13 decision rules are shown. In Fig. 14 one surface fuzzy system that performs the third step in the algorithm for recognition the command TURN RIGHT, are presented.

3.2.1 System Testing

The system has been tested on images obtained by Kinect camera in total time duration of 30 min. Commands are randomly executed by ten people, who did not participate in the training of system. Pose STOP is correctly identified in each

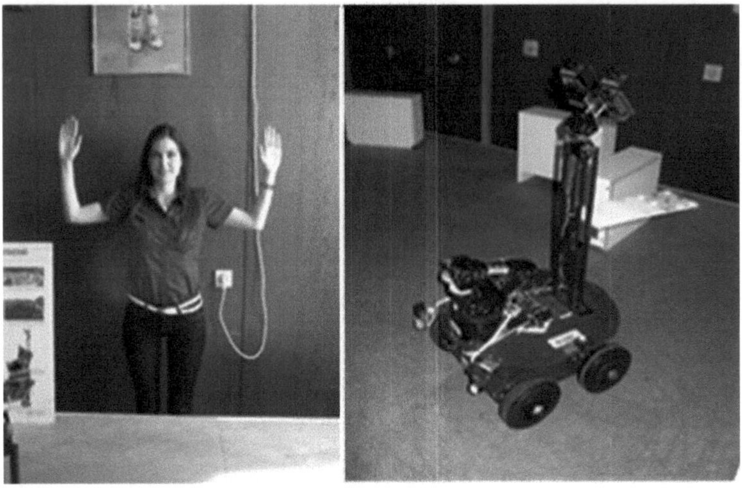

Fig. 15 Gesture command for mobile robot

execution, while the commands that are implemented in the form of gestures, are identified with higher, but still acceptable error classification (under 5 %). During test, algorithm gives a certain number of cases when the time between the executions of two commands some of the gestures are recognized. Implementation of gesture recognition system is realized for remote control of 4WD differentially steered mobile robot (Fig. 15).

4 Conclusions

The result of this work is the development of an algorithm for recognizing user gestures from the video of arbitrary length, made by KINECT camera, their interpretation and dissemination on differentially steered mobile robot on four wheels. The proposed solution has shown satisfactory results for small errors of classification, easy training, providing the customer convenience in using the system. SVM method applied for classification and pattern recognition has given extremely good results in the case of classification one class versus other classes (binary approach). By introducing of fuzzy logic classifier increased the recognition accuracy, but caused additional numerical complexity of the algorithm. It is important to emphasize that the classification error, for order can be reduced by introducing additional constraints and the features in description of precisely executed movements. Further research directions may relate to the extension of existing one and development of new algorithms for multiclass processing. In the development of such multi-disciplinary system, SVM would certainly be elected as a classification method.

Acknowledgments This chapter is supported by Serbian Ministry of Science under the grants TR-35003, III-44008, SNSF "CARE-robotics" project IZ74Z0_137361/1 and by the bilateral Serbia-Portugal "COLBAR" project 451-03-02338/2012-14/12.

References

Burger, B., I. Ferran'e, F. Lerasle, and G. Infantes: Two-handed gesture recognition and fusion with speech to command a robot, Autonomous Robots, vol. 32, pp. 129–147. (2012).

Crammer, K. and Y.Singer: On the algorithmic implementation of multiclass kernelbased vector machines, Journal of Machine Learning Research 2, pp. 265–292.(2001).

Ghobadi, S.E., O.E.Loepprich, F.Ahmadov and J.Bernshausen: Real Time Hand Based Robot Control Using Multimodal Images, IAENG International Journal of Computer Science, Vol.35, No.4, (2008).

Guo, G., Li, S. Z. and K.L.Chan: Support vector machines for face recognition, Image and Vision Computing 19(9-10), pp. 631–638.(2001).

Hanai, M., R.Sato, S.Fukuma, S-I.Mori, T.Shimozawa and N.Hayashi: Physical Motion Analysis System in Driving using Image Processing, Proc. of ISPACS 2009, Kanazawa, Japan, pp. 123–126 (2009).

Hsu, R.CH, Lin, C-C., Lai, C-H. and C-T. Liu: Remotely controlling of mobile robots using gesture captured by the Kinect and recognized by machine learning method. *Proc. SPIE* 8662, Intelligent Robots and Computer Vision XXX: Algorithms and Techniques, (2013).

Iba S., Van de Weghe J.M., Paredis C.J.J. and P.K.K.Khosla:An Architecture for Gesture-Based Control of Mobile Robots, Proceedings of the IEEE/RSJ IROS, pp. 851–857.(1999).

iPiSoft, http://www.ipisoft.com/products.php

Kean S., Hall J. and P.Perry. Meet the Kinect, Technology in Action, (2011).

Lin, C.T. and C. S. G. Lee : Neuro Fuzzy Systems - A Neuro-Fuzzy Synergism to Intelligent Systems, Prentice Hall.(1996)

Microsoft Corporation: Kinect for Windows, http://www.microsoft.com/en-us/kinectforwindows/

Mitra, S. and T. Acharya,: Gesture recognition: A survey, Systems, IEEE Transactions on Man, and Cybernetics, Part C, vol. 37, no. 3, pp. 311–324.(2007).

OpenNI Consortium: OpenNI, The standard framework for 3D sensing, http://www.openni.org/

Pontil, M. and A.Verri: Support vector machines for 3D object recognition, IEEE Trans. Pattern Anal. Machine Intell. 20(6), pp. 637–646.(1998).

Pourmehr, S., Monajjemi, V., Wawerla, J., Vaughan, R., and G.Mori: A Robust Integrated System for Selecting and Commanding Multiple Mobile Robots. Proc. of 2013 IEEE ICRA, Karlsruhe, Germany, pp.2859–2864.(2013).

Raheja, L., R.Shyam, U.Kumar and P.B.Prasad:Real-Time Robotic Hand Control Using Hang Gestures, Machine Learning and Computing, (2010).

Vasilijević, G., Jagodin, N. and Z.Kovačić: Kinect-Based Robot Teleoperation by Velocities Control in the Joint/Cartesian Frames, Proc.of SYROCO 2012, pp.878–883, (2012).

Vicon:http://www.vicon.com/System/TSeries,

Waldherr S., Romero R. snd S.Thrun: A Gesture Based Interface for Human-Robot Interaction, Journal Autonomous Robots, Volume 9, Issue 2, pp. 151–173, (2000).

Yang, H.-D., A.-Y. Park, and S.-W. Lee: Gesture spotting and recognition for human–robot interaction. IEEE Transactions on Robotics. *(2007).*

[illegible]

Recursive Design of Dependable Robot Systems for Safety-Critical Applications

A. Wagner

Abstract Medical systems such as medical and rehabilitation robots need to be highly safe and dependable since they directly influence health and live of patients. Furthermore, modern assistance technology allows the design of highly sophisticated medical devices and the use of medical systems in a more flexible and interactive way. Thus, dependability of the medical system, which is possibly in interaction with the human operator has to be considered additionally to the basic system behavior and functions. A unique view on the overall system can be achieved by modeling the technical system and the human operator on a behavioral description level and its realization as functional descriptions. A methodology for designing dependable robot systems is proposed, which is based on a behavioral modeling of the technical system and the user in the closed control loop. Decomposing the system recursively into behavioral levels leads to well-defined interfaces between the corresponding subsystem and the operator. The closed-loop behavior is evaluated using an integrated measure that combines safety and performance acceptance functions in a unique dependability functional. Defining dynamic safety margins, system behavior and interface parameters can be adopted in real-time in order to ensure the safe operation of the interactive system. The methodology is demonstrated on a surgical robot example.

Keywords Recursive system design · Dependability measure · Dynamical safety control · Safety-critical applications

A. Wagner (✉)
Institute of Computer Engineering, Heidelberg University, 68131 Mannheim, Germany
e-mail: achim.wagner@ziti.uni-heidelberg.de

A. Rodić et al. (eds.), *New Trends in Medical and Service Robots*,
Mechanisms and Machine Science 20, DOI: 10.1007/978-3-319-05431-5_14,

1 Introduction

Medical and service robotics is an emerging application field, where scientists from many disciplines like mechanical and electrical engineering, computer and communication, medical, and live sciences work together. The complexity of such kind of systems increases continuously, which makes them difficult to manage and control. Especially dependability and safety of the system is getting more and more a serious problem, because the dynamics and uncertain environment conditions of such systems play a dominant role.

Standard reliability and safety engineering approaches, which are based on probabilistic component fault modeling, in general do not tackle the dynamic nature of a system. However, system failures often do not occur due to accidently faults during the stationary operation of a system but in the transient phase, where a system changes from one stationary state to another. The classical example of such a system is the light bulb, which is mostly destroyed due to an overshoot of the transient filament current while switching the bulb on. Besides the dynamics of the system the system structure is an important factor. Thus, different system structures can lead to the same desired system functionality. Nevertheless, for achieving the desired behavior and non-functional properties the system structure must be designed accordingly. For instance, a mobile robot with castor wheels has a higher mobility than one with steered wheels, while at higher velocities instable castor-wheel flipping can be expected in general. Hence, the system architecture has a major impact on the dependability in terms of stability, robustness, safety, and fault tolerance.

In this work, a methodology is proposed for the analysis, the design, and the validation of dependable systems based on a rigorous dynamics modeling based on behavioral descriptions, which are suited for hardware-software co-design and human-technology-interaction design. Formerly published concepts for behavior-based dependability modeling (Rüdiger et al. 2007; Willems 1991), dependability measuring (Rüdiger et al. 2007; Wagner et al. 2009), system decomposition (Badreddin 1989; Bartolein et al. 2007; Wagner et al. 2010), system testing (Atkinson 2008; Wagner et al. 2013), monitoring and recovery (Wagner et al. 2010, 2011; Zouaghi et al. 2011) are integrated in the recursive system design methodology. For a simplified example from surgical robotics the approach is demonstrated by applying the Integrated Dependability Measure (IDM) for validation and direct dependability control, the Recursive Nested Behavior-based Control (RNBC) (Badreddin 1989; Wagner et al. 2010) structure as a starting point for system design and the integration of active fault-tolerant mechanism on the local levels.

2 Behavior-Based Concept of Dependability

According to (Willems 1991) dynamical systems can be described by the time-dependent behavior of the system variables in signal space. Other mathematical descriptions, such as input-output or state-space models can be derived from the basic behavioral model as special realizations. Because of the general properties, the behavioral framework is used as the starting point for the description of dynamical systems leading to the following linguistic definition of dependability: "Dependability in general is the capability of a system to successfully and safely fulfill its mission" (Rüdiger et al. 2007). Fortunately, this linguistic informal definition can be formalized in the following way: The capability of a system can be captured using an evaluation measure in the form of a functional over the system mission with weighted coefficients for success (performance function and other specified property functions) and safety. The mission again is defined by a set of prototypical reference actions of the system with overall duration t_m. In software systems, e.g. the mission may be defined by use cases as part of the system specification. The performance is defined as the gradual fulfillment of the expected behavior of the system, while the safety describes the distance from the safety boundary, which can be captures in a dynamic safety margin (Abdel-Geliel 2006).

The dependability concept is illustrated for the one-dimensional case in signal space (Fig. 1). The plot shows the system mission as reference trajectory $y_r(t)$ and the actual system behavior $y(t)$. Furthermore, the safety boundary is plotted as time-dependent signal $y_{max}(t)$. It is assumed that exceeding this boundary by the system variables would lead to a safety-critical system failure. The minimum distance to the safety boundary in the multidimensional space is referred to the dynamic safety margin $\delta_s(t)$ (Abdel-Geliel 2006). Furthermore, the figure shows the deviation $e_p(t)$ between actual and reference trajectory.

2.1 Dependability Measure

A formal dependability definition based on the system behavior description was proposed in (Rüdiger et al. 2007) and an Integrated Dependability Measure (IDM) was worked out in (Wagner et al. 2009), in order to provide a method to evaluate the dependability as an overall dynamical system property.

The IDM is a continuously decreasing functional over the mission time t_m with a range from 1 (totally dependable) to 0 (totally undependable):

$$D(t) = 1 - \frac{1}{t_m}\sum_{j=1}^{d} a_j \int_0^t \left[1 - A_j\big(u(t'), y_r(t'), y(t'), \Theta_j\big)\right] dt' \quad \text{with} \sum_{j=1}^{d} a_j = 1. \quad (1)$$

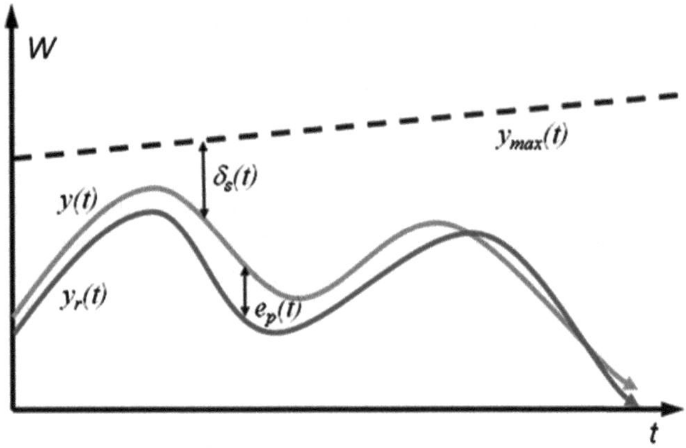

Fig. 1 System behavior in signal space: reference trajectory $y_r(t)$, actual trajectory $y(t)$, and dynamical safety boundary $y_{max}(t)$

The IDM coefficients (acceptance functions) A_j in the integral are time-dependent functions of defined dynamic properties (see below), which are normalized in the interval [0, 1] and weighted by the constant factors a_j, while the sum over all $j = 1 \ldots d$ factors is unity. Further variables are: mission input trajectory $u(t)$, reference output trajectory (reference behavior) $y_r(t)$, and actual system output (actual behavior) $y(t)$. The parameter vector Θ_j includes for example the required performance of the out y_p. Since many safety-critical systems are controlled by digital computers, a time-discrete version of the IDM over n samples can be defined:

$$D_n = 1 - \frac{1}{m}\sum_{j=1}^{d} a_j \sum_{k=1}^{n} 1 - A_j\left(u_k, y_{r,k}, y_k, \Theta_j\right) \quad \text{with} \quad \sum_{j=1}^{d} a_j = 1. \tag{2}$$

The overall mission with duration t_m consists of m samples. The acceptance coefficients are parameterized according to the user requirements and the resulting system specifications. Corresponding to the linguistic definition of Dependability (see above) one acceptance function for success, i.e. the performance, and one for safety can be defined with

$$A_{performance,k} = \exp\left(-\left\|\frac{y_k - y_{r,k}}{y_p}\right\|^2\right) \tag{3}$$

and

$$A_{safety,k} = 1 - \exp\left(-\left\|\frac{\delta_k}{y_s}\right\|^2\right), \tag{4}$$

respectively. The exponential function in the performance definition serves as a normalization function, which reaches unity for no error and zero, if the error approaches infinity. In contrast, the safety is zero (unsafe), if the dynamic safety margin delta approaches zero (system states are reaching their limits) and safety approaches unity (very safe), if delta is large. The parameter y_p and y_s are specified according to the performance and safety requirements. The IDM is a functional (sum) over mission time, which integrates the instantaneous value of the acceptance functions. Thus, it is possible to measure the instantaneous dependability in relation to the past behavior from $t' = 0$ up to the present time t. It is also possible to predict future dependability using behavior predictions from of a $t' = t$ to $t' = t_m$.

It is worth to mention that the IDM is an objective measure, which is free from any human perception and interpretation. All variables and parameters are crisp numbers and uncertainty is modeled as a range of possible deviations in the data. Randomness of stochastic processes is not included explicitly in the basic concept. However, analytical systems with additive stochastic disturbances can be tackled in this framework as well. Unlike traditional acceptance tests, which are built on statistics over passed and failed tests, the IDM describes "how well" the system behavior meets the requirements.

The IDM coefficients describe (in terms of a value in [0, 1]), in which degree a particular behavior of the system is acceptable for the application in hand. The overall IDM constitutes a general concept based on system dynamics modeling, which is open for further extensions. Besides the basic coefficient according to (3) and (4) further coefficients can be defined describing additional success criteria.

Using the IDM with user-specified acceptance functions and weighting factors, the user is enabled to compare different realization of the required system. A further major advantage of the IDM is the easy application of built-in-tests such as TestSheets (Atkinson et al. 2001, 2008; Wagner et al. 2013) to define and apply the tests along the system specification by reusing the same design artefacts as in the functional descriptions.

3 Behavior-Based System Design

Top-down development of complex technical systems begins in general with an analysis and planning phase. As an output of these activities the life-cycle of the product is organized according to the time and resources available. Finally the technical requirements and specifications as well as the constraints are defined as the input knowledge for the system design process, which starts in general with the definition of the system architecture (Maier and Rechtin 2002). A major challenge here is to integrate the dependability aspects right from the beginning. Since design errors in the early stages of the development process are difficult to eliminate in later phases the design process must be very clear and straight forward.

3.1 Generic System Architecture

Behavior-based design is a well-known approach for handling complexity by decomposing the overall system into elementary behavioral entities, so called "autonomous agents". Thus, the overall system behavior is the resulting combination of basic behaviors (Arkin 2000; Brooks 1986; Crowley 1985). Existing behavior-based approaches distinguish in the way how the interaction and communication between the behavioral components is organized.

Multi-Agent Systems yield often a highly decentralized, loosely coupled, and therefore flexible nature (Cook et al. 2003; Vallée et al. 2005). However, most of the known architectures do not consider complexity, which is a draw-back for the design, the implementation, the test, and the operation of such a system. Due to the variable structure the predictability of a system's overall behavior decreases leading to significant restrictions in dependability. A fixed hierarchy is proposed in C@sa (De Carolis 2005), where agents are grouped at different levels according to their role. By defining central agents, however, the system operability depends on single point of failure reducing its overall dependability.

Here, we propose a system decomposition approach, which considers complexity by reducing the number of possible interconnection of a system while dynamical system properties as well as dependability requirements are taken into account. As basis for the Generic System Architecture the Recursive Behavior-based Control (RNBC) structure (Badreddin 1989; Bartolein et al. 2007; Wagner et al. 2010) is proposed, which is based on behavior descriptions (see Sect. 3) to support the design engineers for early decisions while developing dependable systems. The key idea behind this kind of system decomposition is to generalize cascaded control principles originally developed for linear dynamical systems (Antoulas 1986; Goldman et al. 1981). Accordingly, complex computer-controlled systems are decomposed into behavioral components. In contrast to other agent-based structures, for which stability is difficult to be proven, the RNBC structure is a fixed structure making stability investigations applicable. Besides this kind of inherent properties for supporting dependability, further implementation-related properties are provided in order to facilitate the integration of fault-tolerant mechanisms (see Sect. 3.2).

Originally the RNBC structure was developed and successfully applied for mobile robotics (Badreddin 1989) and rehabilitation technology (Bartolein et al. 2007) and subsequently enhanced for multi-robot-interaction and shared human-robot control (Mekacher Zouaghi et al. 2013; Wagner et al. 2010). Since the original behavior specific structure is generalized to many technical fields such as car driver assistant systems (Mekacher Zouaghi et al. 2013) and unmanned air

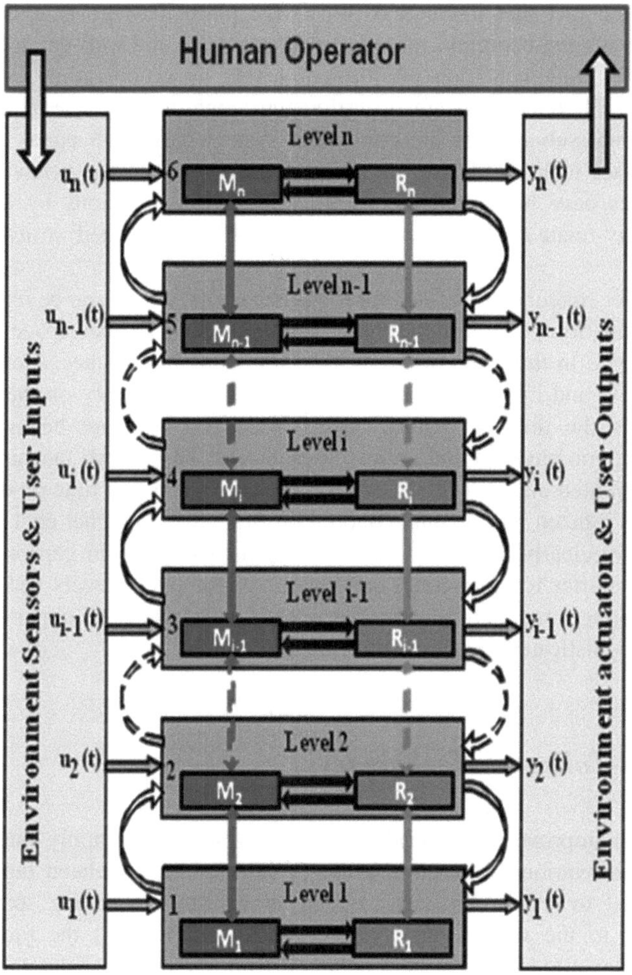

Fig. 2 Generic system architecture based on the recursive nested behavior-based control (RNBC) structure with local monitoring (*red blocks*) and recovery (*green blocks*)

vehicles (Wagner et al. 2010) it is referred here as "Generic System Architecture" (Fig. 2).

The single robot architecture including local Monitoring-Recovery mechanisms is plotted in Fig. 2 showing the n behavioral levels numbered from 1 to *n*. The structure provides nested feedback loops, which increases the robustness against external influenced and which facilitates the stabilization of the behavior on the corresponding level (nestedness). Thus the upper behaviors can be built upon stable local sub-behaviors. Disturbances as well as uncertain conditions from the environment are compensated by dynamics control using local feedback.

Due to the fact that interactions only take place between neighbored levels (recursiveness), the communication effort is moderate and well-defined interfaces facilitate the implementation of different levels by co-operating work groups. Prototypes built bottom-up are operational through-out all development stages. The functional sub-systems are equivalent system parts with equal abstractions which interact with each other by communicating within the behavioral levels. This ensures easy horizontal extensibility with new functions by keeping the dependability-related advantages of the fixed RNBC-oriented structure for the subsystems.

Each level contains one or several robot behaviors, which can be realized using a concise functional description, e.g. transfer functions or state-space models, on the local level. In this way, different local modeling approaches, such as continuous, discrete and hybrid descriptions, can be used separately on the behavioral levels. Thus the different nature of hardware and software behavior can be reflected, e.g. on physical and logical abstractions. The human-machine-interface can be distributed on the levels as well, if the user's reaction time on diverse sub-behaviors is it taken into account (Badreddin et al. 2011; Wagner et al. 2010). The interfaces are clearly defined by its input-output variables. In general, the faster behaviors (shorter reaction time) are located in the lower levels and the slower behaviors (longer reaction time) in the upper levels, while the upper levels yield the more sophisticated behaviors with higher complexity.

3.2 Fault-Tolerance Techniques

One way to improve the dependability of a system is to apply fault-tolerance techniques on various abstraction levels. While reliability related fault-tolerance has the goal to reduce the (static) fault probability by adding space or time redundancy to the system, in dynamic control applications the fault-tolerance avoids the deviation of the system behavior from the desired behavior (Avizienis et al. 2004; Laprie et al. 1992; Siewiorek and Swarz 1998). The deviation of system behavior may origin from different sources: Besides errors due to design faults and incomplete modeling, the system variables are influenced by disturbances from external inputs, uncertain environmental conditions, or internal parameter shifts, e.g. due to component aging. A failure of a component is a special case of an internal fault, which may change the system structure or parameters.

Fault-tolerant control mechanisms detect faults and prevent them from propagation in the system in order to maintain a minimum degree of performance and safety. Two basic approached exist: Passive Fault Tolerant Control (PFTC) and Active Fault Tolerant Control (AFTC) (Abdel-Geliel 2006; Mahmoud et al. 2003; Patton 1997). PFTC utilized a priori known faults without having additional online information during the operation phase. Consequently, the fault-tolerance capability of PFTC is limited. AFTC in general uses a mechanism for fault detection, isolation, diagnosis and recovery.

Both types of fault-tolerance mechanism (PTFC and ATFC) can be integrated in the Generic System Architecture in a recursive way. On the behavior levels the system variables are monitored and diagnosed locally and the corresponding levels are recovered if indicated. In order to facilitate or the improve monitoring and recovery, the results from the neighbored levels can also be used (Wagner et al. 2010; Zouaghi et al. 2011) which is described by the green and red arrows in Fig. 2. Here, a model-based method is proposed, which is based on the direct (online) use of the time-dependent IDM and related coefficients such as safety coefficients in order to adapt the parameters of the system on multiple levels for recovery. The approach is described in detail in the Sect. 4.

3.3 Recursive Behavior-Based Design Process

The design process starts with identifying the fundamental behaviors, corresponding to the user requirements. The basic sub-behaviors are sorted along their reaction times. Behaviors with narrow reaction times are clustered in one behavior level, while the number of levels can be chosen freely or according to given design constraints e.g. the number of groups working separately during the component integration phase. Along with the behavior allocation, the internal level structure including the processing blocks and the input and output signals can be defined straight forward. The behavior levels will be connected recursively corresponding to Fig. 2 building the overall system structure.

In the next design steps, the overall system structure can be reused in the component specification process. Due to the recursiveness of the architecture the components are strictly encapsulated by unique interfaces. The decision, how the behaviors shall be realized, e.g. as hardware or software component, can be made later in the design process, which facilitates the hardware/software co-design.

The behavioral, functional and structural specification can be further elaborated in component-based design models like KobrA (Atkinson et al. 2001), which apply for example UML-profiles and System C language to decompose and to realize the overall system behavior in a recursive way. Furthermore, the resulting description can be reused for the semi-automatic specification of monitoring components (Wagner et al. 2011).

4 Reference Design of a Surgical Robot

The recursive design and dependability-related control concept is demonstrated in this section using a surgical robot application. A general task executed by many of such applications is the resection of tissue in a given area (Pott et al. 2005). In orthopedics, the resected material is e.g. the human bone for preparing a hip or knee implant. Accordingly, the robot milling tool has to remove a preplanned volume of bone in the patient frame with defined processing parameters. Critical structures, such as blood vessels and nerves have to be avoided, which is reflected by geometric constraints. For safety reasons and due to additional physical constraints, further restrictions are put on the velocity and position variables, e.g. in order to avoid internal collisions or overloads.

4.1 System Structuring

Surgical robots belong to the class of dynamical safety-critical systems, which may harm human health and live during operation if the system behaves not as desired. Thus, surgical robots are required to be highly dependable, which must be reflected by the robot control system. The structural design is shown in Fig. 3 on the example of an image-based surgical intervention for orthopedic surgery.

According to the overall task following sub-behaviors can be described top down beginning with the slowest behavior:

- The *Intervention Planning* is a behavior carried out by the surgeon in general based on 3D image patient data, e.g. from Computer Tomography (CT) and the results from former interventions. The activity maybe also supported by graphical systems, which fit processing trajectory into the 3D patient model. The resulting outputs are the way of intervention, the volume for resection, and the required tools.
- The *Mission Control* behavior separates the overall intervention task into sub-mission e.g. system initialization, patient preparation, registration, processing and implantation.
- The *Path Control* behavior is responsible for finding an efficient and safe trajectory for the resection of tissue volume using the predefined tool. The path is controlled by position feedback.
- The *Position Control* behavior conducts the tool on the desired path while position deviations are compensated for.
- The *Collision Avoidance* is a reflexive behavior which prevents for colliding with suddenly occurring object such as the hand of the surgical assistant or other surgical tools.
- The *Velocity Control* behavior adjusts the desired processing velocity considering dynamic constraints and stabilizes the end effector in the processing area.
- The *Force control* behavior generates the desired force on the actuator, e.g. in order to compensate for internal friction.

In the overall view, the dynamical system behavior is a simultaneous execution of sub-behaviors which interact over defined interfaces. Additionally to the signals from the neighbored level, the behavioral blocks receive signals from the environment using suited sensors for the behavioral level under consideration and from the operator, e.g. from the surgeon, via defined human-machine-interfaces.

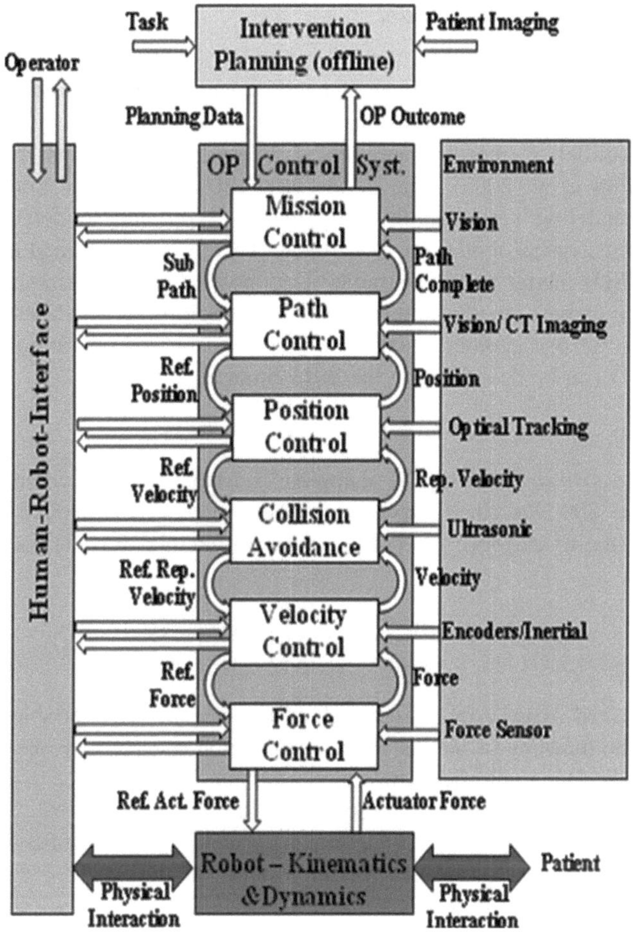

Fig. 3 Proposed control structure for a surgical robot based on the generic system architecture

According to the system resources available and other requirements, now, the design engineer allocates the behavioral levels to the functional components. The actuator-level related force and velocity control levels, for instance, can be implemented on local hardware, while the robot-level related behaviors (task space) can be implemented as separate processes on a real-time control computer. Each level contains its own control model as dynamical description, while the lowest level acts on the robot, which is described by its kinematics and dynamics model.

4.2 Dynamical Robot Model

Corresponding to the huge number of possible surgical interventions, many different mechanical robot structures are utilized in medical applications, e.g. based on serial, parallel or hybrid kinematics. A overview on different robots can be found in (Pott et al. 2005). Due to the different structures the kinematics and dynamics modeling varies significantly and it is difficult to define a general applicable mechanical model for all of them. Therefore a simplified mass-spring-damper (MSD) model with constraints is proposed here for demonstration purposes, which captures the basic relationships between force, acceleration, velocity and position for one geometric axis of a robot in a limited operation range.

The MSD can be described by the differential equation

$$F(t) = m\ddot{x}(t) + d\dot{x}(t) + kx(t) \tag{5}$$

with the mass $m = 2.635$ kg the damping constant $d = 9.18$ Ns/m and spring constant $k = 800$ N/m. In the special case, the force $F(t)$ is excited by an input signal $u(t)$ (motor current). According to the differential Eq. (1) the state space formulation

$$\begin{bmatrix} \dot{x}_1(t) \\ \dot{x}_2(t) \end{bmatrix} = \begin{bmatrix} 0 & 1 \\ -k/m & -d/m \end{bmatrix} \begin{bmatrix} x_1(t) \\ x_2(t) \end{bmatrix} + \begin{bmatrix} 0 \\ 1/m \end{bmatrix} u(t) \tag{6}$$

can be derived with $x_1(t) = x(t)$ and $\dot{x}_2(t) = x_1(t)$. The variables $x_1(t)$ and $x_2(t)$ have the meaning of the instantaneous position and velocity, respectively, of the rigid body. Due to physical constraints, e.g. due to the distance to other objects and maximum friction forces, these values are bounded by $x_{1,max} = 0.28$ m, $x_{1,min} = -0.28$ m, $x_{2,max} = 1.2$ m/s, and $x_{2,min} = -1.2$ m/s. Further bounds may exist in the phase space (see Fig. 5), for instance as the result of the maximum allowed forces at the spring-damper fixture.

4.3 Controller Design

According to the required basic behaviors, the system is decomposed into a velocity control level and into a position control level, which interact in a recursive way (Fig. 4). The input of the position control level is the reference position p_r provided from the next upper levels, i.e. the trajectory control level. Together with the feedback signal p, the position controller produces a reference velocity v_r for the velocity control level. The collision avoidance level is not available (short-cut) in the example. The velocity controller again uses the deviation of the actual velocity v from the reference velocity v_r to generate a reference torque τ_r for the robot actuators. Additional lower control levels, such as force control and motor current behaviors, are possible. However, in the example these lower loop

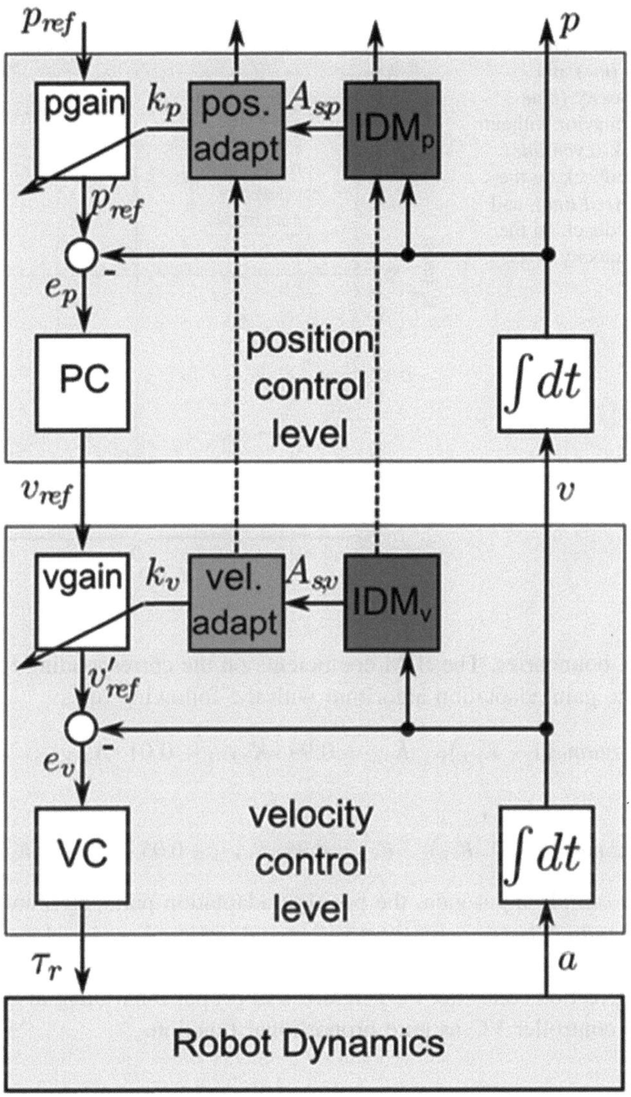

Fig. 4 Control structure for the lower behavior levels, position control level and velocity control level, with integrated local monitoring-recovery mechanisms

behaviors are assumed to have a significant shorter time constant, which can be approximated by a static transfer function for convenience.

A monitoring-recovery mechanism is integrated locally on the behavioral levels. In contrast to other monitoring methods, where the outputs from the actual system and from the fault models are compared, here, the system is assessed by calculating the IDM coefficients directly from the system states and their distances

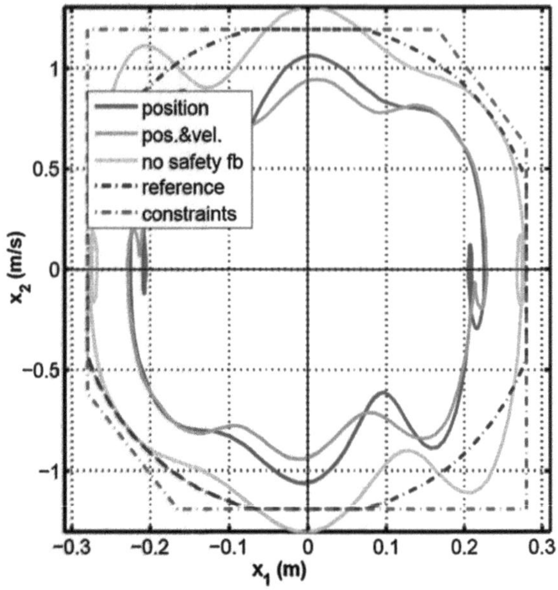

Fig. 5 System behavior in phase space: constraints (*red dashed dotted line*) and reference trajectory (*blue line*), actual behavior without safety feedback (*cyan line*), with safety feedback on the position level (*red line*), and with safety feedback on the position and velocity level (*green line*)

to the safety boundaries. The IDM coefficients on the corresponding level are the inputs for the gain adaptation algorithm with the following rules:

$$pgain_k = pgain_0(1 - K_{p,k}), \quad K_{p,k} = 0.99 \cdot K_{p,k-1} + 0.01 \cdot A_{sp,k-1}, \quad K_{p,0} = 0, \tag{7}$$

$$vgain_k = vgain_0(1 - 0.9 \cdot K_{v,k}), \quad K_{v,k} = 0.95 \cdot K_{v,k-1} + 0.05 \cdot A_{sv,k-1}, \quad K_{p,0} = 0, \tag{8}$$

with the kth sample input gain, the position adaptation parameter, and the safety coefficient $pgain_k$, $K_{p,k}$, $A_{sp,k}$ for the position and $vgain_k$, $K_{v,k}$, $A_{sv,k}$ for the velocity, respectively. As a result the original reference inputs p_r and v_r are alternated to p_r' and v_r'. The position controller PC is realized as proportional-integral structure and the velocity controller VC as pure proportional function.

4.4 System Simulations

The System behavior was simulated using MATLAB (The Mathworks Inc.). As system reference input, the specified overall mission trajectory (sinus: amplitude 0.3 m, frequency 0.65 Hz) was applied and the system actual output was calculated from the dynamics model. According to the limits in the system variables, the input values are clipped to the maximum values. This is illustrated in phase space (Fig. 5) with the position variable x_1 and the velocity variable x_2. While the clipped input trajectory is plotted as blue dash-dotted line, the constraints on the

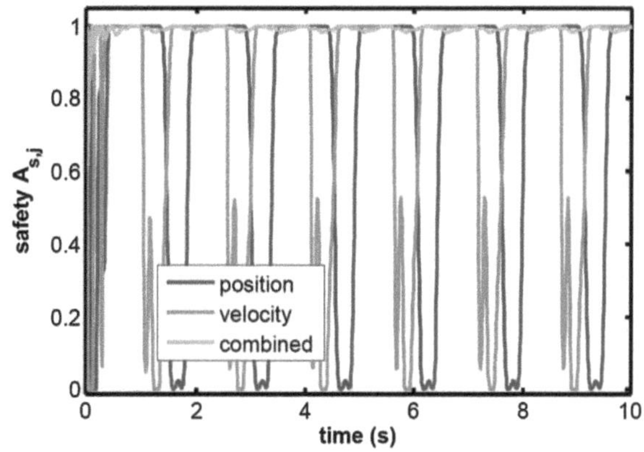

Fig. 6 Safety coefficients over the time: position constraints (*red line*), velocity constraints (*green line*), combined (*cyan line*)

system variable are shown as red dash-dotted line. The system response for the case without input gain adaptation is shown as cyan line, which reaches the position limits at some instances of time or even exceeds the velocity limits at $x_1 = 0$ m.

According to (3) the safety coefficients are influenced over the time, which is plotted in Fig. 6. Here, a safety reduction can be noticed at that instance of time, when approaching the limit. The corresponding variables for the position, velocity and combined constraints are plotted separately as red, green, and cyan line.

If the input gain of the position control level is adapted according to the safety condition, the output trajectory keeps a distance from the limits (see Fig. 5, red line), resulting in a higher safety value in the position dimension (Fig. 7a). An additional velocity gain adaptation according to the velocity constraints and the resulting safety coefficient in the velocity dimension leads to a further increase of the dynamic safety margin (Fig. 7b).

Since the performance of the controller in terms of deviations from the reference behavior decreases in general, if safety conditions are getting active, the overall system design is a trade-off between performance and safety, which is reflected by the overall dependability functional. The resulting time-dependent dependability values for the three cases (1. without gain adaptation, 2. with position gain adaption, and 3. with both position and velocity gain adaptation) are plotted in Fig. 8. It is obvious that the dependability decreases continuously over the time starting a unity until it reaches its final value at mission time $t_m = 10$ s. Without gain adaption the final value is $D(t_m) = 0.10$ (cyan line), with position gain adaption $D(t_m) = 0.58$ (red line), and with both adoptions $D(t_m) = 0.62$ (green line). The example demonstrates how dynamic safety control can be implemented in a nested way by decomposing the system as well as the monitoring-recovery mechanism into local behavioral levels. Furthermore, the example shows how dependability can be increased successively by adding multiple adaptation processes.

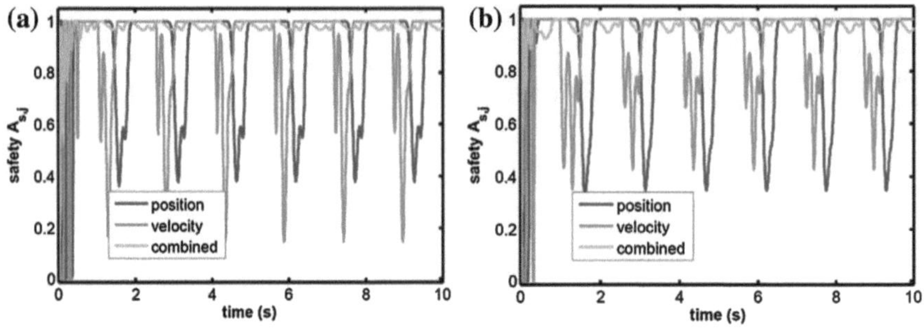

Fig. 7 Safety coefficients over the time with safety feedback on the (**a**) position level (**b**) position and velocity levels: position constraints (*red line*), velocity constraints (*green line*), combined (*cyan line*)

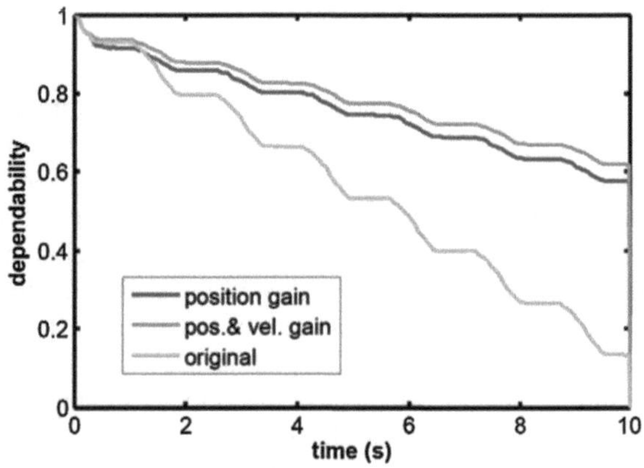

Fig. 8 Overall dependability functional: without safety feedback (*cyan line*), with safety feedback on the position level (*red line*), and with safety feedback on the position and the velocity level (*green line*)

5 Conclusion

A methodology for the recursive design of dependable systems is proposed. The methodology is based on a number of core concepts, such as the behavior modeling, the integrated dependability measure, the generic system architecture, the distributed active fault-tolerant control, and component-based system realization, which were already successfully applied to various kinds of dynamical system types in previous work. According to the methodology the reference design of a simple surgical robot example is worked out, here. The methodology targets the system structure and dynamics modeling in order to achieve inherent robustness against dependability impairments and to facilitate system realization by behavior-based system decomposition rules and universal monitoring-recovery concepts.

Additionally, the online usage of the dependability measure and the related coefficients on multiple behavioral levels is proposed in order to increase the dependability in real-time by closed-loop feedback control.

This approach tackles disturbances and changing environmental condition, which reduce the distance from internal and input/output safety constraints. By measuring dependability relevant dynamical properties in real-time, a tool is available to influence the dependability immediately by system reconfiguration or parameter adaptation. Furthermore, a prediction of the dependability measures based on dynamical models is also plausible enabling system configuration in advance, e.g. by selecting a controller from a controller bank or by setting the control parameters before a critical situation arises. Future work is concentrated on the developing a tool basis for direct dependability control.

References

Abdel-Geliel, M.: Fault Diagnosis and Performance Recovery Based on the Dynamic Safety Margin, doctoral thesis, University of Mannheim, (2006).

Antoulas, T.: On Recursiveness and Related Topics in Linear Systems. IEEE Trans. Automatic Control, Vol. AC-31, No.12, pp.1121–1134, (1986)

Arkin, R. C.: Behavior-Based Robotics. MIT Press: Massachussetts Institute of Technology, (2000)

Atkinson, C., Brenner, D., Falcone, G., Juhasz, M.: Specifying High-Assurance Services. IEEE Computer, vol. 41, no. 8, pp. 64–71, (2008)

Atkinson, C.; Bayer, J.; Bunse, C.; Kamsties, E.; Laitenberger, O.; Laqua, R.; Muthig, D.; Paech, B.; Wüst, J.; Zettel, J: Component-based product line engineering with UML, Addison-Wesley, London (2001)

Avizienis, A., Laprie, J.-C., Randell, B., Landwehr, C.: Basic concepts and taxonomy of dependable and secure computing. IEEE Trans. on Dependable and Secure Computing, 1 (1):11–33, (2004)

Badreddin, E.; Wagner, A.: Real-Time Level of Autonomy Adaptation for Human-Machine-Interaction Based on the Reaction Time, 18th IFAC World Congress, Milano, Italy, (2011)

Badreddin, E.: Recursive Control Structure for Mobile Robots. International Conf. on Intelligent Autonomous Systems 2 (IAS.2), Amsterdam, pp. 11–14, Dec. (1989)

Bartolein, C.; Wagner, A.; Jipp, M.; Badreddin, E.: Multilevel Intention Estimation for Wheelchair Control, in Proc. of the European Control Conference 2007, Kos, Greece, July 2–5, (2007)

Brooks, R.: A robust layered control system for a mobile robot. IEEE Journal of Robotics and Automation, vol. 2(1), pp. 14–23, (1986)

Cook, D.J. et al.: An Agent-Based Smart Home, In proceeding of the Conference on Pervasive Computing, (2003).

Crowley, J. L.: Navigation for an intelligent mobile robot. IEEE Journal of Robotics and Automation, vol. 1, pp. 31–41, (1985)

De Carolis, B.: Adapting Home Behavior to Its Inhabitants, Lecture Notes in Computer Science, 2005.3538: p. 282–286, (2005)

Goldman, M.J.; Porras, W.J.; Leondes, C.T.: Multivariable system reduction via Cauer forms. Int. J. Control, Vol. 34, No. 4, 623-650, (1981)

Laprie, J. C.: Dependability: Basic Concepts and Terminology. Ed. Springer, (1992)

Mahmoud, M.; Jiang, J.; and Zhang, Y.: Stabilization of Active Fault Tolerant Control systems with imperfect fault detection and diagnosis, Stochastic Analysis and Application, Vol. 21, No. 3, pp. 673–701, (2003).
Maier M. W. and Rechtin, E.: The Art of Systems Architecting, sec. edition, CRC Press, Boca Raton, (2002).
Mekacher Zouaghi, L.; Wagner, A.; Badreddin, E.: Design of Fault-Tolerant and Dependable Assistance Systems with Degree of Autonomy Adaptation. International Conference on Advanced Logistics and Transport, Sousse, Tunisia, 29–31 May, (2013)
Patton, R. J.: Fault-tolerant Control: the 1997 situation, Proc. of IFAC Symposium SAFEPROCESS'97, Hull, UK, pp. 1033–1055, (1997).
Pott, P.P.; Scharf, H-P; Schwarz M.L.R.: Today's State of the Art of Surgical Robotics. Journal of Computer Aided Surgery, 10(2), 101–132. (2005)
Rüdiger, J., Wagner A., Badreddin E.: Behavior Based Definition of Dependability for Autonomous Mobile Systems, in Proc. of the European Control Conference, Kos, Greece, July 2–5, WeD11.4, (2007)
Siewiorek, D. P., Swarz, R. S.: Reliable Computer Systems: design and evaluation. 3rd ed., A K Peter Ltd. Massachusetts, USA, (1998)
Vallée, M.; Ramparany, F.; and Vercouter, L.: A Multi-Agent System for Dynamic Service Composition in Ambient Intelligence Environments, Doctoral Colloquium - Pervasive 2005, Munich, Germany, (2005).
Wagner, A.; Mekacher Zouaghi L.; Barth, F.; Atkinson, C. and Badreddin, E.: Behavior-Based Built-in Testing and Monitoring for Dependability Assessment of Dynamical Systems. Competitiveness through maintenance and Asset Management (COMADEM 2013), Helsinki, Finland (2013)
Wagner A., Zouaghi, L., Barth, F., Atkinson, C., Badreddin, E.: A Unified Design Approach for Component-Based Dynamical Systems Monitoring. IEEE/SICE International Symposium on System Integration (SII), pp.1137–1142, (2011)
Wagner, A., Atkinson, C., and Badreddin, E.: Towards a Practical, Unified Dependability Measure for Dynamic Systems. in Proceedings of the International Workshop on the Design of Dependable Critical Systems, Hamburg, (2009)
Wagner, A.; Jipp, M.; Kandil, A.; Eck, C.; Badreddin, E.: Generic system architecture for dependable interactive systems: A flying robot example. IEEE Intern. Conf. on Systems, Man and Cybernetics, Istanbul, Turkey (2010)
Willems, J.C.: Paradigms and puzzles in the theory of dynamical systems. IEEE Transactions on Automatic Control, 36(3): 259–294, March (1991)
Zouaghi, L, Wagner, A., and Badreddin, E.: Monitoring of Hybrid Systems using Behavioral System Specification. IFAC World Congress, (2011)

Some Applications of Biomimetics and Fractional Calculus in Control and Modeling of (Bio)robotic Systems

M. Lazarević

Abstract Rapid development of biological science and technologies will further improve the active applications of control engineering by advanced biomimetic and biologically inspired research. First of all, it has promoted a biologically inspired control synergy approach that allows the resolution of redundancy of a given robotized system. In particular, the actuator redundancy control problem has been stated and solved by using Pontryagin's maximum principle, where control synergy was established at the coordination level. Besides, fractional calculus (FC), is a mathematical topic with more than 300 years old history, in recent years there have been extensive research activities related to applications of FC in many areas of science and engineering. Here, they are presented by the advanced algorithms of PID control based on FC, tuned by genetic algorithms, in the position control of robotic system with 3 DOFs driven by DC motors. Also, a chattering-free fractional PD^{α} sliding-mode controller in the control of a given robotic system has been proposed and realized. The effectiveness of the proposed optimal fractional order controls are demonstrated by the given robot. Finally, it is shown that one can obtain analytical expressions for generalized forces of the magnetorheological damping elements of fractional order which are used for obtaining better model of (bio)robotic systems.

Keywords Biomimetic · Actuator redundancy · Biologically inspired control · Fractional order PID controller · Fractional order sliding mode controller

M. Lazarević (✉)
Faculty of Mechanical Engineering, University of Belgrade,
street Kraljice Marije 16, Belgrade, Serbia
e-mail: mlazarevic@mas.bg.ac.rs

A. Rodić et al. (eds.), *New Trends in Medical and Service Robots*,
Mechanisms and Machine Science 20, DOI: 10.1007/978-3-319-05431-5_15,

1 Introduction

It is well known that biological systems possess significant capabilities in their specialized functions perfected through long evolutionary processes whereby they were developed to optimize themselves under the long lasting selective pressures (Webb 2001). The field of biomimetics and biologically inspired principles for the application of methods and systems, found in nature, to engineering and technology, has spawned a number of innovations far superior to what the human mind alone could have devised (Bar-Cohen et al. 2006). Also, the fast growing interest in flexible, versatile, and mobile robotic manipulators demands for robots with an inherent high passive safety suited for direct human–robot interaction, especially in the field of medical and service robotics (Karas and Baig 2008). On the other hand, the system control theory, which forms the core foundation for understanding, designing, and operating of many technical systems, is still limited and insufficient to handle complex large-scale systems in real time, like biological systems (Lathash 1994). Biologically inspired approaches have recently succeeded in the processes of design and control in robotics (Bar-Cohen et al. 2006; Klug et al. 2008; Vepa et al. 2009). Moreover, general biomechanical systems, including human body as well as the bodies of mammals and insects, are also redundantly actuated and, consequently, redundant actuation can be also found in many robotic applications (Harkegard et al. 2005).

Firstly, a biologically inspired control synergy approach that allows the resolution of redundancy of a given (bio)robotized system is proposed. In particular, the actuator redundancy control problem has been stated and solved by using Pontryagin's maximum principle, where control synergy is established at the coordination level. On the other hand, typical behaviors of biomimetic actuators in (bio)robotic systems include the anisotropy, elasticity, viscoelasticity and other memoryless nonlinearities. The authors (Chen et al. 2004) introduce fractional calculus (FC) in biomimetic actuator control and reveal the possibility of FC to model the dynamics of biomimetic materials. FC is a mathematical topic with more than 300 years old history, and there have been extensive research activities related to applications of FC in many areas of science and engineering, in recent years (Podlubny 1999; Sabatier et al. 2007). The fractional integro-differential operators present a generalization of the integration and derivation of non-integer order (fractional) operators. The interest in fractional order dynamic systems and controllers has been increasing in many areas of science and engineering in the last few years (Sabatier et al. 2007). In most cases, the objective of using FC is to apply the fractional order controller to enhance the system control performance, as well as obtaining better robotic fractional model, by using FC. For example, the authors (Oh and Hori 2008) proposed impedance control based on using FC to control power assistive devices in more human friendly way or in Romanovas et al. (2013) recursive Bayesian estimation algorithms for human motion tracking using FC models is presented.

Here are presented the advanced algorithms of PID control based on FC, tuned by genetic algorithms, in the position control of robotic system with 3 DOFs driven by DC motors (Lazarević et al. 2013). Also, a chattering-free fractional PD^{α} sliding-mode controller in the control of a given robotic system (Lazarević 2012) is proposed. Finally, an analytical expression of the generalized force of the damping element (viscoelastic element of fractional order) will be determined (Cajić et al. 2013). In that way, one can obtain values in the region of changing fractional order of the derivative which is unavailable by using the integer order models of magnetorheological damping elements.

2 Fundamentals of Biologically Inspired Control

Recent rapid development of the biological science and technologies will further improve the active applications of control engineering. Meanwhile, system control theory itself will also be promoted by advanced biomimetic and biologically inspired control researches (Bar-Cohen et al. 2006). The mathematical analysis and clarification of functions of complex biological systems at the system level, and imitation of them in engineering, will lead to a deeper understanding of ourselves and will be significant for constructing the next generation of advanced artificial systems such as human friendly robots (Wu and Geng 2012; Klug et al. 2008) e.g., self-organization of the environmental adaptive motor function is one of the most interesting characteristics that we should learn through biomimetic control research. Nervous system takes advantage of the kinematic and multi-muscle redundancies to control actions in a flexible way so that, e.g., the same motor goal can be reached differently depending on our intentions and external environmental (e.g. obstacles) or intrinsic (neural) constraints. Despite this flexibility, the central control of actions is unambiguous: each time the body moves, a unique action is produced despite the possibility of using other actions leading to the same goal. It is amazing how these seemingly opposite aspects—flexibility and uniqueness—are combined in the control of actions. Following Bernstein (Bernstein 1961), we refer to these aspects of action production as the "redundancy problem". In other words, it was observed in the execution of functional motions that certain trajectories, from the infinite number of options (Bernstein 1961; Latash et al. 2008), are preferred. Such behavior of organisms can be explained only by the existence of inherent optimization laws in the self-organized systems governing the acquisition of motor skills. Existence of invariant features in the execution of functional motions indicates that central nervous system (CNS) uses synergy (i.e. rule(s) that can be developed by the CNS based on some principles) (Grinyagin et al. 2004).

2.1 Control of Robotic System-Synergy Approach

Here we focus on the resolved redundant actuation of a given robotic system applying a biologically inspired synergy approach together with an optimization procedure. First of all, we are going to use the term 'synergy', as suggested by Bernstein (1961), in order to denote a set of rule(s) which unite the central control signal and other control signal(s) to the given redundant bio-robotic system. One may obtain additional equation(s) helping to solve the problem of redundancy. The redundancy control problem has been discussed within the framework of optimal control problem which is solved by Pontryagin's maximum principle. The joint actuator synergy approach established by optimization law at the coordination level is proposed, where a central control, as suggested Bernstein, is introduced. In that way, one may obtain a specific constraint (or constraints) on the control variables (Lazarević et al. 2012), i.e. control synergy where a central control is used, now acting upon the joints of the redundant robotic system at the actuator level. The proposed biologically inspired optimal control is illustrated by the simulation results of a cylindrical Autolemec ACR robot with 3 DOF's and 4 control variables (Fig. 1), (see Gering et al. 1986), where $M = 0.65$ kg m^2, $B = C = D = 8.3$ kg and the control weighting matrix is $R = diag(1,1,2,3)$. The covariant coordinates of the basic metric tensor $[a_{\alpha\beta}]_{\alpha,\beta=1,2,3}$ are

$$[a_{\alpha\beta}] = [M + B q_2^2\; 0\; 0; 0\; C\; 0; 0\; 0\; D] \tag{1}$$

and the potential energy due to gravitational forces is given by $\Pi = Dgq_3 + \text{const}$ where g is gravity acceleration.

Dynamic model of the robot can be described by the set of the $2n$ Hamiltonian equations in terms of Hamiltonian phase variables q_i, p_i (Hilfer 2000). For a global optimization, a performance criterion is introduced at the coordination level as the energy quadratic criterion in the form of the functional sum of weighted controls of the robot:

$$J = 0.5\int_{t_0}^{t_k} u^T(t)Ru(t)dt \to min, \quad R = diag\{r_j\}, \quad j = 1,2,\ldots,\dim(u) \tag{2}$$

where t_o, t_k are the initial and final times of an end-effector movement, which are known and fixed, and control weighting matrix R is a symmetric positive definite matrix. Control $u(t)$ must be entry of a given subset U of admissible controls, $u(t) \in U \subset R^m$, it is assumed that there is no constraint on the control vector and admissible controls belong to an open set. Generalized forces can be presented as functions of the components of control u as

$$Q_i = u_i + \alpha_i u_c, \quad i = 1,2,3, \tag{3}$$

where all generalized forces are introduced as superposition of the two control signals—central control u_c and the corresponding additive control u_i, where

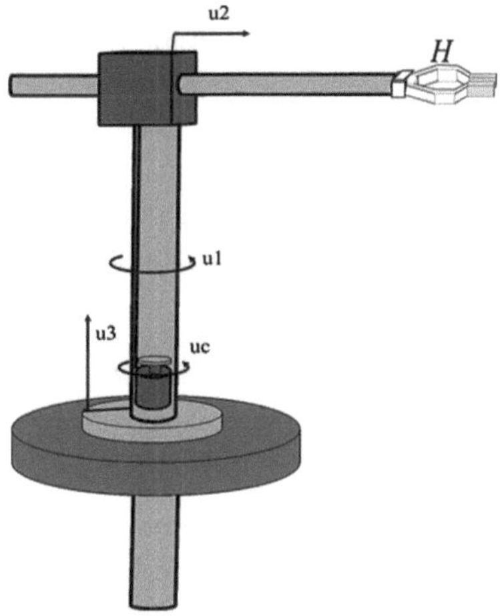

Fig. 1 Model of ACR robot with 3 DOF's and 4 control variables

coefficients $\alpha_i = \text{const},\ i = 1, 2, 3$ are introduced due to different dimensions of the control variables. In that way, one of the possible control strategies is established. The necessary conditions are presented by Theorem 1 and obtained by applying Pontryagin's maximum principle, where the corresponding Pontryagin's Function, $\aleph(\mu_0, \mu, \lambda, q, p, u)$ is introduced.

Theorem 1 *If there is $u^*(t),\ t \in [t_0 t_k]$ optimal control of the given optimal control problem and if $q^*(t), p^*(t)$ are the corresponding optimal trajectories, then the dimension vector $(\mu_0, \mu(t), \lambda(t))$ ($\mu_o \in R^1, \mu \in R^n, \lambda \in R^n$ are Lagrange multipliers) different from zero exists, and it satisfies the following expressions: $q^*, p^*, u^*, \mu^*, \lambda^*$, in interval $t \in [t_0, t_k]$, satisfying the following system of equations*

$$\text{a)} \quad \dot{q}^i = \sum_{\alpha=1}^{n} a^{i\alpha} p_\alpha, \dot{p}_i = -\frac{1}{2}\sum_{\alpha=1}^{n}\sum_{\beta=1}^{n} \frac{\partial a^{\alpha\beta}}{\partial q^i} p_\alpha p_\beta - \frac{\partial \Pi}{\partial q^i} + Q_i(u), \quad i = 1, 2, \ldots, n \tag{4}$$

$$\dot{\mu}_i = -\sum_{\alpha=1}^{n}\sum_{\beta=1}^{n} \mu_\beta \frac{\partial a^{\alpha\beta}}{\partial q^i} p_\beta + \frac{1}{2}\sum_{\alpha=1}^{n}\sum_{\beta=1}^{n}\sum_{\gamma=1}^{n} \lambda^\gamma \frac{\partial^2 a^{\alpha\beta}}{\partial q^\gamma \partial q^i} p_\alpha p_\beta + \sum_{\gamma=1}^{n} \lambda^\gamma \frac{\partial^2 \Pi}{\partial q^\gamma \partial q^i} \tag{5}$$

$$\dot{\lambda}^i = -\sum_{\alpha=1}^{n}\sum_{\beta=1}^{n} \mu_\beta a^{i\beta} + \sum_{\alpha=1}^{n}\sum_{\beta=1}^{n}\sum_{\gamma=1}^{n} \lambda^\alpha \frac{\partial a^{\beta i}}{\partial q^i} p_\beta \tag{6}$$

where the contravariant coordinates $a^{\alpha\beta}(q)$ denote the basic metric tensor $[a_{\alpha\beta}] \in R^{n\times n}$.

$$\text{b)} \quad \mu_o^* = \text{const} \leq 0 \tag{7}$$

$$\text{c)} \quad \left(\frac{\partial \aleph}{\partial u}\right)_{u^*} = 0, \left(\frac{\partial^2 \aleph}{\partial u_\alpha \partial u_\beta}\right) u_\alpha u_\beta \leq 0, \quad \alpha, \beta = 1, 2, \ldots m \tag{8}$$

or in a more explicit form

$$\mu_0 \frac{\partial f_0}{\partial u} - \frac{\partial Q^T(u)}{\partial u} \lambda_{|u^*} = 0 \tag{9}$$

Applying the matrix theory to solve (9) implies that the condition must be fulfilled, that there is a unique solution for the vector λ

$$\det \begin{bmatrix} 1 & 0 & 0 & u_1^* r_1 \\ 0 & 1 & 0 & u_2^* r_2 \\ 0 & 0 & 1 & u_3^* r_3 \\ \alpha_1 & \alpha_2 & \alpha_3 & u_c^* r_0 \end{bmatrix} = 0 \Rightarrow u_c^* r_0 = \alpha_1 u_1^* r_1 + \alpha_2 u_2^* r_2 + \alpha_3 u_3^* r_3. \tag{10}$$

Equation (11) presents an invariant of control variables "control synergy". The obtained synergy control and the proposed approach differ from the recently suggested rivaling controls introduced in (Schanzer and Callies 2008) by splitting up one original control into two independent and additive controls. The two-point boundary value problem has been solved for the following boundary conditions (Lazarevic et al. 2012), where the proposed initial and final positions for three different values of $t_1 = 1, 1.5, 2$ s (see Fig. 2a–d).

$$\begin{aligned} t_0 = 0 \text{ s}, \quad & q_1(t_0) = 0 \text{ rad}, \; q_2(t_0) = 0.1 \text{ m}, \; q_3(t_0) = 0 \text{ m}, \\ & p_1(t_0) = p_2(t_0) = p_3(t_0) = 0 \left(\text{kg m}^2/\text{s}, \; \text{kg m/s},\right) \end{aligned} \tag{11}$$

$$\begin{aligned} t_1 = 1, 1.5, 2 \text{ s} \quad & q_1(t_1) = \pi/4 \text{ rad}, \; q_2(t_1) = 0.25 \text{ m}, \; q_3(t_1) = 0.2 \text{ m}, \\ & p_1(t_1) = 0 \text{ kg m}^2/\text{s}, \; p_2(t_1) = 0 \text{ kg m/s}, \; p_3(t_1) = 0 \text{ kg m/s}. \end{aligned}$$

3 Fractional Order Control and Modeling of (Bio)robotic Systems

FC has attracted attention of researchers from different fields in the recent years and the fractional integro-differential operators are generalization of integration and derivation operators of an arbitrary order (Kilbas et al. 2006; Oldham and Spanier 1974; Podlubny 1999; Sabatier et al. 2007; Webb 2001). Interest in fractional order dynamic systems and controllers has been increasing in many areas of science and engineering in the last few years. Here, our objective of using FC is to apply a fractional order controller to enhance the system control performance especially in the field of medical and service robotics and applications. Fractional-order PID (FOPID) controller is a generalization of a standard (integer) PID controller due to its five controller parameters (instead of the standard three) (Astrom and Hagglund 1995; Lazarević 2006; Podlubny 1999). An advanced algorithm of PID control based on FC, tuned by genetic algorithms, in the control of robotic system driven by DC motors has been proposed and realized here.

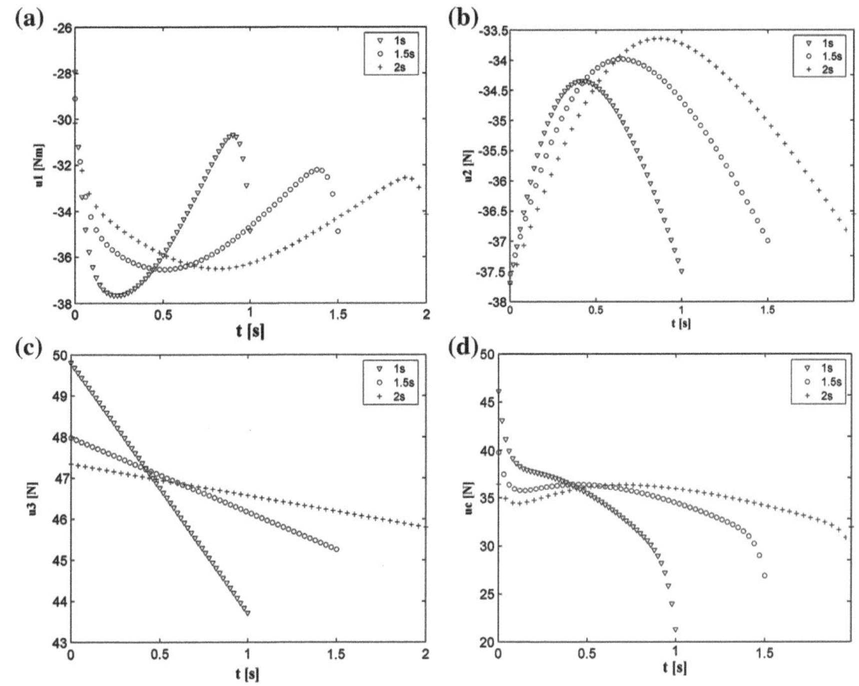

Fig. 2 Optimal controls u, **a** Optimal control u^1. **b** Optimal control u^2. **c** Optimal control u^3. **d** Optimal control u^c

A sliding-mode controller (SMC) is a powerful tool to robustly control incompletely modeled or uncertain systems (Edwards 1998) which has many attractive features such as fast response, good transient response and asymptotic stability. However, an SMC has some disadvantages related to the well-known chattering in the system which must be eliminated from the SMC system (Hace and Jezernik 2000). Recently, a fractional-order sliding mode control technique (Monje et al. 2010) has been successfully applied for a robot manipulator. In this chapter, we propose and realize a chattering-free fractional PD$^\alpha$ sliding-mode controller in the control of a robotic system driven by DC motors. The three most frequently used definitions for the general fractional differintegral are: Grunwald-Letnikov (GL), Riemann-Liouville (RL), and Caputo definitions (Hilfer 2000; Oldham and Spanier 1974; Podlubny 1999). Grunwald definition, (Podlubny 1999) suitable for numerical calculation, is given by

$$^{GL}D_a^\alpha f(t) = \lim_{h\to 0}\frac{1}{h^\alpha}\sum_{j=0}^{[(t-a)/h]}(-1)^j\binom{\alpha}{j}f(t-jh), \tag{12}$$

where a, t are the limits of operator and [x] means integer part of x. The left Riemann-Liouville (RL) definition of fractional derivative is given by

$$ {}_{a}^{RL}D_{t}^{\alpha}f(t) = \frac{1}{\Gamma(n-\alpha)}\frac{d^n}{dt^n}\int_{a}^{t}\frac{f(\tau)}{(t-\tau)^{\alpha-n+1}}d\tau, \quad (13) $$

for $(n-1 \leq \alpha < n)$ and for the case of $(\alpha > 0)$; the left fractional integral is defined by

$$ {}_{a}^{RL}D_{t}^{-\alpha}f(t) = \frac{1}{\Gamma(\alpha)}\int_{a}^{t}\frac{f(\tau)}{(t-\tau)^{1-\alpha}}d\tau, \quad (14) $$

where $\Gamma(.)$ is the well known Euler's gamma function. Also, there is another definition of the left fractional derivative introduced by Caputo (Kilbas et al. 2006; Podlubny 1999) as follows:

$$ {}_{a}^{C}D_{t}^{\alpha}f(t) = \frac{1}{\Gamma(n-\alpha)}\int_{a}^{t}\frac{f^{(n)}(\tau)}{(t-\tau)^{\alpha-n+1}}d\tau, \quad n-1 < \alpha < n. \quad (15) $$

3.1 FOPID Control for Robotic System

Our objective of using FC is to apply the fractional order controller to enhance the system control performance especially in the field of medical and service robotics and applications. For example, neurosurgery was one of the first organ systems in which robotic surgery was introduced, due to the high precision required to localize and manipulate within the brain and the relatively fixed landmarks of the cranial anatomy. Several robotic systems which serve in surgery are: Puma, Neuromate, Minerva, Rams, NeuroRobot, Unimation PUMA 200, CyberKnife, as well as the Neuro Arm Robot which is the world's first Magnetic Resonance Imaging (MRI) compatible surgical robot designed to work inside the powerful magnet of an MRI (Karas and Baig 2008). Also, one of these robotic systems capable of operating in human friendly environments is *NeuroArm Manipulator System*, Fig. 3.

In particular, it is used here as a basic robotic system with 3 DOF's, driven by DC motors, where an end-effector orientation will not be considered, but only its position in space. Simulation studies have been carried out to verify the effectiveness of the proposed fractional order PID (FOPID) controller tuned by genetic algorithms (GA) for robot control. Both, the FOPID and the integer order IOPID, controllers are designed on the basis of the proposed GA. Rodriguez' method (Čović and Lazarević 2009) is proposed for modeling kinematics and dynamics of

Fig. 3 Laboratory Robot—NeuroArm MS, Department of Mechanics, Fac. of Mech. Eng., UB

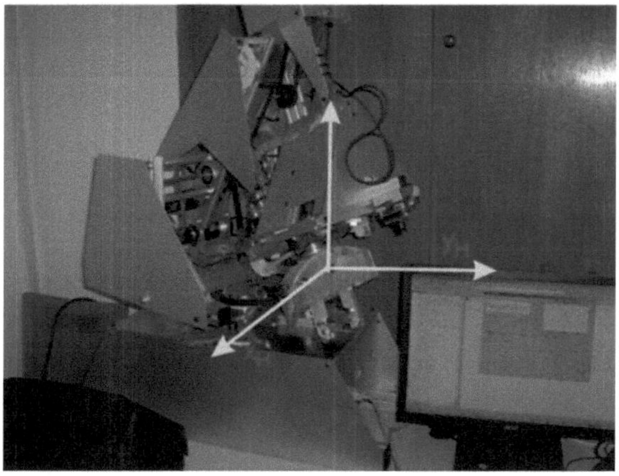

the holonomic (bio)robotic system which possesses n degrees of freedom $(q) = (q_1, q_2, \ldots, q_n)^T$. For automated setting of analytical expressions dedicated to equations of motions of (bio)robotic system can be obtained using modified Lagrange's equation of second kind in the identical covariant form as follows

$$\sum_{\alpha=1}^{n} a_{\alpha\gamma}(q)\ddot{q}^{\alpha} + \frac{\partial}{\partial q^{\beta}}\left[E_{k(\gamma)} - E_{k(n-\gamma)}\right] + \sum_{\beta\neq\gamma}^{n}\frac{\partial}{\partial q^{\beta}}\left(\sum_{\alpha=1}^{n} a_{\alpha\gamma}\dot{q}_{\alpha}\right)\dot{q}^{\beta} = Q_{\gamma},\ \gamma = 1, 2, \ldots, n \tag{16}$$

where $E_{k(\gamma)}$ is kinetic energy of a system (with 1 DOF's where $\dot{q}_\alpha = 0,\ \alpha \neq \gamma$) and $E_{k(n-\gamma)}$ is kinetic energy of a sub-system with $n - 1$ DOF's from the whole system with n DOF's, $(\dot{q}_\gamma = 0)\gamma = 1, 2, \ldots n$ as well as coefficients $a_{\alpha\beta}$ denote covariant coordinates of basic metric tensor $[a_{\alpha\beta}] \in R^{n\times n}, \Gamma_{\alpha\beta,\gamma};\ \alpha, \beta, \gamma = 1, 2, \ldots, n$ present Christoffel's symbols of first kind and Q_i are generalized forces. The time equation of the FOPID controller is given by:

$$u(t) = K_p e(t) + K_{d0} D_t^{\alpha} e(t) + K_{i0} D_t^{-\beta} e(t), \tag{17}$$

where it is proposed to use GA for determination of the five optimal parameters $K_p, K_d, K_i, \alpha, \beta$ of fractional order PID controllers. The optimality criterion, which involves besides steady state error e, i.e. IAE, integral of absolute value of the error, overshoot P_o, as well as settling time T_s, is introduced (Lazarević et al. 2013).

$$J = |P_0| + T_s + \int |e| dt \rightarrow min. \tag{18}$$

All GA parameters are arranged as follows: population size: $N = 100$; cross-over probability: $p_c = 0.75$; mutation probability: $p_m = p_{m0}\min(1, l/g)$, $p_{m0} = 0.1$—initial mutation probability, $l = 25$—generation threshold, g—current number of generation, generation gap $gr = 0.35$. As the selection method,

Table 1 The optimal parameters of the FOPID, IOPID

Controller		K_p	K_i	K_d	β	α	J_{opt}
PID	1.	199	2	24	–	–	0.98651
	2.	212	2	26	–	–	0.84875
	3.	246	1	28	–	–	0.68718
FOPID	4.	199	2	24	0.020	0.965	0.69887
	5.	212	2	26	0.145	0.933	0.72954
	6.	246	1	28	0.135	0.932	0.56187

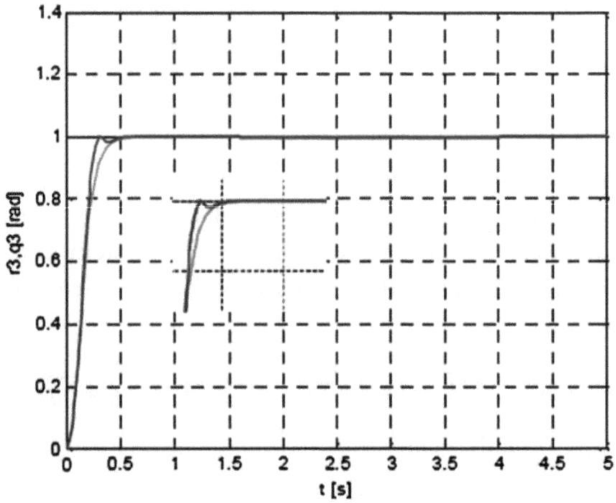

Fig. 4 The step responses of the $q_3(t)$ $[rad]$

remainder stochastic sampling with replacement is used. For calculation of fractional derivatives and integrals the Crone approximation of the second order was used (Monje 2010).

In Table 1, the optimal parameters of the FOPID as well as IOPID controller using GA are presented. In the simulations, step responses of these two optimal FOPID/IOPID controllers are compared.Here they are presented only for $q_3(t)$ in Fig. 4, where one can observed better performance of the robot control using FOPID.

Also, a chattering-free fractional PD$^\alpha$ sliding-mode controller in the control of an RS driven by DC motors is proposed (Batalov et al. 2012). It is well-known that the sliding-mode control is used to obtain high-performance robust control insensitive to disturbances and parameter variations. A nonlinear MIMO (bio)robotic system is represented in a more general form:

$$\dot{x} = f(x) + \tilde{f}(x) + \left[G(x) + \tilde{G}(x)\right]u, \tag{19}$$

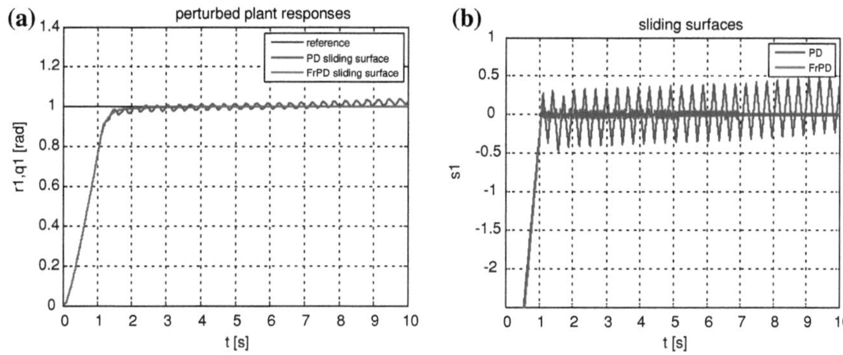

Fig. 5 Stabilization by using the sliding mode control PD and fractional PD^{α}. **a** Perturbed plant response q_1[rad]. **b** Sliding surface s_1 (perturbed case)

where $\tilde{f}(x)$ and $\tilde{G}(x)$ represent uncertainties or unknown plant dynamics. General sliding mode control law is (Edwards 1998)

$$u = -[\Lambda G(x)]^{-1}\Lambda[f(x) - \dot{x}_d] - [\Lambda G(x)]^{-1}Q\text{sgn}(s), \tag{20}$$

where switching surfaces s are defined as $s = \Lambda(x - x_d), x_d$ being the vector of the desired states and Q is positive definite diagonal matrix. In most cases, this leads to good results, but there are some disadvantages such as the chattering phenomenon. To overcome this problem, application of the fractional sliding surface is suggested in order to decrease output signal oscillations. For a 3-DOF's RS, a conventional sliding manifold is of the first order PD structure $s_i = d\tilde{x}_i/dt + \lambda_i\tilde{x}_i$, $i = 1, 2, 3$ where $\tilde{x}_i = x_i - x_{id}$ and here we propose a fractional PD^{α} structure as follows:

$$s_i = d^{\alpha}\tilde{x}_i/dt^{\alpha} + \lambda_i\tilde{x}_i,\ i = 1, 2, 3. \tag{21}$$

The simulations were performed for $\alpha = 0.95$, with matrix $Q_{nom} = diag(5, 5, 5)$ as well as $\lambda = (5, 2.5, 2.5)^T$. To verify the robustness of the proposed fractional sliding/mode control, we have applied the parameter variations as follows:

$$\frac{\Delta m_i}{m_i}, i = 1, 2, 3 \sim [9.5\,\% - 10\,\%],\ \frac{\Delta K_i}{K_i} \sim [5\,\% - 20\,\%],\quad \frac{\Delta J_i}{J_i} \sim [9\,\% - 18\,\%]. \tag{22}$$

The simulation results are shown in Fig. 5. It presents the comparison of the results obtained for the first coordinate q_1 responses to perturbation with the *PD* and fractional PD^{α}, with all other conditions being the same.

It can be seen from the previous figures that the sliding mode control with fractional sliding surface is more robust to parameter perturbations. It is most important to emphasize that the output oscillations are almost completely attenuated and the overall quality of the transient response is much better.

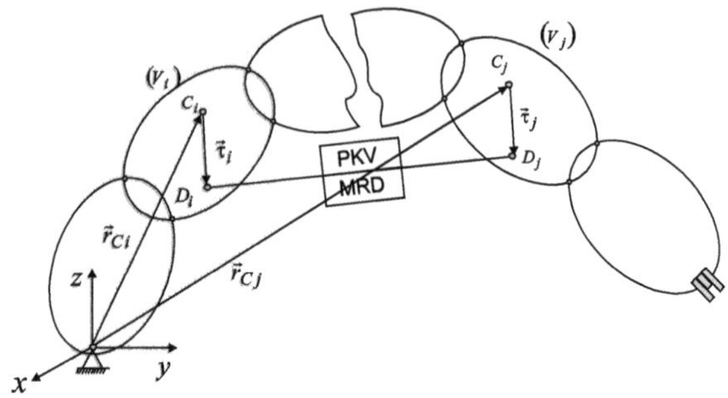

Fig. 6 Multibody robotic system with an MRD element

Table 2 Values of parameters of the MR element

MRD	Value
l_o	70 cm
u	1 V
μ_o	50 Ns/cm
μ	10 Ns/cm · V
E_c	25 N/cm

3.2 Fractional Order Modeling of (Bio)robotic System

Recently, some efforts have been devoted to obtaining better models of (bio) robotic systems by applying FC (Cajić et al. 2013; Lazarević and Bucanović 2012). Spring, damper, or actuator elements are often used in multibody systems to improve their characteristics. Such systems can be found in (bio)robotics. In particular, generalized forces of the robotic system (see Fig. 6) in which two different bodies in the system are connected with magnetorheological damping element (MRD) are considered and obtained. MRD is described by fractional order derivative model, where the force of viscoelasticity is given by force-dilatation relation of Kelvin-Voigt type by introducing the RL fractional order derivative $D^{\lambda}(x)$ (Cajić et al. 2013)

$$F_{mr} = E_c \cdot x + E_m D^{\mu}(x), \quad E_m = (\mu_o + u \cdot \mu), \tag{23}$$

where x is dilatation of the element, F_{mr} is force of the MRD element, E_c, E_m are coefficients, u is the voltage applied to MRD element, μ_o is the initial constant of the MR fluid, and $\mu = \mu(u)$ is parameter of MR fluid which varies linearly with u, see Table 2.

Dilatation of the MRD element $x\left(q^i(t), q^{i+1}(t), \ldots, q^k(t)\right)$ is equal to the difference of the instantaneous length l of the elements and constant initial length l_0. It is a composite function depending on the generalized coordinates $q^j(t)$, $j = 1, 2, 3\ldots$ which are time-dependent functions. Generalized forces of the MRD element can be determined as follows

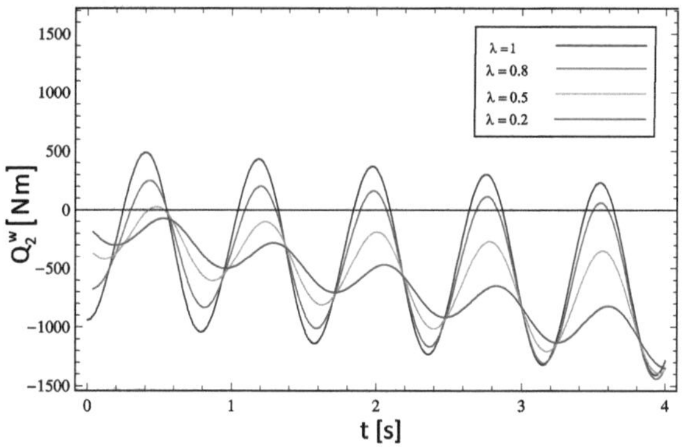

Fig. 7 Generalized force Q_2^w of the MRD element for different values of fractional order λ

$$Q_\beta^w = -\left[E_c x \frac{\vec{l}}{l}\frac{\partial\left(\vec{l}\right)}{\partial q^\beta} + E_m \cdot \frac{\vec{l}}{l}\frac{\partial\left(\vec{l}\right)}{\partial q^\beta} \cdot D^\lambda(x)\right]; \quad \vec{l} = \overrightarrow{D_i D_j} \tag{24}$$

In Fig. 7 one can see values of Q_2^w of the MRD element for different values of fractional order λ. It can be seen that by changing the fractional order of derivative one can obtain values in the region which is unavailable if using the integer order derivative models.

4 Conclusions

A kind of biologically inspired control of a redundant robotic system which allows resolving actuator redundancy is presented. A suggestion is given for obtaining a class of control synergy, arising from the theory of optimal actuator behavior. The actuator redundancy control problem has been discussed within the framework of the optimal control problem which is solved by Pontryagin's maximum principle. Usefulness of the idea of biologically inspired control synergy has been tested by its applications to a suitable redundant actuation robot with 3DOF's and 4 control variables. Also, advanced fractional order PID controllers are introduced and proposed for control of robotic system with 3 DOFs. From the comparison made, we conclude that the optimal FOPID controller, tuned by genetic algorithms, gives better performance for robot control compared to the optimal IOPID controller method. It is shown that a sliding mode control with the fractional sliding surface is more robust to the parameter perturbations and output oscillations, which are almost completely attenuated, and the overall quality of the transient response is much better. Finally, in the case of modeling of (bio)robotic system with MRD elements, it is possible to investigate the influence on the generalized forces of MRD by changing the system parameters, including fractional order parameter.

Acknowledgments The support of the Ministry of Education, Science and Technological Development of the Republic of Serbia through projects TR 35006, 41006 is gratefully acknowledged.

References

Astrom, K. and T. Hagglund: PID controllers: theory, design, and tuning, Instrument Society of America, North Carolina (1995)

Bar-Cohen,Y.: Biomimetics-Biologically Inspired Technologies, CRC Press, Taylor & Francis Group, Boca Raton:FL, pp.399–425 (2006)

Batalov S.A, M. Lazarevic,A.Hace, K. Jezernik,A Chattering-free Fractional PDa Sliding-mode Control of a 3-DOF Robot System Driven by DC motors, 5'th FDA2012, pp.77,Nanjing, China,May 20, (2012)

Bernstein,A.:The Coordination and Regulation of Movements,Oxford Perg., 77–92 (1961)

Cajić,M. Lazarević,M.,and T.Latinović: Equations of motion of robotic system with piezo-modified viscoelastic and magnetorheological elements of fractional order,S.7.1,-GAMM2013,Novi Sad,Serbia,(2013)

Chen, D. Xue, H. Dou:Fractional calculus and biomimetic control, in Proc. IEEE International Conference on Robotics and Biomimetics,Shenyang, China, Aug., pp. 901–906 (2004)

Čović, V., Lazarević, M.: Mechanics of robots, Faculty of Mechanical engineering, University of Belgrade, (in Serbian), (2009)

Edwards,C., Spurgeon,S.K.:Sliding mode control theory and applications, Taylor & Fran., NewYork, (1998)

Geng Fan Wu,Zhi-Yong:Coordinating control of multiple rigid bodies based on motion primi tives, Acta Mech. Sin., 28(2):482–489 (2012)

Gering,H., Guzzella,L., Hepener,S., Onder,C.: Time optimal motions of robots in assembly tasks, IEEE Transactions on Automatic Control, AC-31,(6):512–518 (1986)

Grinyagin,I.V., Biryukova,E.V., Maier,M.A.: Kinematic and Dynamic Synergies of Human Precision-Grip Movements, J Neurophysiol.,94: 2284–2294 (2004)

Hace,A., Jezernik,K.,: Robust position tracking control for direct drive motor, Industrial Electronics Society, 2000. IECON 2000. 26th Annual Confjerence of the IEEE, (2000)

Harkegard O, S. T. Glad:,Resolving actuator redundancy-optimal control vs. control allocation, Automatica 41, pp.137–144 (2005)

Hilfer R: Applications of Fractional Calculus in Physics,World Scientific, NJ, USA, (2000)

Karas and Baig: Robotic Neurosurgery,in Medical Robotics, ISBN: 978-3-902613-18-9, InTech Europe,(2008)

Kilbas, A.A., Srivastava, H.M., Trujillo, J.J. Theory and Applications of Fractional Differential Equations. Elsevier, Amsterdam (2006)

Klug,S.,Lens,T.,Von Stryk,O, Mohl,B.,Karguth,A.: Biologically Inspired Robot Manipulator for New Applications in Autom. Eng. Proc.of Robotik 2008,Munich,Germany,11–12 (2008)

Lathash,M.: Control of human movement, Human Kinetics Publishers (1994)

Latash,M.L.: Synergy, Oxford University Press US, pp.432 (2008)

Lazarević,M.P.: Finite time stability analysis of PD^{α} fractional control of robotic time-delay systems, Mech. Resch.Commun., 33, pp.269–279 (2006)

Lazarević M.,A.Obradović,T. Latinović:Bio-Inspired Control of Redundant Robotic Systems Optimization Approach, Scientific Technical Review,Vol.62,No.3-4,pp.45–54 (2012)

Lazarević, M. :Fractional Order Control of a Robot System Driven by DC Motors, Scientific Technical Review,Vol.62,No.2,pp.20–29 (2012)

Lazarević P.M., Lj. Bucanović: Contribution to modeling and dynamical analysis of fractional order systems with basis of fractional calculus, Monograph (in Serbian) (Mechanical Engineering Faculty, University of Belgrade, Belgrade (2012).

Lazarević M., S.Batalov, T.Latinović, Fractional PID Controller Tuned by Genetic Algorithms for a Three DOF's Robot System Driven by DC motors, 6th Workshop on Fractional Differentiation and Its Applications Part of 2013 IFAC Joint Conference SSSC Grenoble, France, February 4-6, pp.380–385 (2013)
Monje,C.A., et al.: Fractional-order Systems and Controls, Springer - Verlag, London, (2010)
Oldham K B and J. Spanier:The Fractional Calculus: Theory and Applications of Differentiation and Integration to Arbitrary Order, Academic Press,New York, NY,USA (1974)
Podlubny, I.,: Fractional Differential Equations, Academic Press,San Diego,(1999)
Romanovas,M. Traechtler, M. L. Klingbeil and Y. Manoli: On fractional models for human motion tracking, Journal of Vibration and Control, DOI: 10.1177/1077546313479637,(2013)
Sabatier J., O.Agrawal, J.Atenreiro Machado: Advances in Fractional Calculus, Theoretical Developments and Applications in Physics and Engineering,Springer (2007)
Schanzer,G, Callies,R.: Multiple constrained rivaling actuators in the optimal control of miniaturized manipulators, Multibody System Dynamics, 19:21–43 (2008)
Sehoon, Oh and Yoichi Hori: Fractional Order Impedance Control by Particle Swarm Optimization International Conference on Control, Automation and Systems,Oct. 14–17, 2008 in COEX, Seoul, Korea (2008)
Vepa,R.: Biomimetic Robotics-mechanisms and control, Cambridge University Press, (2009)
Webb,B.: Can robots make good models of biological behaviour? Behav. Brain Sci. 24, 24:1033–1094 (2001)

Towards Sensor-Less Haptic Teleoperation

A. Hace and M. Franc

Abstract This chapter presents an approach that leads toward sensorless haptic teleoperation. Such implementation requires no external sensor that can deteriorate system dynamics and performance. The position information, as well as force information, that are required in order to provide high-performance bilateral control, is provided by using miniature analog Hall sensors. Such sensors might be already built within the motor housing. The $\alpha\beta$-tracker has been applied in order to provide velocity information. The motion data estimation has been furthermore improved by introducing PLL concept into the $\alpha\beta$-tracker. The enhanced $\alpha\beta$-tracker provides not only better noise insensitivity but also simplified calculation algorithm that presents significant contribution for implementation. The force information is provided by external force observer that requires no force sensor and extends the sensing bandwidth. The applied algorithms were validated by the 1-DoF experimental system for bilateral control. It has been shown that the proposed pseudo-sensorless implementation enables haptic-based teleoperation.

Keywords Haptic teleoperation · Bilateral control · Pseudo sensor-less · Motion data acqusition · Force observer

1 Introduction

Robotic surgery has been strongly developing in practice in last decade. It aims to so-called Minimal Invasive Surgery (MIS), i.e. performing surgery with minimal injury to the body. In practice, MIS robotic systems are widely used worldwide by

A. Hace (✉)
University of Maribor, Mežica, Slovenia
e-mail: ales.hace@uni-mb.si

M. Franc
Isomat d.o.o, Mežica, Slovenia
e-mail: marko.franc@uni-mb.si

A. Rodić et al. (eds.), *New Trends in Medical and Service Robots*,
Mechanisms and Machine Science 20, DOI: 10.1007/978-3-319-05431-5_16,

hospitals, though they do not provide the force reflection. However, force feedback and haptic information are highly desirable during robotic surgery. They could be assured by so called bilateral teleoperation that generally denotes the control of remotely located machines (Sheridan 1992). In practice, it is widely used when humans are unable to perform certain tasks, or if human operators want to improve a manual task execution (Hokayem and Spong 2006). Such teleoperation aims to give the human operator a feeling of being physically present at the remote place by providing haptic feedback (Lawrence 1993). However, the remote place is not always physical distant, it may mean a place that is from some reason inaccessible for human operator.

Haptic fidelity during the bilateral teleoperation is strongly desired. This property is highly related to the quality of the position and force information (Yokokohji and Yoshikawa 1994). Typically, these data are acquired by external sensors. In practice, low-cost external sensors, i.e. force sensor or optical encoders, may be applied. They generally provide low-resolution measurement and/or low sampling rate that will inherently reduce sensing bandwidth. Though dedicated sensors may be applied (Puangmali et al. 2012), they present additional costs and also complicate mechanical design. Nevertheless, such sensor-based system configuration can deteriorate the teleoperator performance.

In this chapter we focus on a pseudo-sensorless implementation of a bilateral teleoperation system that contains no external sensor, neither for position/velocity nor external force information that are, however, all required for high performance bilateral control; hence the size and mass of the slave device can be reduced and the teleoperator performance enhanced. In order to obtain pseudo-sensorless operation, we propose the use of analog Hall sensors that are built within the electrical motor housing, along with the algorithm for position computation (Hace and Franc 2014). Furthermore, we propose the use of $\alpha\beta$ tracker for velocity estimation from the position information since traditional methods for velocity estimation could introduce control delay and inaccuracy, and may involve computational load, difficulty in preserving transients and in tuning, and therefore prevent to achieve high bilateral control performance required for haptic-based teleoperation. The information for the external forces is obtained by disturbance observer structure (Katsura et al. 2007). We also present the control algorithm for bilateral teleoperation that is derived using sliding mode control design and modal decomposition. The control algorithm and data acquisition algorithms are implemented by FPGA (Hace and Franc 2013). The presented implementation is experimentally validated.

2 Bilateral Control in Virtual Modes

In this chapter, a robust algorithm for bilateral teleoperation was utilized in order to cope with uncompensated disturbance and model perturbations. The control is performed in the virtual modal space that enables the design within the independent

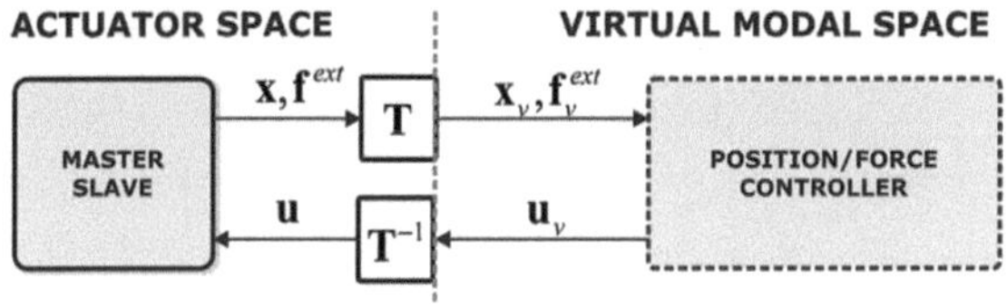

Fig. 1 Modal transformation

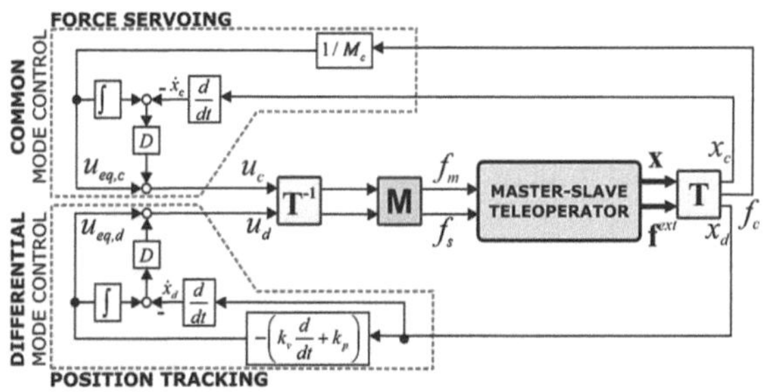

Fig. 2 The control algorithm block scheme for bilateral teleoperation

coordinates (see Fig. 1). The actuator signals are transformed into the virtual modes that involve a common mode and a differential mode for force servoing and position tracking, respectively (Ohnishi 2010).

The robust bilateral control algorithm block scheme is depicted by Fig. 2. It has been derived by sliding mode control design procedure (Hace and Franc 2013). Efficient disturbance rejection is assured by the practically model-free robust controller. The control law is governed by

$$\mathbf{f} = \mathbf{M}\mathbf{T}^{-1}\mathbf{u} \tag{1}$$

$$\mathbf{u} = \mathbf{u}_{eq} + D\left(\int_0^t \mathbf{u}_{eq} dt - \dot{\mathbf{x}}_v\right) \tag{2}$$

where $\mathbf{u} = [u_c, \quad u_d]^T$ and $\mathbf{u}_{eq} = [u_{eq,c}, u_{eq,d}]^T$, $u_{eq,c} = f_c/M_c$ and $u_{eq,d} = -(k_v \dot{x}_d + k_p x_d)$, $\mathbf{x}_v = \mathbf{T}\mathbf{x}$, $\mathbf{x} = [x_m, x_s]^T$,

$$\mathbf{T} = \begin{bmatrix} 1 & 1 \\ 1 & -1 \end{bmatrix}, \tag{3}$$

and $\mathbf{M} = \text{diag}(m_m, m_s)$ is the mass matrix of the bilateral teleoperator. m_m, m_s, x_{m}, x_{s}, f_m, and f_s are the masses, positions, and control forces of the master and the slave devices, respectively. x_c, x_d, f_c, and f_d depicts positions and forces in virtual modal space. u_c and u_d depicts control output that is given in acceleration dimension. Indexes $(.)_c$, and $(.)_d$ apply the common mode and the differential mode. The control

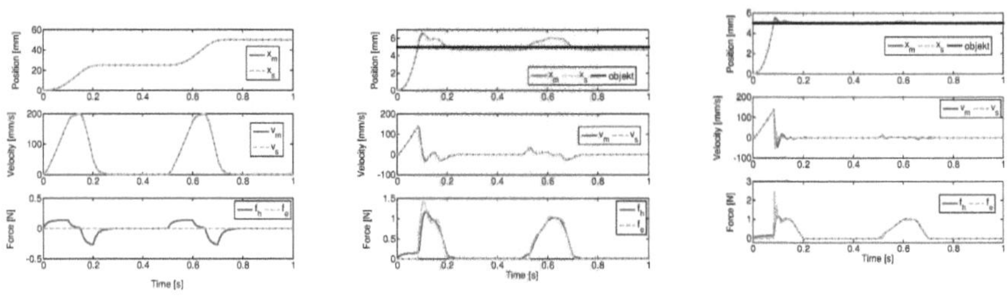

(a) (b) (c)

Fig. 3 Simulation results for free motion (**a**), soft object touching (**b**) and hard object touching (**c**)

parameters M_c, D, k_p, and k_v depict virtual mass, disturbance rejection parameter, position gain, and velocity gain, in virtual modes, respectively.

Figure 3 shows simulation results for bilateral teleoperation for free motion (Fig. 3a), soft environment touching (Fig. 3b), and hard environment touching (Fig. 3c). It is clearly shown that the presented bilateral control allows high performance bilateral teleoperation for unconstrained and constrained teleoperation. Moreover, such teleoperator enables remote haptic sense that is strongly desired for challenging task execution, i.e. robotic surgery.

3 Data Acquisition for Pseudo-Sensorless Bilateral Control

Bilateral control requires motion information as well as force information. The data acquisition regarding position, velocity, and force impacts on the teleoperator performance, i.e., poor or noisy signals can deteriorate the system performance. This section describes the data acquisition of the robot positions and velocities, and the external action and reaction forces, respectively.

Digital sensors are often used for position measurements, such as an incremental encoder or a digital Hall sensor. Incremental encoders may increase complexity of mechatronic design, and furthermore are sensitive to dust. Thus the performance may be deteriorated. The drawbacks of using external mechanical position sensor such as incremental encoder can be listed also in more detail: (1) numbers of connections between the motor and the controller, (2) interference increases, (3) limitations in accuracy of the sensor because of environmental factors such as temperature, humidity, vibration, (4) additional system cost including sensor and electronic circuit which is most meaningful when compared with a given level of resolution of the sensor, (5) volume and the moment of inertia increase. These problems can be avoided or significantly reduced with position (pseudo-) sensorless operation, e.g. by using built-in digital Hall sensors that are insensitive to severe environments like dust, water, oil, vibration and others; however, they suffer from low resolution. In order to overcome low resolution problem, analog Hall sensors present more advanced solution. Such a solution retains low-cost design and can provide sufficiently high resolution measurement (Hace and Franc 2014). Furthermore, analog Hall sensors may be integrated within the electrical motor housing. Then, such simplified mechanical structure eliminates framework friction and also solves the problem of performance degradation. In bilateral teleoperation, such design significantly contributes towards applications, such as MIS. This chapter presents pseudo-sensorless bilateral teleoperation without external sensor for position as well as force measurement.

3.1 Motion Data Acquisition

Servo linear motors can used as an advanced approach for laparoscopic devices (Navarro et al. 2010). A servo linear motor consists of a moving shaft with permanent magnets that are aligned to the pole pairs by the magnetic pitch τ_m. The Hall sensors may be integrated within the motor housing in order to measure the magnetic fields produced by the permanent magnets. The analog Hall sensor output three signals, u_1, u_2, and u_3.

$$\begin{aligned} u_1 &= \sin(\varphi) \\ u_2 &= \sin(\varphi + 2\pi/3) \\ u_3 &= \sin(\varphi - 2\pi/3) \end{aligned} \tag{4}$$

where $\varphi = 2\pi x_\tau/\tau_m$. The signals u_1, u_2, and u_3 are used for determining the shaft position by the following technique. The signals are transformed into the two phases u_a and u_b by using Clarke transformation

$$\begin{aligned} u_a &= \frac{2}{3}\left(u_1 - \frac{1}{2}u_2 - \frac{1}{2}u_3\right) \\ u_b &= \frac{2}{3}\left(\frac{\sqrt{3}}{2}u_2 - \frac{\sqrt{3}}{2}u_3\right) \end{aligned} \tag{5}$$

3.1.1 Direct Method

From u_a and u_b it is possible to calculate position information x_τ

$$x_\tau = \frac{\tau_m}{2\pi} \operatorname{a}\tan 2(u_a, u_b) \tag{6}$$

that refers to the absolute value within a magnetic pitch τ_m.

The algorithm (4)–(6) enables calculation of the linear motor shaft position within a single magnetic pitch. To calculate the motor's shaft position in a full range, the transitions between the magnetic pole pairs must be tracked such that position x is given by (7).

$$x = x_\tau + k\tau_m, \quad k = 0, \pm 1, \pm 2, \ldots \tag{7}$$

Motion control algorithms such as (1)–(3) besides position require also velocity information. In our case, position obtained by analog Hall sensors is combined with $\alpha\beta$-tracker in order to provide velocity information (Hace and Franc 2014).

The $\alpha\beta$-tracker is a simplified steady-state closed-form of the Kalman observer (Cunningham et al. 1992) that gives optimal state estimates for linear stochastic systems with additive Gaussian errors. The $\alpha\beta$-tracker can give sub-optimal estimates. It can also be viewed as a recursive filter and provides position as well as velocity estimation output. Furthermore, the $\alpha\beta$-tracker can provide satisfactory average characteristics over a wide-range. The simplicity and computational efficiency justify its use in many practical real-time engineering applications such as motion control.

The $\alpha\beta$-tracker assumes constant velocity during a single sampling interval. Thus, the position prediction $\tilde{x}_k$ $\hat{v}_k$ are given by the model

$$\tilde{x}_k = \hat{x}_{k-1} + T_s \hat{v}_{k-1} \tag{8}$$

$$\tilde{v}_k = \hat{v}_{k-1} \tag{9}$$

where $\hat{x}_{k-1}$ and $\hat{v}_{k-1}$ represents the estimated position and estimated velocity at past sample instance $k - 1$, respectively, and T_s is the sampling interval. The predicted position and predicted velocity are corrected by

$$\hat{x}_k = \tilde{x}_k + \alpha(x_k - \tilde{x}_k) \tag{10}$$

$$\hat{v}_k = \hat{v}_{k-1} + \beta/T_s(x_k - \tilde{x}_k) \tag{11}$$

where x_k, $\tilde{x}_k$, α, and β denote the measured position, predicted position, the position correction gain, and the velocity correction gain, respectively (Fig. 4).

The α and β correction gains are defined as positive constants and values are chosen such that the $\alpha\beta$ tracker addresses the limit Kalman filter ($0 < \alpha$ and $0 < \beta < \alpha^2/(2 - \alpha)$) (Cunningham et al. 1992). The choice of the gain values is a trade-off optimization problem between tracking accuracy and noise suppression capability. In order to guarantee an asymptotically stable response, α and β are selected within the range $0 < \alpha < 1$ and $0 < \beta < 4 - 2\alpha$, respectively, and for smooth convergence, selection of β can be further limited to $0 < \beta < 2 - \alpha$. The values in practice are typically adjusted empirically. In this chapter, the values are decided by the poles that the root-locus method provides for the transfer functions (12), and the desired cut-off frequency. The poles can be either real or complex.

$$\hat{v} = \frac{\beta z^2}{z^2 + (\alpha + \beta - 2)z + (1 - \alpha)} \frac{\Delta x}{T_s} \tag{12}$$

where Δx can be described in time domain as a position change in the past sampling interval $\Delta x = x_k - x_{k-1}$. Figure 5 shows total block scheme for motion data acquisition by direct method that involves position calculation and velocity estimation by $\alpha\beta$-tracker. It enables both position and velocity estimation outputs, respectively.

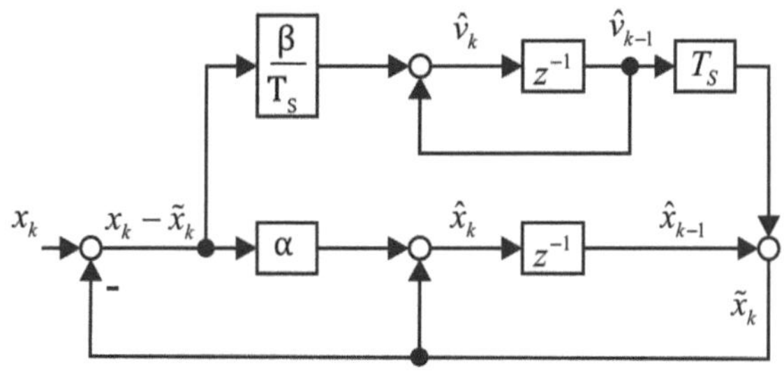

Fig. 4 Block scheme of the $\alpha\beta$-tracker for position and velocity estimation

3.1.2 PLL Method

The direct method for position and velocity estimation might be enhanced by combination of the PLL concept with the $\alpha\beta$-tracker (see Fig. 6). The PLL concept is known for excellent noise-rejection capability and has been utilized in motion control applications to achieve high-precision speed control (Hoang and Jeon 2011; Emura and Wang 2000). Thus, we involve the PLL concept in order to improve insensitivity to the signal noise.

We derive the so called PLL $\alpha\beta$-tracker from the general $\alpha\beta$-tracker structure presented in previous section. It is modified such that most salient features of the PLL concept is incorporated within its structure. The position input x of the $\alpha\beta$-tracker is replaced by sine and cosine waveforms u_{a} and u_{b}. Figure 7 depicts the PLL $\alpha\beta$-tracker block scheme. It has similar structure as the ordinary quadrature PLL block scheme in Fig. 6, which consist of: Phase Detector (PD), Low-pass Filter (LPF), and Voltage Controlled Oscillator (VCO).

PD in Fig. 6 implements a cross-product between the input pair of sinusoidal signals $[u_a, u_b]$ and the output pair of sinusoidal signals $[\sin(\tilde{x}), \cos(\tilde{x})]$. It consists of two multipliers and an adder that compute

$$x_e = u_a \cos(\tilde{x}) - u_b \sin(\tilde{x}) = \sin(x)\cos(\tilde{x}) - \cos(x)\sin(\tilde{x}) = \sin(x - \tilde{x}) \quad (13)$$

such that it provides error signal x_e that involves information about the phase correspondence. When $\tilde{x}$ follows x, such that $\tilde{x} \approx x$, the loop is said to be locked. In this case, x_e can be approximated by phase difference $x_e \approx x - \tilde{x}$.

The position velocity estimator (PVE) outputs position estimation $\hat{x}_k$, velocity estimation $\hat{v}_k$, and position prediction. Consequently, Eqs. (10) and (11) turns to (14) and (15).

$$\hat{x}_k = \tilde{x}_k + \alpha x_e \quad (14)$$

$$\hat{v}_k = \hat{v}_{k-1} + (\beta/T_s)x_e \quad (15)$$

The design of α and β can be selected similarly as within the Direct method. The cut-off frequency of the PVE has to be sufficiently high in order to provide the loop to be able to track the input signal. Otherwise, the loop would not be able to track the input signal and may fall out of the locked state. The VCO outputs sine

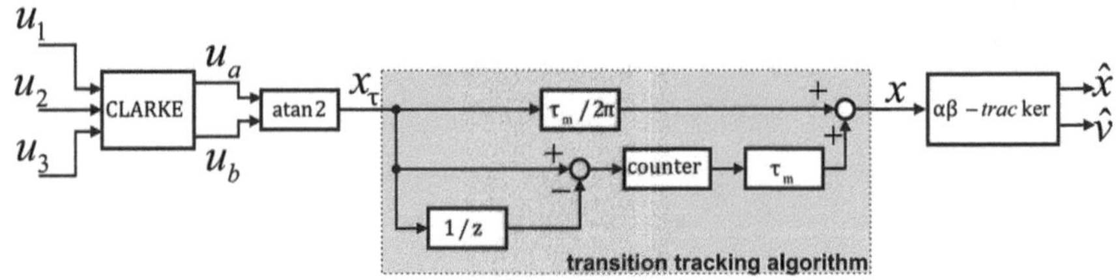

Fig. 5 Block scheme for motion data acquisition by direct method

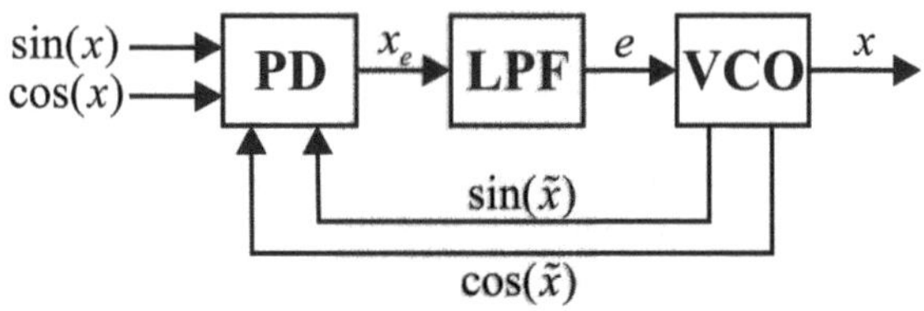

Fig. 6 Ordinary PLL block scheme

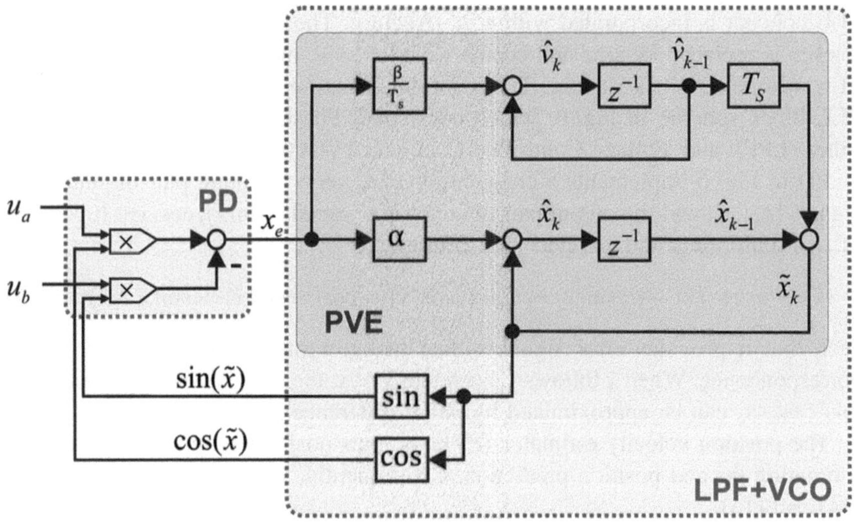

Fig. 7 PLL $\alpha\beta$-tracker block scheme

and cosine waveforms of its position argument $\tilde{x}_k$ such that output pair $[\sin(\tilde{x}), \cos(\tilde{x})]$ are locked on the input pair [sin(x), cos(x)]. When this is fulfilled, the PLL $\alpha\beta$-tracker can retain the locked state ($\tilde{x}$ is kept locked on x). It can retain locked state even in case of magnetic pole transition though signal is contaminated by noise. Therefore, the transition tracking algorithm is not necessary and the

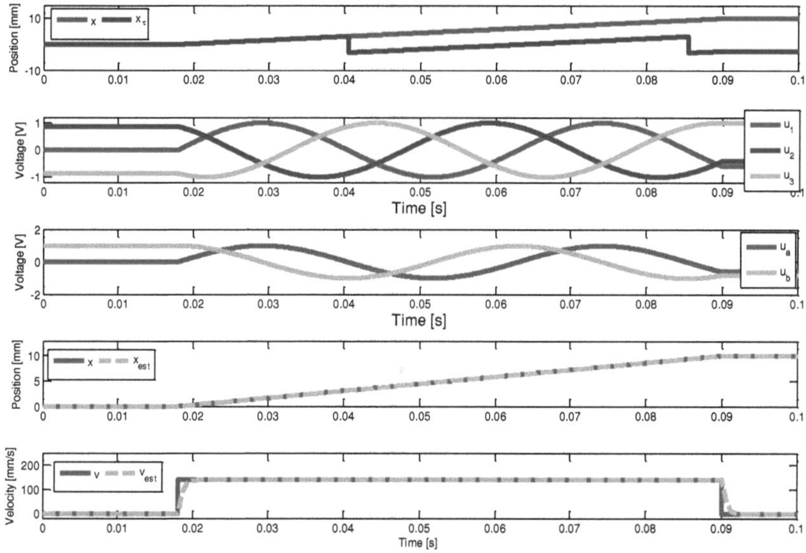

Fig. 8 Position and velocity estimation of the PLL $\alpha\beta$-tracker

dithering problem with multiple transitions is avoided. Consequently, the cut-off frequency of the $\alpha\beta$-tracker can be increased. Position and velocity information can be obtained with effective noise-rejection capability. Thus, it is possible to provide sufficiently wide sensing bandwidth in order to be able to achieve high-performance bilateral teleoperation. However, in order to provide correct position information, proper initial position value has to be set prior an effective operation (Fig. 8).

3.1.3 Comparison of the Methods

The PLL $\alpha\beta$-tracker offers important advantages over the direct method. A significant advantage is elimination of the transition tracking algorithm that is required for determination of shaft position in full range. Consequently, multiple transitions due to the noisy signals are avoided. Moreover, that also means less computing operations; they can cause severe computing noise in case of fixed point calculus by limited FPGA hardware resources (Franc and Hace 2013); position data that is contaminated by noise drastically deteriorates system performance. Hence, the PLL-based approach provides less computing noise and consequently improved system performance.

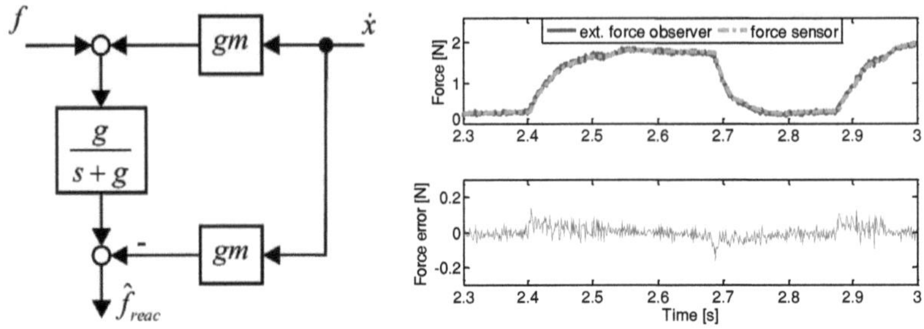

(a) (b)

Fig. 9 General disturbance observer block scheme (**a**) and observed and measured force (**b**)

3.2 Force Data Acquisition

The action operator force and the environment reaction force can be observed by the external force observer. Such an observation does not require a force sensor. Furthermore, it can also significantly widen the sensing bandwidth in comparison to external force sensor with strain gauge (Katsura et al. 2007).

The external force observer is based on the disturbance observer, which provides an estimation of the disturbance force using a low-pass filter. The estimation algorithm is described by

$$\hat{f}_{ext} = \frac{g}{s+g}(f - f_{dist} + gm\hat{v}) - gm\hat{v} \qquad (16)$$

where $f, \hat{f}_{ext}, f_{dist}, \dot{x}, m$, and g denote the control force, the estimated external force, the disturbance force, the velocity, the nominal mass, and the cut-off frequency, respectively. Figure 9a depicts a general external force observer block scheme. It can be applied on the master side, to estimate the operator action force, and on the slave side, to estimate the environment reaction force.

Figure 9b shows comparison between observed force (solid red line) and measured force using force sensor (dashed green line). It has been proven that the proposed PLL $\alpha\beta$-tracker provides sufficient velocity information for external force observation with relatively low error.

4 Results

In this section, validation of presented approach for bilateral teleoperation is presented. The presented approach was validated by both, simulation and experiments, respectively. Simulation includes comparison between direct method and PLL $\alpha\beta$-tracker. Experiments include unconstrained and constrained teleoperation.

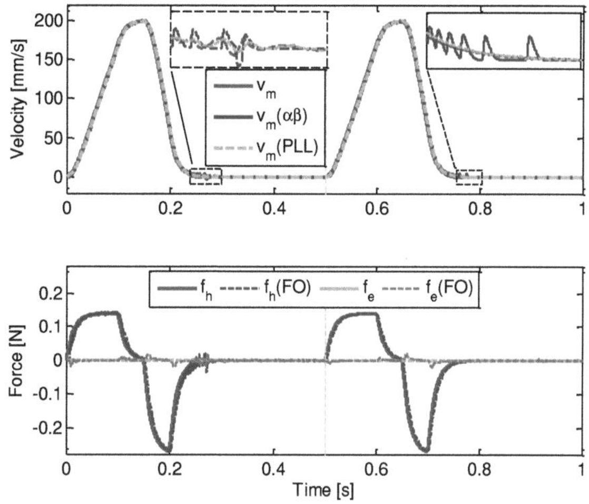

Fig. 10 Comparison results for bilateral teleoperation

4.1 Simulation Results

Figure 10 depicts simulation results of bilateral teleoperation for control parameters in Table 1. The top diagram shows true velocity signal and velocity signals computed by $\alpha\beta$-tracker and enhanced PLL method, respectively. The bottom diagram shows true external forces and computed external forces by the external force observers, respectively. The simulation case applies the $\alpha\beta$ tracker within the loop until 0.5 s and then switches to the enhanced PLL method. It is clearly shown that computing noise significantly deteriorates system performance in case of the $\alpha\beta$ tracker. Thus, the PLL $\alpha\beta$-tracker can provide better control stability and improved performance.

4.2 Experimental Setup

The performance of PLL $\alpha\beta$-tracker was experimentally validated by 1-DoF laboratory bilateral teleoperation system (Fig. 11). It consists of two identical 1-DoF robot mechanisms, the master device and the slave device. Each consists of a linear motor Faulhaber LM1247-080-01. The linear motor is equipped with three analog Hall sensors that are used for position and velocity estimation. The control force is applied to the input of the motor driver. The bilateral controller and data acquisition was implemented by NI PXI-7841R with FPGA Virtex-5. The logic configuration circuit and user interface was designed by LabVIEW using fixed point representation. FPGA design methodology has been presented in (Franc and Hace 2013).

Table 1 Manipulator and control parameters

Parameter	Value	Parameter	Value
Master device mass m_m	80 g	Position gain k_p	65,000 $1/s^2$
Slave device mass m_s	35 g	Velocity gain k_v	200 1/s
PLL $\alpha\beta$-tracker cut-off freq.	350 rad/s	Virtual mass M_c	35 g
Force observer cut-off freq. g	350 rad/s	Control period T_c	20 μs

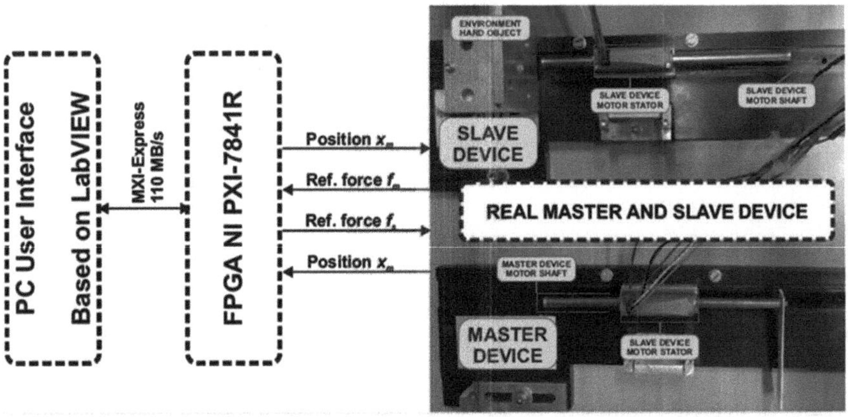

Fig. 11 Experimental test bed

4.3 Experimental Results

The validation of the achieved bilateral teleoperation performance includes the following experiments: free motion, touching the soft object, and touching the hard object. The manipulator and bilateral control parameters are depicted by Table 1.

The experimental results in time domain are displayed in Fig. 12. Figure 12a shows the results for the free motion, whereas Fig. 12b and c depict results for constrained motion in contact with a soft object and a hard object, respectively. As shown in Fig. 12a, excellent position tracking was achieved in the free motion. However, low action and reaction forces were observed, due to non-compensated friction. When the slave device was in contact with the soft object (Fig. 12b), excellent force tracking was achieved simultaneously with position tracking.

In case of hard object contact (Fig. 12c), the slave position trajectory follows the master position trajectory with low position tracking error. On the other hand, excelent force tracking was achieved. The main causes for position tracking error are: (1) limited bandwidth of the commercially available motor driver that was applied in the experimental setup, which allows only relatively low sampling rate of the control input signal, and (2) the imperfect measurement of the input signals that are contaminated with the system noise. Consequently, the relatively low internal actuator force dynamics, that has not been considered within our control

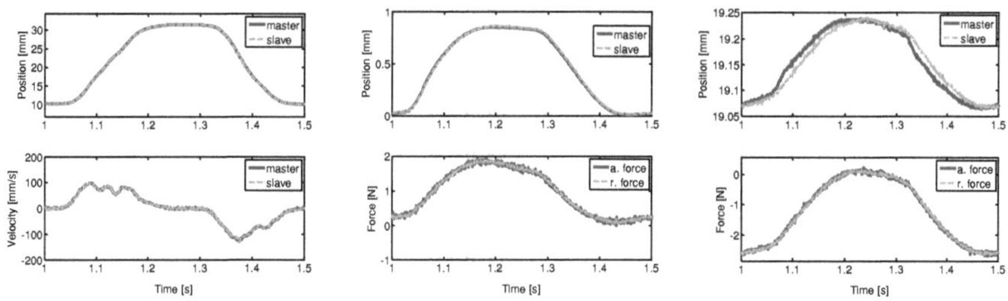

Fig. 12 Bilateral teleoperation experiment for free motion (**a**), touching the soft object (**b**) and touching the hard object (**c**)

design, prevents high-dynamic transmission of the environmental impedance that is required in the case of hard object contact in order to provide haptic sense with high-fidelity. The maximum transmitted impedance of the teleoperator is thus lower then the stiffness of the hard object. Therefore, the teleoperator is not perfectly transparent; mainly due to the relatively low internal driver-actuator dynamics. Thus, the human operator feels the hard object softer than it is. Nevertheless, the teleoperator is highly transparent in case of soft objects.

5 Conclusions

The chapter studies a bilateral control method implementation that leads toward sensorless-based haptic teleoperation. Position was obtained by using miniature analog Hall sensors, velocity by a PLL $\alpha\beta$-tracker and force by the force observer. In comparison with the conventional $\alpha\beta$-tracker, the PLL $\alpha\beta$-tracker provides simplification and elimination of the transition tracking algorithm; thus, dither was avoided. The enhanced approach provides better signal-noise ratio. This is important in high-performance control design; it leads to less delay in a feedback signal and thus higher control bandwidth that is strongly desired. Furthermore, the proposed algorithm leads towards more optimal hardware resources consumption that is extremely important where hardware resources are limited. The proposed algorithm was validated by a simple experimental system with no external sensor for position, velocity or force acquisition. Experimental results showed that the proposed approach allows bilateral teleoperation with high haptic performance.

References

E. P. Cunningham, "Digital Filtering: An Introduction," Houghton Mifflin Company, Boston 1992.

T. Emura, and L. Wang, "A high-resolution interpolator for incremental encoders based on the quadrature PLL method", IEEE Trans. on Industrial Electronics, vol. 47, no. 1, pp. 84–90, feb. 2000.

M. Franc, and A. Hace, "A Study on the FPGA Implementation of the Bilateral Control Algorithm Towards Haptic Teleoperation", Automatika, vol. 54, no. 1, pp. 49–61, 2013.

A. Hace, and M. Franc, "Pseudo-Sensorless High Performance Bilateral Teleoperation by Sliding Mode Control and FPGA", in IEEE Trans. Mechatronics, vol. 19, no. 1, 2014.

A. Hace, and M. Franc, "FPGA Implementation of Sliding Mode Control Algorithm for Scaled Bilateral Teleoperation," IEEE Trans. Industrial Informatics, vol. 9., no. 3, pp. 1291–1300, 2013.

H. V. Hoang, and J. W. Jeon, "An Efficient Approach to Correct the Signals and Generate High-Resolution Quadrature Pulses for Magnetic Encoders" IEEE Trans. Industrial Electronics, vol. 58, no. 8 pp. 3634–3646, aug. 2011.

P. F. Hokayem, and M. W. Spong", Bilateral teleoperation: An historical survey," Automatica, vol. 42, pp. 2035–2057, Dec. 2006.

S. Katsura, Y. Matsumoto, and K. Ohnishi, "Modeling of Force Sensing and Validation of Disturbance Observer for Force Control," IEEE Trans. Industrial Electronics, vol. 54, no. 1, pp. 530–538, Feb. 2007.

D. A. Lawrence, "Stability and transparency in bilateral teleoperation", IEEE Trans. on Robotics and Automation, vol. 9, no. 5, pp. 624–637, 1993.

J. S. Navarro, N. Garcia, C. Perez, E. Fernandez, R. Saltaren, M. Almonacid, "Kinematics of a robotic 3UPS1S spherical wrist designed for laparoscopic applications", Int. J. of Medical Robotics and Computer Assisted Surgery, vol. 6, pp. 291–300, May 2010.

K. Ohnishi, "Real world haptics and telehaptics for medical applications", Proc. of IEEE Int. Symposium on Industrial Electronics ISIE 2010.

P. Puangmali, H. Liu, L. D. Seneviratne, P. Dasgupta, and K. Althoefer, "Miniature 3-Axis Distal Force Sensor for Minimally Invasive Surgical Palpation," IEEE/ASME Trans. Mechatronics, vol. 17, no. 4, pp. 646–656, Aug. 2012.

T. B. Sheridan, "Telerobotics Automation & Human", MIT Press, 1992.

Y. Yokokohji, and T.Yoshikawa, "Bilateral Control of Master-Slave Manipulations for Ideal Kinesthetic Coupling – Formulation and Experiment," IEEE Trans. on Robotics and Automation, vol.10, no.5, pp.605–620, Oct. 1994.

Brain Incorporation of Artificial Limbs and Role of Haptic Feedback

A. Sengul, S. Shokur and H. Bleuler

Abstract We—as humans—can learn to use tools like hammers, tennis rackets, scalpels or robotic arms. Learning curves to become proficient in using the tools can be very different. Typical questions for learning use of a new tool are the level of complexity in manipulation, i.e. learning time and the ergonomy. We ask here these questions from a cognitive neuroscience perspective: How can we promote fast and natural embodiment of a tool? What are the neuronal mechanisms underlying quick and "natural" incorporation of a tool into the sensory-motor system, with the purpose of gaining proficiency rapidly and efficiently? This approach could benefit practically e.g. design of surgical telemanipulators and at the same time advance knowledge about the sensori-motor control system and learning mechanisms, a topic of interest in neuroprosthetics. We review both behavioral and neurophysiological data and show the importance of a coherent haptic feedback for the emergence of embodiment. We will also present a test platform for studying the mechanisms of incorporation by using advanced haptic interfaces on the master-side and VR environments on the slave side of a telemanipulator aimed at endoscopic surgery.

Keywords Embodiment · Tool incorporation · Haptic interface · Telemanipulation · Force feedback

A. Sengul (✉) · S. Shokur · H. Bleuler
STI IMT, Ecole Polytechnique Fédérale de Lausanne, Lausanne, Switzerland
e-mail: ali.sengul@epfl.ch

S. Shokur
Edmond and Lily Safra International Institute of Neuroscience of Natal, Natal, Brazil

A. Rodić et al. (eds.), *New Trends in Medical and Service Robots*,
Mechanisms and Machine Science 20, DOI: 10.1007/978-3-319-05431-5_17,

1 Introduction

One of the fundamental roles of the human brain is the self-representation of the subject's body (Gallese et al. 2004). There are two different notions about body representation, body image and body schema (Hoffmann et al. 2010). Body image refers to perceptual representation of one's own body, while body schema refers to spatial representations of one's own body, such as length of limb segments and the position of the limb in space. Body representation is plastic and can be changed over time. Examples from neurological disorders that show disembodiment of body parts as well as experimental manipulation of body perception or incorporation of tools, and prostheses illustrate that the unitary sense of one's body can be modified or manipulated (Giummarra et al. 2008). A classical multisensory illusion, known as the rubber hand illusion, shows the plasticity of body representation. Simultaneous tactile stimuli to a visible rubber hand and to the hidden subject's hand induce the feeling that the rubber hand was in someway one's own hand (Botvinick and Cohen 1998).

The rubber hand illusion shows a change in the brain's body representation that occurs to accommodate the new fake arm. This mechanism is also called neuroplasticity. An MRI study by Ehrsson et al. (2005) showed that multisensory areas like intraparietal sulcus and ventral premotor cortex were more active in the case of the illusion. Recent neurophysiological study by our groups showed in addition implication of sensory-motor area in the genesis of the rubber hand illusion (Shokur et al. 2013; Ifft et al. 2013). These studies suggest that the rubber hand illusion induces cortical reorganization. We believe that this method can be used for increasing the ownership of the neuroprostethetics devices for amputee patients. Simultaneous stroking with visual stimuli would trick the brain into embodying the prosthetic arms.

Ehrsson et al. (2008) showed how to increase embodiment of prosthetic arms with simultaneous stroking. They studied whether upper limp amputees could feel the rubber hand illusion. Based on the findings of this study, new prostheses could be designed in a way to integrate a touch sensor on the stump, which would help integrate the artificial arm into body image by creating an illusion. Marasco et al. (2011) showed that robotic touch helps amputee patients to restore the feeling of prosthetic limbs as their arms. O'Doherty et al. (2011) have proposed intra–cortical micro–stimulation (ICMS) of hand sensory representation areas to convey tactile feedback.

Previous studies showed that in humans and in monkeys, there is multisensory representation of peripersonal space and this representation can be changed with tool use: peripersonal space extends to include the space reachable by the tool, indicating a kind of incorporation of the tool into the body schema (Berti and Frassinetti 2000). Iriki et al. (1996) showed that multimodal neurons in the monkey's intraparietal areas that usually respond to tactile stimuli and to visual stimuli presented near the tactile receptive field change their visual response after the monkey has used a long tool to reach far food pellets for a while: after tool-use, visual stimuli near the end of the tool activate intraparietal bimodal neurons. In this study it has been shown that monkeys extend their visual receptive field into the extrapersonal space reached by the tip of a tool when it is actively used. After training with the tool, the visual response from these neurons is stronger for visual stimuli far from the body. Such stimuli were unable to elicit any response before training with the tool. This finding is interpreted as "*tool incorporation.*"

2 Tool Incorporation in Rhesus Monkeys

In a series of experiments recorded at Duke University, NC we have tested the rubber hand illusion paradigm with rhesus monkeys. The monkeys are implanted with multichannel electrodes in the sensorimotor cortex (Shokur et al. 2013; Ifft et al. 2013; O'Doherty et al. 2011). The experiment was conducted with two rhesus monkeys with recording of a large number of single neurons. The monkeys were observing a virtual 3D arm mimicking the position and size of their own arm. Their actual arm was gently restrained under the monitor on which the avatar arm was shown. A virtual sphere was touching the virtual arm in synchrony with a physical touch—performed by a robotic brush—of the forearm of the monkey.

Our experiment revealed that after a period of synchronous touching of the real arm and observed touching of the avatar arm, a subset of neurons in the sensory-motor cortices starts to modulate to the observed touch of the avatar arm. This activation happens even in absence of actual physical touch and is robust over the session (approx. 1 h) and subjects. No such modulation is observed if the physical touch and the observed touch are asynchronous. These results suggest that brain representation of the monkey's arm can expand to include a sur-numerary virtual arm. For this to happen it is necessary to have a congruent visuo-tactile stimulation. Results of this experiment are reported in detail in Shokur et al. (2013).

2.1 Experiment

We implanted two adult monkeys (*Macaca mulatta*) with four 96-microwire arrays constructed of stainless steel 304 (two per hemisphere one for upper limb sensory motor area and one for lower limb). Procedure is described in (O'Doherty et al. 2011).

We have recorded 62 neurons in S1 and 82 neurons in M1 for one monkey and 15 S1 and 34 M1 neurons in a second one. We will show here data from the first monkey.

We started every session with 100 trials where the monkey only observed the virtual touch on the avatar arm (V*only*). We continued the session with 100 V*only* trials intermingled with 900 synchronous virtual and physical touches (V + P). Figure 1a shows an example of an S1 and an M1 neuron. Both neurons significantly increase their firing rate over the baseline activity ($p < 0.001$, Wilcoxon Test) when a virtual and a physical touch are presented (V + P).

Neural modulation under V + P condition is expected, but while S1 responses to a tactile stimulus are well-known since long time (Meyer 1898), M1 responses might appear surprising to the reader. However they have been equally reported in numerous studies (Albe-Fessard and Liebeskind 1966; Evarts and Tanji 1976; Flament and Hore 1988; Hatsopoulos and Suminski 2011).

We observe significant responses [cumulative sum method (Nicolelis and Chapin 1994)] in 73 % of recorded neurons in S1 and 85 % of M1 neurons. Interestingly, after V + P is introduced both neurons are significantly modulated when only an observed touch of the avatar occurs (V*only—after*). The same is not true before V + P was introduced. We found 50 % of S1 and 70 % of M1 neurons to significantly modulated their firing rate after V + P. In the other hand, only 2 % of S1 and 2 % of M1 had modulation to V*only* before V + P. Figure 1b shows normalized (z-score) average of firing rate of the neurons responding to V + P. The reader can notice that mean response of the population for V*only—after* is smaller then V + P but significantly higher then V*only—before*.

The same experience was reproduced by replacing V + P trials with asynchronous physical and virtual touches (asyc V + P). Here no modulation was observed in V*only* : neither before, nor after async V + P was introduced (see Fig. 1c).

3 Tool Incorporation in Healthy Humans

To study tool incorporation in healthy human subjects, several groups used a behavioral task developed in the context of crossmodal attention study by the group of Jon Driver in late nineties, called 'crossmodal congruency task' (CCE). This task allows measuring multisensory interactions in different sectors of space. Since peripersonal space representation is based on multisensory integration of vision, touch and auditory cues, behavioral studies are used to study the interaction of visual and tactile cues (Spence et al. 2004) auditory and tactile cues (Zampini et al. 1869).

CCE experiments typically involve participants holding foam blocks in both hands with vibrators and LEDs placed on the tips of the thumbs and index fingers. Participants are asked to make speeded elevation judgment (up vs. down) of the vibrotactile stimulus while ignoring the LED stimuli. CCE magnitude is calculated as the reaction time difference between incongruent conditions (light and vibration in opposite position (up vs. down)) and congruent conditions (light and vibration both either up or down). The CCE can be used as an index of the perceived spatial proximity between visual and tactile stimuli. Furthermore, it allows quantifying the contributions of visual, tactile and proprioceptive cues to the multisensory representation of peripersonal space (Spence et al. 2004). CCE was used to investigate the role of proprioception in the multisensory representation of the

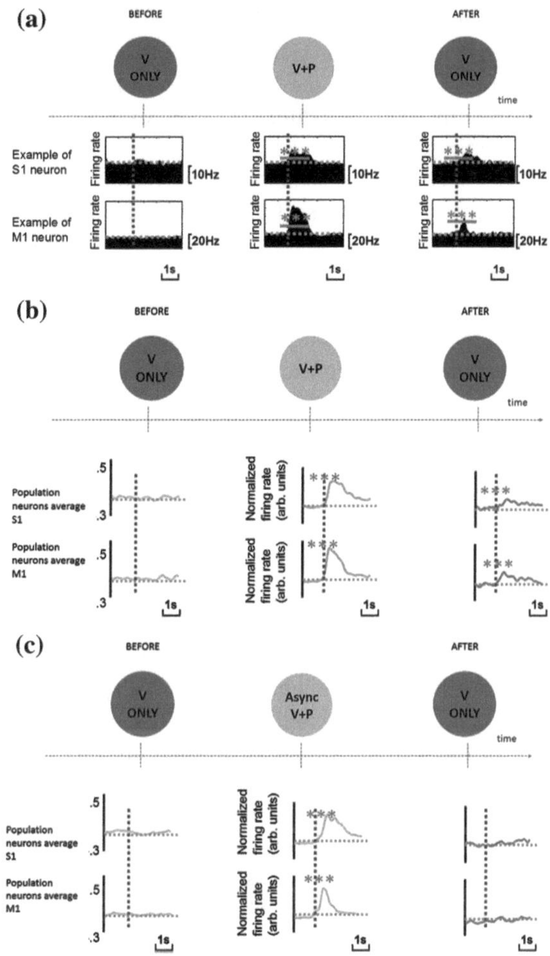

Fig. 1 **a** Example of single neurons in S1 and M1. Y axis represent firing rate in Hz for binned data (50 ms). X axis represents time window around the stimulus. Stimulus onset is shown with green dashed line. Dashed magenta line represents baseline firing rate calculated as mean firing rate 1 second before the stimuli. Significance is reported with ***, for $p < 0.001$, Wilcoxon Test. "Before" and "After" corresponds to "before V + P was introduced" and after. **b** Mean firing rate of normalized neurons (only neurons responding to V + P were selected) for S1 and M1 neurons. **c** Same as **b**, but for a session with V + P async

peripersonal representation when they are placed close to the body and CCEs were shown to be modulated by body ownership (Pavani et al. 2000). Additionally, CCEs were used to assess the changes in the peripersonal space when body parts were seen via a mirror (Maravita et al. 2002) or whether shadows of the body parts are incorporated into the body schema (Pavani and Castiello 2004). CCE was also used to assess bodily self-consciousness (Aspell et al. 2009). Recently, the cross modal congruency task has also been used to study the effect of tool-use, and in particular, whether peripersonal space can be extended or somehow dynamically modified by tool-use (Maravita 2006; Holmes 2012).

Tool use studies with healthy subjects analyzed the changes in the representation of peripersonal space using the CCE and they were all done with simple physical tools such as golf clubs, rakes or sticks (Maravita 2006; Holmes 2012). Maravita et al. (2002) tested association of visual stimuli at the end of the tools with simultaneous vibrotactile stimuli on the handle (Maravita et al. 2002). Holmes et al. (2004) investigated the effect of tool use in different sectors of space, by testing CCE along the tip, middle and end of the tool. They found that, after tool-use, the spatial modulation of the CCE varied at the tip of the tool, but not in the middle of the tool.

With advances in technology new sophisticated tools are emerging. Haptic devices, master/slave systems and surgical robotic systems are some of the advanced tools that link peripersonal space with extrapersonal space, as these tools are used in the workspace space of hands, but operate in a far space or even in VR (computer screen) (Bassolino et al. 2010) or, further yet, on a different planet. In the next section we analyze whether virtual tool use (haptic device) can extend peripersonal space representation from near to far space (or to the virtual space).

3.1 Experiments

We aim to measure multisensory integration of vision and touch in haptic devices and to evaluate the potential of emerging multimodal interaction at the level of the perception of the tool by the human brain. Designing new interfaces will require adequate integration of the different sensory modalities. This promises to improve the performance of the whole man-robot system. The experiments described here have been done on a modified haptic man-robot interface designed for the simulator of the well-known surgical robot *daVinci*® (Sengül 2013).

The users interact with such a telemanipulator to perform complex tasks. Ideally, this interaction should be as natural and as intuitive as possible and should give the operator the impression of physically being at the point of interaction (telepresence, immersion). Sensory modalities such as force, touch (texture), temperature etc. could be included at the master console to increase the realism of an interaction. Simply displaying these signals on a computer screen is however not a good solution, it would just increase the cognitive load and might thus be more of a drawback than an advantage. However, multimodal physical haptic interaction directly at the handle of the control console could bring the desired result (Sengül 2013).

There is large number of tool-use studies that measure such changes in the representation of peripersonal space by CCE done with simple tools such as golf clubs, rakes or sticks. Advanced robotic tools such as haptic devices and master-salve systems have, to our knowledge, not yet been used in this context. Recently, haptic and even multi-modal man-robot interfaces are emerging in research. The human operator is facing new interaction challenges. Either, as e.g. with present-day "classical" commercial surgery robotics, using the tool relies exclusively on visual feedback. Or, in case other interaction modalities are measured, the unintuitive presentation (on screens, scales, with alarms) will lead to a cognitive overload of the operator (Sengül 2013).

As the focus is on learning, through experimental studies with test subjects, how the brain integrates a telemanipulated robot as a tool, it would be highly desirable to control precisely, in a very repeatable manner, the actual interaction on the slave side. Telemanipulators offer the possibility to replace the physical part of the slave-robot by a manipulation in VR. This will enable the neuroscience community to perform studies with very precisely definable and reproducible experimental conditions, as would be difficult to realize with actual tools.

3.2 Experimental Setup

We employed a robotic system that is a training device for use of the da Vinci® surgery system. The details of this setup are presented in (Sengül 2013).

Open source platform, CHAI 3D, and a set of C++ libraries have been used for the modeling and simulation of the haptics and visualization of the virtual world. This platform supports several commercial haptic devices and it is possible to extend it to support new custom Force Feedback (FFB) devices. We have extended this platform by adding the drivers and libraries of our FFB device.

Two vibrotactile target stimulators (microdrive shaftless vibration motors) are attached to the participants' thumb and index finger. Vibrotactile stimuli are driven by electrical signal generated by a desktop computer. The participants see two virtual tools through a head mounted display. Visual distractor stimuli are 5 mm in diameter virtual LEDs, positioned in upper and lower locations of the tip of the virtual tools.

3.3 Study 1: Incorporation of Virtual Tools

The experimental setup, the protocols and the results are described in detail (30). Ten participants (two female, ages 21–24, mean age (SE) 22.3 1.2 years) were recruited. This experiment is a three within-subject design. The three within-subjects factors were congruency of the elevation of the vibrotactile stimuli with respect to the visual distractors (congruent vs. incongruent), the vibrotactile target side to the visual distractor side (same vs. different), and the type of posture (uncrossed vs crossed). After each posture CCE was performed.

Data from all trials that resulted in correct responses were analyzed by using a repeated-measures three-way analysis of variance (ANOVAs) on the mean values of reaction times (RTs).

Congruency effects derived from RT data from the first experiment are represented in Fig. 2. The ANOVA performed on RTs from Experiment 1 revealed a main effect of congruency ($F(1, 9) = 32.90$, $p < 0.001$) and a significant interaction between congruency and side ($F(1, 9) = 9.07$), $p < 0.05$) confirming that CCEs were significantly larger in the same side conditions compared to the

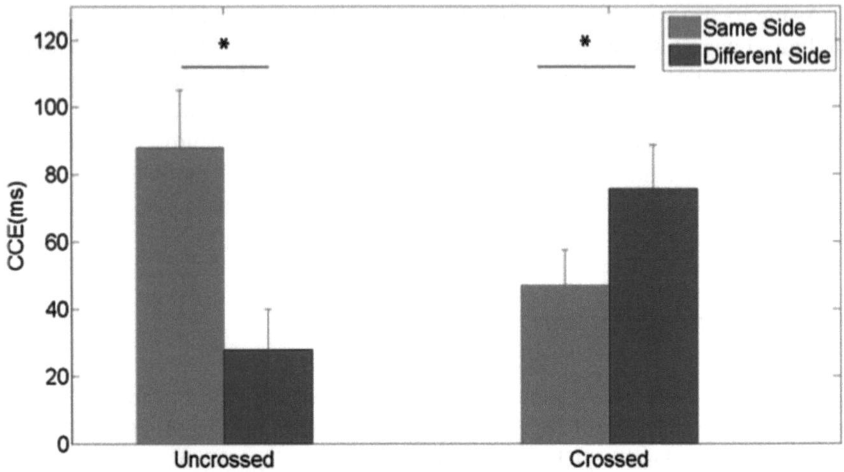

Fig. 2 Crossmodal congruency effect with standard error for reaction time in Study 1. CCE was calculated as incongruent reaction time minus congruent reaction time. Red bar are for the trials in which visual stimuli is in the same visual hemifield with tactile stimuli. The bars on the left side are for the uncrossed posture and on the right side for the crossed posture. The difference between "same" and "different" side is significant for both uncrossed and crossed posture (Sengül 2013)

different side conditions ($t(9) = 3.02$; $p < 0.05$). Crucially, we also found a three-way interaction between Congruency, Side and Tool Posture ($F(1, 9) = 37.88$, $p < 0.001$) (Sengül 2013).

To determine the driving factor of this three-way interaction, we performed post hoc comparisons between the same side CCE versus the different side CCE for the RT measures for each tool posture. This analysis revealed that the CCE differed significantly between same side and different side for the uncrossed ($t(9) = 5.80$; $p < 0.001$) and crossed condition ($t(9) = 3.30$; $p < 0.01$) (see Fig. 2). As inspection of Fig. 2 reveals, the direction of these effects differed for uncrossed versus crossed conditions. In line with data obtained with physical tools, for the uncrossed condition the same side CCEs were larger than the different side CCEs, whereas for the crossed condition the different side CCEs were larger than the same side CCEs. These data indicate that active tool use results in a remapping of peripersonal space, depending on the position of the tools (Sengül 2013).

Our results show that active virtual-robotic tool use changes the spatial modulation of the CCEs, comparable to changes in the representation of peripersonal space observed during real-world tool use. Moreover, when the virtual-robotic tools are held in a crossed position, the visual distractors interfer strongly with tactile stimuli connected to the hand by the tool, reflecting a remapping of peripersonal space. Such remapping is not only observed when the virtual-robotic tools are actively used, but also when the tools are passively held. The present study expands on earlier findings on the extension of peripersonal space from physical and pointing tools to virtual-robotic tools using haptics and VR. We discuss our data with respect to learning and human factors in the field of surgical robotics in (Sengül 2013).

We show with this experiment how the virtual tools change the peripersonal space representation. Our results show that in order to change the representation of peripersonal space, it is not necessary to have a physical connection between the space where the tool is held and the space where the tool operates. This finding illustrates that the peripersonal space representation can be extended to a virtual world. Similar mechanisms likely also apply to the use of robotic tools, such as a surgical telemanipulator robot, where the surgeon may use a bimanual haptic interface to control manipulation at a remote workspace (Sengül 2013).

3.4 Study 2: Role of Force Feedback in Incorporation of Virtual Tools

After showing that the peripersonal representation is extended with the use of a virtual tool use (surgical simulator) in the previous section, we will focus on the role of the signals (feedbacks) in the representation of peripersonal space that should be sent from the slave (workspace) to the master (control console). More specifically we will focus on the role of the force feedback (FFB) in multisensory representation of the peripersonal space.

The experimental protocols and the findings are described in detail (Sengül et al. 2013). The CCE is measured using the same apparatus and procedures as in (Sengül et al. 2012). In this study the same robotic system has been used as before.

In this experiment there are two main tasks: the tool–use task and the cross-modal congruency task. Instructions relating to these two tasks were given to the test-subject prior to testing. In the tool–use task, participants used the robotic tool to interact with a deformable object for a duration of 40 seconds. There were three conditions: 'static', 'without FFB' and 'with FFB'. In the 'static' case, which was used as a baseline condition, participants did not move the robotic tool. During the 'without FFB' condition, participants were required to use the tools to virtually grasp the red boxes and pull them. While they were interacting with the boxes, the pulling of an elastic rope was visualized but no FFB was provided during that interaction. In the 'with FFB' condition, while participants pulled the red boxes, in addition to visualization of the pulling of an elastic rope, FFB was provided. After performing one of the three tool-use tasks, participants were instructed to perform the second task, the crossmodal congruency task (Sengül 2013).

We found a three-way interaction between the factors Condition, Side and Congruency ($F(2, 11) = 4.9$, $p < 0.05$). Posthoc analysis revealed that the same side CCEs in the with FFB condition was significantly larger than same side CCE for the static condition ($t(1,11) = 2.17$; $p < 0.05$) and the without FFB

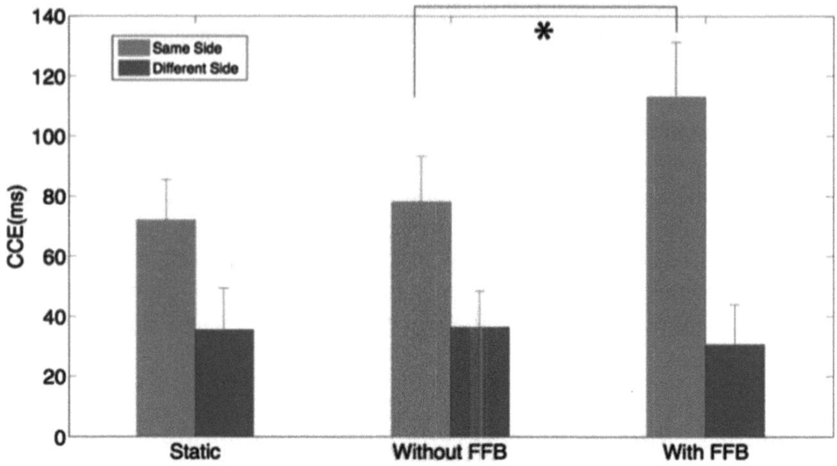

Fig. 3 Result of the force feedback experiment. The graph shows the crossmodal congruency effect (CCE) in milliseconds in Study 2. The CCE was calculated by subtracting congruent from incongruent reaction times. Same side CCEs (*red bars*) were significantly different than the different side CCEs (*blue bars*). Moreover, same side CCE for the FFB condition (*left bars*) was significantly higher than the CCE for both the no-feedback (*middle bars*) and the static condition (*right bars*). Error bars represent standard errors (Sengül 2013)

condition($t(1, 11) = 3.03$; $p < 0.05$), whereas no such difference between conditions was found for different side CCEs ($p > 0.61$; see Fig. 3) (Sengül 2013).

The ANOVA result of study 2 showed that spatial interaction of vision and touch depends on feedback type (three-way interaction of congruency, side and feedback type). A comparison of this interaction revealed that the same side CCE was the largest for the FFB condition and it was significantly different than other two conditions (static and without FFB) same side CCEs, see Fig. 3.

In the previous tool-use studies, researchers used physical tools to analyze the multisensory integration of vision and touch. These studies did not investigate the role of FFB since it was not possible to manipulate FFB systematically with a physical tool. As we used a haptic robot in the current study, it was possible to manipulate and investigate its effect on multisensory integration in peripersonal space. We showed that FFB plays a crucial role in the integration of vision and touch (measured by the CCE). Our findings about the effect of FFB measured by the CCE may also be useful for the fast growing field of surgical robotics. Although the role of FFB is being intensively studied in surgical robotics (Bethea et al. 2004; Okamura 2009), there are no studies investigating it with CCEs. Our result showed that CCEs could be used to clarify the role of FFB from a cognitive perspective. Moreover, CCEs could provide an objective method to measure telepresence/usability for different surgical robotic systems (Sengül 2013).

4 Conclusions

A new type of experimental setup for the study of tool incorporation (or embodiment) has been introduced into the field of cognitive neurosciences. Robotic devices such has telemanipulators, haptic man-machine interfaces, force feedback and virtual reality have been adapted and newly developed for this purpose. A first series of experiments hints at the potential of this new approach. Experiments testing for paradigms such as intracortical recording with rhesus monkeys, the cross-modal congruency effect or the rubber hand illusion confirm earlier results obtained without robotic tools and open up entirely new possibilities for the study of dexterous manipulations and its working within the motor control system. It is hoped that this kind of research will not only advance cognitive neuroscience research, but also development of improved neuroprosthetics and telemanipulators such as e.g. surgical robots.

Acknowledgments The research work reported here was partially supported by the SAFROS FP-7 project of the European Union and by Grant No. 900 of MESROB Research Council (Swiss National Science Foundation SNF).

References

A. Berti, F. Frassinetti, When far becomes near: Remapping of space by tool use. *J Cognitive Neurosci* **12**, 415 (May, 2000).

A. Iriki, M. Tanaka, Y. Iwamura, Coding of modified body schema during tool use by macaque postcentral neurones. *Neuroreport* **7**, 2325 (Oct 2, 1996).

A. M. Okamura, Haptic feedback in robot-assisted minimally invasive surgery. *Current opinion in urology* **19**, 102 (Jan, 2009).

A. Maravita, C. Spence, C. Sergent, J. Driver, Seeing your own touched hands in a mirror modulates cross-modal interactions. *Psychological science* **13**, 350 (Jul, 2002).

A. Maravita, C. Spcncc, S. Kcnnctt, J. Drivcr, Tool-usc changcs multimodal spatial intcractions between vision and touch in normal humans. *Cognition* **83**, B25 (Mar, 2002).

A. Maravita, *From body in the brain, to body in space: sensory and intentional aspects of body representation*. I. G. K. M. S. M. Grosjean, Ed., The human body: perception from the inside out (Oxford University Press, Oxford, 2006).

A. Meyer, Critical review of the data and general methods and deductions of modern neurology. *Journal of Comparative Neurology* **8**, 249 (1898).

A. Sengül, EPFL (2013).

A. Sengül *et al.*, Extending the body to virtual tools using a robotic surgical interface: evidence from the crossmodal congruency task. *PloS one* **7**, e49473 (2012).

J. E. O'Doherty *et al.*, Active tactile exploration using a brain-machine-brain interface. *Nature* **479**, 228 (2011).

B. T. Bethea *et al.*, Application of haptic feedback to robotic surgery. *Journal of Laparoendoscopic & Advanced Surgical Techniques* **14**, 191 (2004).

C. Spence, F. Pavani, J. Driver, Spatial constraints on visual-tactile cross-modal distractor congruency effects. *Cognitive, affective & behavioral neuroscience* **4**, 148 (Jun, 2004).

D. Albe-Fessard, J. Liebeskind, Origin of somato-sensitive messages activating the cells of the motor cortex in monkeys]. *Experimental brain research. Experimentelle Hirnforschung. Expérimentation cérébrale* **1**, 127 (1966).
D. Flament, J. Hore, Relations of motor cortex neural discharge to kinematics of passive and active elbow movements in the monkey. *Journal of neurophysiology* **60**, 1268 (1988).
E. V. Evarts, J. Tanji, Reflex and intended responses in motor cortex pyramidal tract neurons of monkey. *Journal of neurophysiology* **39**, 1069 (1976).
F. Pavani, C. Spence, J. Driver, Visual capture of touch: out-of-the-body experiences with rubber gloves. *Psychological science* **11**, 353 (Sep, 2000).
F. Pavani, U. Castiello, Binding personal and extrapersonal space through body shadows. *Nature neuroscience* **7**, 14 (Jan, 2004).
A. Sengül *et al.*, Force feedback facilitates multisensory integration during robotic tool use. *Exp Brain Res*, 1 (2013).
H. H. Ehrsson, N. P. Holmes, R. E. Passingham, Touching a rubber hand: feeling of body ownership is associated with activity in multisensory brain areas. *J Neurosci* **25**, 10564 (Nov 9, 2005).
H. Ehrsson, B. Rosén, A. Stockselius, C. Ragnö, P. Köhler, G. Lundborg, Upper limb amputees can be induced to experience a rubber hand as their own. *Brain*, **131**(12), 3443–3452 (2008).
J. E. Aspell, B. Lenggenhager, O. Blanke, Keeping in touch with one's self: multisensory mechanisms of self-consciousness. *PloS one* **4**, e6488 (2009).
M. Bassolino, A. Serino, S. Ubaldi, E. Ladavas, Everyday use of the computer mouse extends peripersonal space representation. *Neuropsychologia* **48**, 803 (Feb, 2010).
M. Botvinick, J. Cohen, Rubber hands 'feel' touch that eyes see. *Nature* **391**, 756 (Feb 19, 1998).
M. Hoffmann *et al.*, Body Schema in Robotics: A Review. *IEEE Transactions on Autonomous Mental Development* **2**, 304 (2010).
M. J. Giummarra, S. J. Gibson, N. Georgiou-Karistianis, J. L. Bradshaw, Mechanisms underlying embodiment, disembodiment and loss of embodiment. *Neuroscience and biobehavioral reviews* **32**, 143 (2008).
M. Nicolelis, J. K. Chapin, Spatiotemporal structure of somatosensory responses of many-neuron ensembles in the rat ventral posterior medial nucleus of the thalamus. *The Journal of neuroscience* **14**, 3511 (1994).
M. Zampini, D. Torresan, C. Spence, M. M. Murray, Auditory-somatosensory multisensory interactions in front and rear space. *Neuropsychologia* **45**, 1869 (Apr 9, 2007).
N. G. Hatsopoulos, A. J. Suminski, Sensing with the motor cortex. *Neuron* **72**, 477 (2011).
N. P. Holmes, Does tool use extend peripersonal space? A review and re-analysis. *Exp Brain Res* **218**, 273 (Apr, 2012).
N. P. Holmes, G. A. Calvert, C. Spence, Extending or projecting peripersonal space with tools? Multisensory interactions highlight only the distal and proximal ends of tools. *Neurosci Lett* **372**, 62 (Nov 30, 2004).
P. D. Marasco, K. Kim, J. E. Colgate, M. A. Peshkin, T. A. Kuiken, Robotic touch shifts perception of embodiment to a prosthesis in targeted reinnervation amputees. *Brain* **134**, 747 (Mar, 2011).
P. Ifft, S. Shokur, M. Lebedev, Z. Li and M.A.L Nicolelis. Brain-Machine Interface Enables Bimanual Arm Movements in Monkeys. Accepted for publication in Science Translational Medicine. 20 September 2013.
S. Shokur *et al.*, Expanding the primate body schema in sensorimotor cortex by virtual touches of an avatar. *Proceedings of the National Academy of Sciences* **110**, 15121 (2013).
V. Gallese, C. Keysers, G. Rizzolatti, A unifying view of the basis of social cognition. *Trends Cogn Sci* **8**, 396 (2004).

Offline Imitation of a Human Motion by a Humanoid Robot Under Balance Constraint

K. Munirathinam, C. Chevallereau and S. Sakka

Abstract This chapter analyzes the offline imitation of a reference whole-body human motion by a humanoid robot. The study uses the systems dynamics models and focuses on the management of the balance constraint. A hybrid approach based on simultaneous time-scaling and joint modification is introduced and takes advantage of both approaches (time-scaling and joint modification) while solving some of their respective drawbacks. The hybrid approach was implemented with two techniques for offline motion imitation: Control approach and Optimization approach. The control approach defines the second derivative of the time-scaling factor from the dynamics equations, and uses it as a control variable to constraint the ZMP inside the support polygon. Time-scaling is predominant in the control approach: the joint trajectories modification will occur only if no solution is found by time-scaling alone. The optimization approach uses a multi-objective function where the mean square difference between the imitating time and joint trajectories with respect to its reference is minimized. The balance (ZMP) criterion is included as an inequality constraint in the optimization process. The joint path is described as function of a spline whose parameters are optimized. In both control and optimization approaches, a feasible solution for the robot joint trajectories is found: the imitator can track the reference trajectories to achieve a natural-looking imitation of the human motion with optimum delay (time-scaling) and joint angle error (joint modification). The results are validated with captured human data converted for the 25-dof NAO humanoid robot with a kick motion.

K. Munirathinam · C. Chevallereau (✉) · S. Sakka
IRCCyN, Ecole Centrale de Nantes, CNRS, Nantes, France
e-mail: christine.chevallereau@irccyn.ec-nantes.fr

K. Munirathinam
e-mail: karthick.munirathinam@irccyn.ec-nantes.fr

S. Sakka
University of Poitiers, Poitiers, France
e-mail: sophie.sakka@irccyn.ec-nantes.fr

A. Rodić et al. (eds.), *New Trends in Medical and Service Robots*,
Mechanisms and Machine Science 20, DOI: 10.1007/978-3-319-05431-5_18,

Keywords Humanoid robot · Motion imitation · Time-scaling · Control · ZMP · Optimization

1 Introduction

The human body is a magnificent physical structure which enables making complex movements such as locomotion and manipulation. The recent advancements in technology especially in miniaturized electronics, artificial intelligence, hybrid materials and efficient motors, have led to a major turning point in the development of humanoid robots. They may indeed, in a short future, have the ability to work in the human environment in real-time and execute even complex defined tasks with good reactivity. To attain this objective, humanoid robots should inculcate the capability to imitate human motion and reproduce it identically to reach a given objective (Schall 1999).

Motion imitation plays a dominant role in robot social learning (Breazeal and Scassellati 2002). By imitation learning, the robot can possess efficient motor learning (Saegusa et al. 2007), modular motor control and autonomous task execution. If this capability is embedded in the action-perception loop, the humanoid robot will speed up learning to perform a task in complex higher dimensional motor system. However, the motion imitation from human beings to humanoid robots should respect the kinematics and dynamics differences between the two.

The main challenge for motion transposition from human beings to humanoid robots is balance. When human joint motion is directly applied to the robot, the humanoid robot may or may not maintain equilibrium. Therefore, the joint trajectories obtained from the human motion need being modified such that the humanoid balance is maintained throughout the complete motion to be imitated.

Numerous research works have been carried out to map offline human motion to humanoid motion. Pollard et al.'s kinematic joint velocity filtering approach (Pollard et al. 2002) first served for the upper body motion imitation, and then was associated to motion primitives to include balance management (Nakaoka et al. 2003) and extended to whole body offline imitation. Many other offline approaches were carried in human to humanoid motion imitation by optimization (Suleiman et al. 2008; Do et al. 2008), by control (Kim et al. 2009) or by machine learning using hidden Markov models (Ott et al. 2008).

Online approaches based on inverted kinematics have also been developed for whole body imitation (Dariush et al. 2009; Sakka et al. 2014) with balance management using the projection of the center of mass on the ground as balance criterion. These approaches can only be applied for slow motions as dynamics is not taken into account.

The motion imitation techniques above are all based on the modification of the joint angles and their derivatives to ensure the balance of the imitating system. The technique we propose is called *time-scaling*. It is based on modifying the time distribution along the human reference motion to accelerate or decelerate the entire motion and therefore influence the ZMP position. The joint accelerations of the imitating system are modified, whereas its joint paths are left untouched: the motion coordination of the reference is exactly reproduced.

According to literature, time-scaling was used in torque control for manipulators (Dahl and Nielsen 1990; Hollerbach 1983; Arai et al. 1998), for proper coordination between the systems (Samson 1995), and for planar biped control (Chevallereau 2003; Holm et al. 2007; Djoudi and Chevallereau 2006; Munirathinam et al. 2012).

With time-scaling, the tracking of a reference path is enabled but with different time distribution: only the velocity and the acceleration profiles of the reference motion are modified. Time-scaling is an effective approach for fast motions to ensure the balance of the system, but in some scenarios, balance cannot be achieved. For example, when the motion is slow enough and the velocity tends to zero, time-scaling has no effect (Munirathinam et al. 2012). In these cases, the joint trajectories should be modified to meet the balance constraint.

We introduce in this chapter a hybrid approach using simultaneously both time-scaling and joint modification. As a consequence, we take advantage of both approaches for balance management while solving some of their respective drawbacks. Moreover, we will compare two ways of solving the human imitation problem: one is based on control and the other one uses optimization. The choice of the manner to imitate depends on what is aimed for imitation. The optimization algorithm deals with the complete motion at once, and therefore benefits from anticipation on the future movements. It also uses high computation time. On the other hand, the control algorithm only uses the current state of the robot. As such, no anticipation on the future movement is made, but the calculation time is much lower than for optimization. This approach may be used for online applications.

This chapter is organized as follows: we first explain in Sect. 2 the basics for time-scaling alone in a simple 2D case with the control approach. Then the control approach is extended to three dimensional cases. Section 3 details the hybrid algorithm using the control approach and Sect. 4 focuses on the hybrid algorithm using the optimization approach. To compare the results using either control or optimization, a similar experiment is used, where an actor performs a kick motion which is successfully reproduced by NAO humanoid robot. Section 5 discusses the plus and minus of both hybrid algorithms and Sect. 6 concludes the chapter.

2 Time-Scaling Approach Based on Control

Time-scaling is defined as modifying the time distribution. Let us consider a reference trajectory $q^r(t)$. The derivatives of $q^r(t)$ are scaled by a scaling factor, whereas the components of $q^r(t)$ are not modified. Let $s(t)$ be the scaling factor and $q(t) = q^r(s(t))$ be the joint trajectories of the imitating system. The imitator joint velocities and accelerations are function of the scaled reference motion as follows.

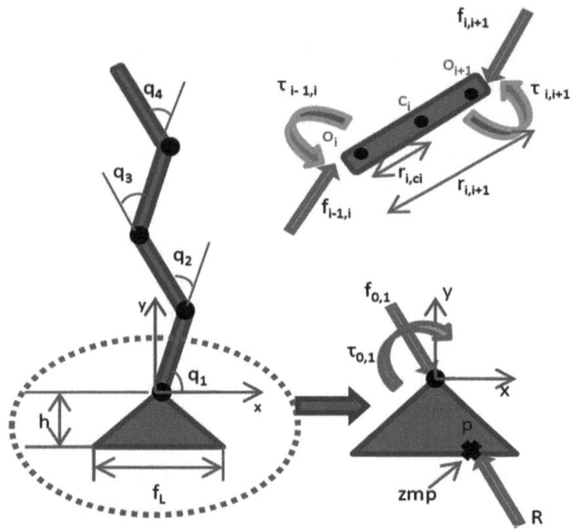

Fig. 1 2D model—foot attached to n-serial links

$$\begin{aligned} q(t) &= q^r(s(t)) \\ \dot{q}(t) &= \tfrac{\partial q^r(s)}{\partial s}\dot{s}(t) \\ \ddot{q}(t) &= \tfrac{\partial q^r(s)}{\partial s}\ddot{s}(t) + \tfrac{\partial^2 q^r(s)}{\partial^2 s}\dot{s}(t)^2 \end{aligned} \quad (1)$$

By using the scaling factor as a prime variable, and by choosing freely its second derivative $\ddot{s}(t)$, the dynamics of the system can be modified. Hence, the balance of the imitating system can be achieved. Time-scaling is performed globally for all the joint angles. This way we can retain the same shape (or joint coordination) for the imitating and the reference systems. The imitating system slows down its motion when balance is at stake and speeds up the motion to catch up with the reference motion when balance is guaranteed.

2.1 Time-Scaling Control in 2D

In this section we explain the general principle of time-scaling alone, using the control approach. Let us consider the reference redundant multi body system described in Fig. 1. This system is an open kinematic chain of n rigid bodies, attached to a massless foot at its lower extremity. The foot is in planar contact with the ground, and the reference motion of the kinematic chain will be dynamically stable.

A second system with similar kinematics but different inertia characteristics is considered as the imitator. The objective of the imitator is to replicate the motion of the reference while ensuring the balance throughout its motion, i.e. essentially to satisfy the constraint on the ZMP due to the difference in foot size with the reference.

To ensure balance, the ZMP position $\ell(t)$ must be constrained within the support polygon limited by $[\ell_{\min}, \ell_{\max}]$ during the entire motion:

$$\ell_{\min} < \ell(t) < \ell_{\max} \tag{2}$$

This objective will be satisfied by scaling the time at which the reference joint trajectories are performed. The ZMP position can be expressed as a function of the ground reaction forces and torques. These quantities depend on the joint accelerations and thus on $\ddot{s}(t)$. The ZMP position can be written as follows (Chevallereau 2003).

$$\ell = \frac{A\ddot{s} + B}{C\ddot{s} + D} \tag{3}$$

where A, B, C and D are functions of q^r and its derivatives and of q, $\dot{q}$, and the dynamics parameters of the robot (Chevallereau 2003). The scaling factor $s(t)$ must remain as close as possible to the reference time t to have a good imitation. Let us introduce the error on time: $e = s(t) - t$, and its derivative $\dot{e} = \dot{s} - 1$. The desired closed loop behavior for the error is the following.

$$\ddot{e} + k_v\dot{e} + k_p e = 0 \tag{4}$$

where k_p and k_v are gains chosen such that the error will converge to zero. The corresponding desired value for the second derivative of the scaling factor is:

$$\ddot{s_d} = -k_v(\dot{s} - 1) - k_p(s(t) - t) \tag{5}$$

If the desired acceleration $\ddot{s_d}$ described by (5) satisfies the balance condition, i.e.:

$$\ell_{\min} < \frac{A\ddot{s_d} + B}{C\ddot{s_d} + D} < \ell_{\max}, \tag{6}$$

it will be used to control the robot. In other cases, the new value of $\ddot{s}$ will be chosen in order to maintain the imitator balance. Based on (2), the set of possible values for $\ddot{s}$ is:

$$\ddot{s} = \frac{-D\ell + B}{C\ell - A} \quad \text{for } \ell_{\min} < \ell < \ell_{\max} \tag{7}$$

The value of $\ddot{s}$ belonging to this set and closest to $\ddot{s_d}$ will be chosen. The control algorithm for the time-scaling based imitation is summarized in Fig. 2.

Figure 3 illustrates a simulation case of the time-scaling control. The solid line on the left figure represents the ZMP trajectory resulting from a direct mapping of the reference joint trajectories. The horizontal bold lines located at −1.4 and +1.4 represent the limits of the support polygon. Therefore, we can see that a direct mapping of the reference trajectories to the imitator does not make it keep its balance.

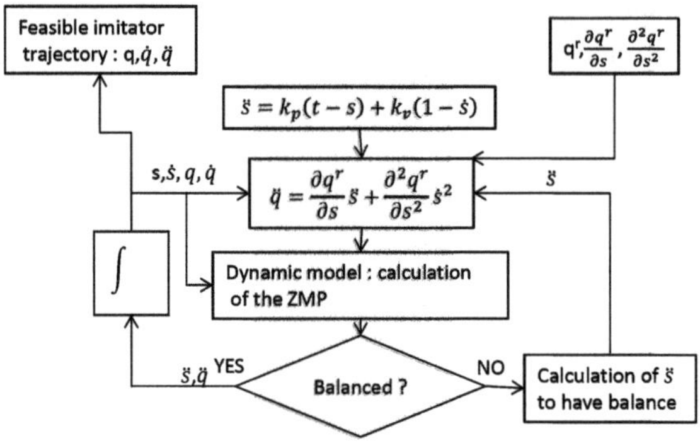

Fig. 2 Time scaling control algorithm

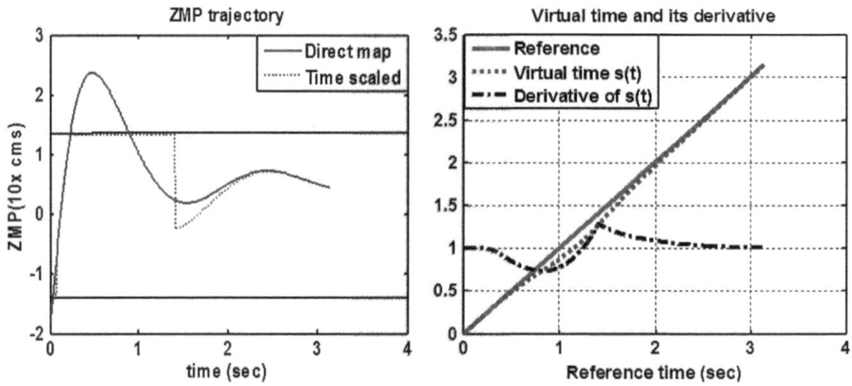

Fig. 3 ZMP trajectory modified by time-scaling (*left*); scaling factor with respect to time (*right*)

After time-scaling control, the ZMP is constrained inside the support polygon and hence the balance is maintained. As was mentioned previously, the control algorithm has no anticipation. It can be observed in the ZMP graph that the reference ZMP is tracked until the ZMP reaches the limits of the support polygon at around 0.2 s. Having reached the limit, the motion of the imitator is slowed so that the ZMP follows the limit of the support area to avoid an unbalance situation. As soon as it is possible, the motion is accelerated again to catch up with the reference time. Then the ZMP trajectory finally tracks the reference trajectory again when the tracking offers safe balance from around 2.5 s.

Figure 3-right shows the evolution of the virtual time $s(t)$ with respect to the reference time for this imitation. The previous observations may be reproduced here: a slight delay between the reference and the virtual times appears from 0.2 s, and increases as the motion remains slowed in comparison with the reference motion. At around 1.4 s, the virtual time accelerates to catch up with the reference, and from around 2.5 s the two are synchronized again: both reference and imitation display the motion at same velocity and acceleration until the end of the observed motion. These points are better observed in the plot of the derivative of $s(t)$. Considering the virtual time, we can point out three cases:

- Case 1: $\dot{s} < 1$: the imitator motion lags behind the reference motion in order to compensate for the violation in ZMP;
- Case 2: $s(t) = t$: imitator and reference motions are perfectly synchronized;
- Case 3: $\dot{s} > 1$: the imitator accelerates its motion to catch up with the reference and at the same time the ZMP constraint is satisfied.

Let us recall that the values of the joint angles were not modified using this approach: the reference path is performed exactly by the imitator, only with a different time distribution. As such, the motion coordination of the reference is reproduced. Cartesian tasks may also be reproduced with this approach. These are some advantages of time-scaling. The possibility to extend the control approach to applications involving online motion imitation is another great advantage of this algorithm.

2.2 *Time-Scaling Control in 3D*

The extension of this time-scaling control to 3D is not so obvious. In 2D, the control variable $\ddot{s}$ has a one-to-one mapping function with the ZMP. In 3D, the ZMP is mapped along the plane of the support area, which leads to two conditions along the two horizontal axes y and z and involving only one control variable $\ddot{s}$. Hence, we have a many-to-one mapping.

The problem with many-to-one mapping is the possibility of inconsistency: a feasible solution for $\ddot{s}$ may not be obtained in some cases which involve violation in ZMP along both y and z axes. Another situation where time-scaling approach fails inevitably may also occur: if the projection of the CoM is outside the support polygon and the velocity of the motion tends to zero, then time-scaling has no more effect on balance. This is the major drawback of time-scaling. To counter this, a hybrid approach is introduced, involving the combination of joint modification and time-scaling to generate a feasible (safe) motion in all cases.

3 Hybrid Approach Based on Control

Hybrid imitation includes time-scaling and joint modification. In the control approach, let $\ddot{q}$ and $\ddot{s}$ be the control variables. Their desired values are defined similarly to (5) to reach the reference motion whatever deviation the system may encounter.

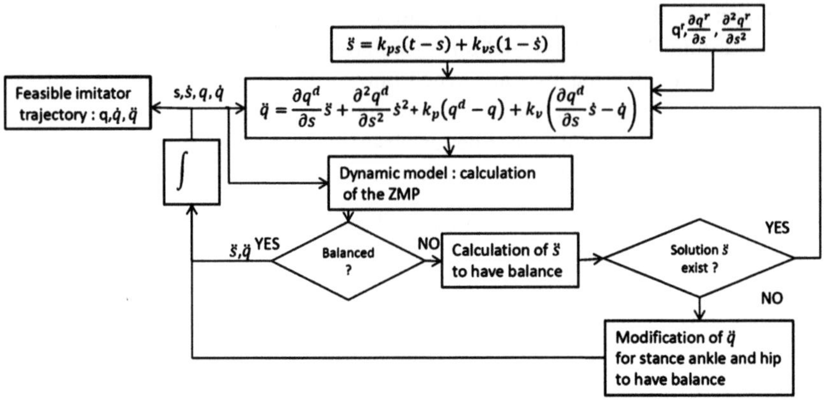

Fig. 4 Hybrid control algorithm

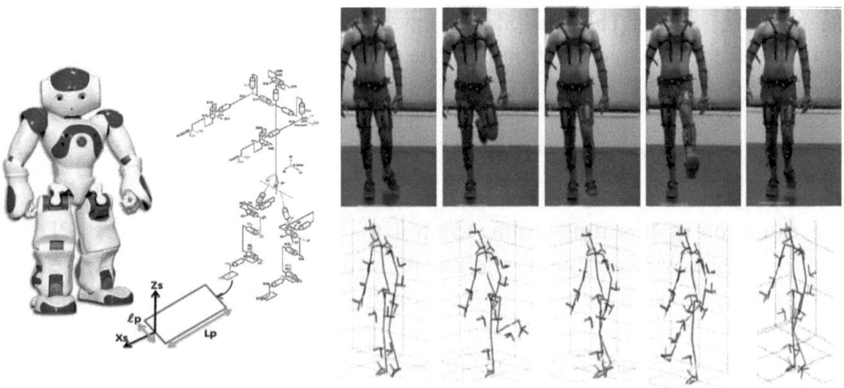

Fig. 5 Kinematics of NAO robot (*left*) and a human kick motion (*right*)

$$\begin{aligned} \ddot{q}_d &= \frac{\partial q^r(s)}{\partial s}\ddot{s} + \frac{\partial^2 q^r}{\partial^2 s}\dot{s}^2 - k_v\left(\frac{\partial q^r(s)}{\partial s}\dot{s} - \dot{q}\right) - k_p(q^r - q) \\ \ddot{s}_d &= -k_{vs}(\dot{s} - 1) - k_{ps}(s - t) \end{aligned} \tag{8}$$

where k_v, k_p, k_{ps}, k_{vs} are positive gains. As previously in the time-scaling algorithm, the scaling factor will modify the joint accelerations of the robot all together to insure that the reference motion synchronization is replayed by the imitator. But in the hybrid case, the joints paths may also be modified if, *and only if*, time-scaling finds no feasible solution. Though, it is not necessary in the joint modification phase to modify all the joint angles of the robot. We will focus on modifying only the most influent joints for balance: the stance ankle (roll and pitch) and hip (roll, pitch and yaw). The detailed block diagram of the hybrid approach is shown in Fig. 4. Comparing this diagram with the one in Fig. 2, the joint modification was added and will be used only in case time-scaling fails.

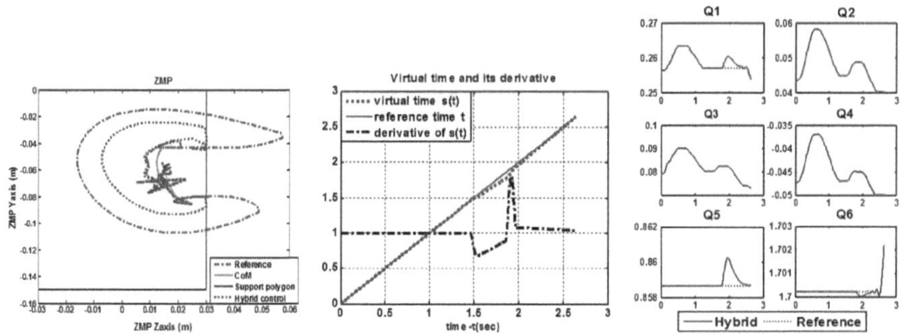

Fig. 6 *Left* ZMP trajectory before (*dashed*) and the after hybrid control (*dotted*). *solid line* is the CoM projection; *middle* the virtual time and its first derivative; *right* Stance ankle (joints 1, 2 and 3) and hip (joints 4, 5 and 6) joint paths obtained from hybrid control. The reference motions are expressed as functions of time t, and the real motions are expressed as functions of virtual time s

The hybrid control for motion imitation was validated using the 25-dof NAO robot (Aldebaran Robotics, Fig. 5). The sample motion was obtained from human motion capture (8 infrared cameras with Dtrack optical system). The human body was segmented in 12 segments similarly to NAO. Human data were registered at the frequency of 60 Hz in a file and post-treated to be mapped according to NAO kinematics and mechanical constraints, leading to our reference motion (the input of the algorithm).

A kick motion (Fig. 5) was performed by an actor in 2.6 s. This motion is hard to perform by a humanoid robot because of high accelerations with reduced support area (the robot is standing on one foot). If the reference trajectories are directly applied to the robot joints, the ZMP would go out of the support polygon as illustrated in Fig. 6-left by the red curve. This example motion was also chosen because time-scaling alone cannot find a feasible solution for the imitation with the control approach.

The hybrid control gives a feasible solution restricting the ZMP (blue line) within the robot support area for the complete motion. We can see that this approach is efficient from the way the ZMP trajectory follows the border of the support polygon.

In Fig. 6-middle, the time scaling effect is confirmed with the plot of the scaling factor and its first derivative, showing that the virtual time gets different from the reference time between 1.4 and 2.4 s. For the implementation, $\ddot{s}$ was also restricted within a tolerance value in order to meet the joint torque limits of the robot. Indeed, if $\ddot{s}$ is very big when catching up with the reference time, the joints accelerations will also be very high.

We can remark that only one delay can be observed on the scaling factor plot in Fig. 6-middle, whereas the ZMP in Fig. 6-left clearly goes along the boundaries of the support area at two occasions. This is due to the fact that time-scaling allows dealing only with the first unbalance situation (around 1.5 s). During the second unbalance situation, the constraints on the ZMP in the sagittal and frontal planes are incompatible thus the joint paths are modified. The joint angles selected as control variables for joint modification control are the stance ankle roll and pitch, and the stance hip pitch, roll and yaw. The ankle and hip pitch (joints 1 and 5, respectively, see Fig. 6-right), were modified between around 1.8 and 2.2 s. The imitating joint paths are almost always superposed to the reference: time-scaling was mostly used to perform the motion meeting the balance constraint, but the use of time-scaling alone would not have allowed performing the kick and keeping the balance of the imitating system.

4 Hybrid Approach Based on Optimization

The hybrid approach via optimization technique is implemented as a weighted multi-objective function. It incorporates the parameters pertaining to the joints and the time evolution of the motion. The objective function minimizes the difference between the virtual time $s(t)$ and the reference time t, and also the difference between the chosen reference joint paths and the performed ones. The time and joint variables are two different entities which will be balanced by a weighting factor α.

The optimization problem consists in finding s and q minimizing $\forall\ t_i \in [t_1, t_N]$ the objective function C.

$$C = \sum_{i=1}^{N} (s(t_i) - t_i)^2 + (0.1)^{\alpha} \sum_{i=1}^{N} (q(t_i) - q^r(t_i))^2 \tag{9}$$

where t_1 and t_N denote respectively the starting and ending instants of the observed motion. The first term of the criterion penalizes the error between virtual time and time; the second term penalizes the error on the joint paths. The variable t_i is the time or virtual time, it is the variable used to express the joint configuration. The optimization is subjected to the following inequality constraints: ZMP within its limits; positive reaction force; physical limits of the robot respected and virtual time monotonically increasing (the derivative of the virtual time should never be negative).

The optimization variables are the cubic spline parameters of the virtual time and of the selected joint trajectories (Munirathinam et al. 2012). The resolution of the polynomial depends upon the number of knots in the spline interpolation. 15 knots, or control points, were defined between the initial and final instants for the kick motion. The Matlab function *fmincon* was used to perform the sequential quadratic programming (SQP) for the constrained nonlinear optimization.

The higher the value of α, the greater influence will the time-scaling criterion have and reciprocally. $\alpha = 4$ is chosen so the result obtained should greatly favor the use of the time-scaling criterion.

The same kick motion presented in Fig. 5 is treated by the optimization algorithm. Figure 7 illustrates the results in terms of ZMP (left) and virtual time

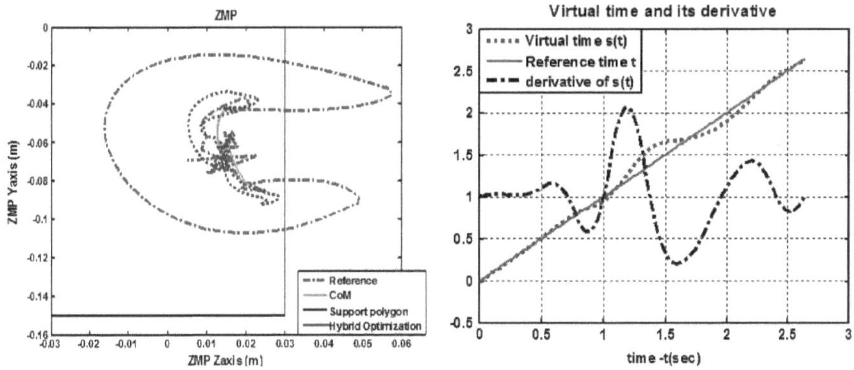

Fig. 7 *Left* ZMP before (*dashed*) and the after hybrid optimization (*dotted*). *Solid line* is the CoM projection; *right* the virtual time and its first derivative

(right). There is no error on the joints trajectories: reference and imitation joint trajectories were identical as expected when setting a high value for α. In this approach, contrarly to the control approach, a feasible ZMP trajectory was found: the ZMP remains within the support area during the complete motion. The ZMP trajectory is continuous and smooth-looking, although far from the limit most of the time. The virtual time remains close to the reference and its derivative results in a smooth curve oscillating around the value 1. The total duration of the kick motion is the same as for the reference motion, which means that virtual and real times were synchronized at the end of the motion.

5 Discussions

In both algorithms, time-scaling was favored as main way of solving the balance problem: in the control part, joint modification occurs only when time-scaling fails. In the optimization part, the weight of the time-scaling criterion is much greater than the one for joint modification, resulting in identical joint trajectories for the reference and the imitated motions in the chosen sample motion.

The behaviors of the two algorithms are very different from the effect of anticipating or not the future movements. Indeed, the optimization algorithm deals with the complete motion as whole, whereas the control approach deals with the balance problem when it occurs. As a result, the ZMP trajectories that can be observed in Figs. 6-left and 7-left show different behaviors: hybrid control tracks the reference trajectory as long and as close as possible, and stops abruptly the tracking when the robot balance is threatened, i.e. when reaching the boundary of the support area. Then, it follows the limit of the support area and gets back to tracking the reference as soon as balance is no more threatened. The ZMP trajectory is continuous but shows some angles illustrating a not so smooth path.

Hybrid optimization proposes a solution that keeps the ZMP farther from the boundaries as much as possible and therefore farther from the ZMP reference even when balance is safe. The reference is not exactly tracked, but this approach generates a smooth ZMP trajectory for the whole observed motion. The solution provided by the optimization approach only involves time-scaling, while the control approach has not been able to find a solution using only time-scaling due to its lack of anticipation. The calculation cost for the hybrid optimization is about 100 times greater than for the hybrid control.

Two of the greatest advantages of the control approach are its potential to be used for online applications and its respect of the reference movement coordination. One of the greatest advantages of the optimization approach is its potential for anticipating the motion. The human beings traditionally use motion anticipation they acquired from their experience (learning) and adapt their behavior to a current context (Sakka and Yokoi 2005). This dual human process anticipation/adaptation is offered by the two approaches, respectively associated to optimization/control. We can conclude that the two discussed algorithm are dual in terms of the way they deal with the imitation problem under balance constraint. Their complementarity could be used in the future, for example to learn online from human motion using the control approach and improve offline the motion by optimization.

We could observe that the hybrid characteristics are used differently by control or by optimization. In the control approach, time-scaling is predominant and joint modification is used only when time-scaling does not find a feasible solution. In the optimization approach, both time-scaling and joint modification are active even though the weighting factor α was chosen high enough to favor time-scaling.

6 Conclusions

A hybrid approach in motion imitation from human beings to humanoid robots was presented, using either control or optimization formulation. Hybrid holds for mixing time-scaling and joints modification in order to take advantage of both while solving some of their respective drawbacks. Several key observations were made on the hybrid approach based on control or on optimization: (1) Hybrid imitation leads to satisfactory results in terms of offline imitation under balance constraint, using either control or optimization approach; (2) Control approach may be used for online imitation whereas optimization may be used for motion anticipation; (3) Time-scaling respects the reference motion coordination; 4) Control and optimization are dual approaches. Their complementarity could be grouped in a learning-by-observation process.

Both approaches were compared and illustrated by a kick motion performed by a human actor, and successfully replayed by NAO humanoid robot.

In our future work, the current control approach will be extended for online motion imitation. A second perspective will be to couple the two approaches to set an autonomous motion learning process based on human imitation.

References

Arai, H. Tanie, K. and Shiroma, N. Time-scaling control of an underactuated manipulator. IEEE International Conference on Robotics and Automation (1998).

Breazeal,C. and Scassellati, B. Robots that imitate humans. Trends in Cognitive Sciences, **6**, 481–487 (2002).

Chevallereau, C. Time-scaling control for an under actuated biped robot. IEEE Transactions on Robotics and Automation, **19**(2), 362–368 (2003).

Dahl, O. and Nielsen, L. Torque-limited path following by online trajectory time-scaling. IEEE Transactions on Robotics and Automation, **6**(5), 554–561 (1990).

Dariush, B. Gienger, M. Arumbakkam, A. Zhu,Y. Jian, B. Fujimura, K and Goerick, C. Online transfer of human motion to humanoids. International Journal on Humanoid Robotics, **6**(2), 265–289 (2009).

Djoudi, D and Chevallereau, C. Feet can improve the stability property of a control law for a walking robot. IEEE International Conference on Robotics and Automation (2006).

Do, M. Azad, P. Asfour, T and Dillmann, R. Imitation of human motion by a humanoid robot using non-linear optimization. IEEE-RAS International Conference on Humanoid Robots (2008).

Hollerbach, John M. Dynamic Scaling of Manipulator Trajectories. American Control Conference (1983).

Holm, H. Lee, D and Spong, M. Time-scaling trajectories of passive dynamic bipedal robots. IEEE International Conference on Robotics and Automation (2007).

Kim, S. Kim, C. You, B and Oh, S. Stable whole-body motion generation for humanoid robots to imitate human motions. IEEE/RSJ International Conference on Intelligent Robots and Systems (2009).

Munirathinam, K. Sakka, S and Chevallereau, C. Dynamic motion imitation of two articulated systems using nonlinear time scaling of joint trajectories. IEEE International Conference on Intelligent Robots and Systems (2012).

Nakaoka, S. Nakazawa, A. Yokoi, K. Hirukawa, H and Ikeuchi, K. Generating whole body motions for a biped humanoid robot from captured human dances. IEEE International Conference on Robotics and Automation (2003).

Ott, C. Lee, D and Nakamura, Y. Motion capture based human motion recognition and imitation by direct marker control. IEEE-RAS International Conference on Humanoid Robots (2008).

Pollard, N. Hodgins, J. Riley, M. and Atkeson, C. Adapting human motion for the control of a humanoid robot. IEEE International Conference on Robotics and Automation (2002).

Saegusa, R. Nori, F. Sandini, G. Metta, G. and Sakka, S. Sensory prediction for autonomous robots. IEEE-RAS International Conference on Humanoid Robots (2007).

Sakka, S. Poubel, L. Cehajic, D and Creusot, D. Tasks prioritization for whole-body IK-based online imitation of human motion by humanoid robots. International Journal of Humanoid Robotics (2014-to appear).

Sakka, S. and Yokoi, K. Humanoid vertical jumping based on force feedback and inertial forces optimization. IEEE International Conference on Robotics and Automation (2005).

Samson, C. Control of chained systems: application to path following and time-varying point-stabilization of mobile robots. IEEE Transactions on Automatic Control, **40**(1), 64–77 (1995).

Schall, S. Is imitation learning -the route to humanoid robots? Trends in Cognitive Sciences, **3**, 233–242 (1999).
Suleiman, W. Yoshida, E. Kanehiro, F. Laumond, J.-P and Monin, A. On human motion imitation by humanoid robots. IEEE International Conference on Robotics and Automation (2008).

Contributions on the Modeling and Simulation of the Human Knee Joint with Applications to the Robotic Structures

D. Tarnita, M. Catana and D. N. Tarnita

Abstract The main objective of this chapter is to develop a three-dimensional solid finite element model of the healthy knee joint to predict stresses in its individual components and to study the effects of the frontal plane tibio–femoral angle on the stress distribution in the knee cartilages and menisci. It was developed the geometric models of the joint which shows different tilt in varus and valgus with 5°, the joint being affected by osteoarthritis in the medial and lateral compartment. For geometric modeling of the human knee joint was used the embedded applications: Design Modeler, SpaceClaim under Ansys Workbench 14.5 software package. For each model a non-linear analysis was performed. The non-linearities are due to the presence of the contact elements modeled between components surfaces. The applied force was equal with 800 N. Finally the results obtained for normal knee and for OA knee joint are compared.

Keywords 3D model · Finite element analysis · Osteoarthritis · Varus · Valgus

1 Introduction

In last years several humanoids robots are able to walk and perform human-like movements, several humanoid friendly robots that assist human activities in human daily environments such as in homes, offices, and hospitals, have been developed (Bae 2012; Fening 2005; Bahraminasaba 2011; Sandholm 2011).

D. Tarnita (✉) · M. Catana
University of Craiova, Craiova, Romania
e-mail: tarnita.daniela@gmail.com

M. Catana
e-mail: marius_catana79@yahoo.com

D. N. Tarnita
University of Medicine and Pharmacy, Craiova, Romania
e-mail: dan_tarnita@yahoo.com

A. Rodić et al. (eds.), *New Trends in Medical and Service Robots*,
Mechanisms and Machine Science 20, DOI: 10.1007/978-3-319-05431-5_19,

Anyhow, the structure of such robots significantly differs from the human's one. Among the most skilled robots are Asimo (Mohammad 2011), produced by Honda, Wabian-2R (Kazemi 2011), produced by Waseda University and LARP (Bahraminasaba 2011; Sandholm 2011), the biped robot of Politecnico di Milano.

An emergence of humanoid robots is strongly expected because of anthropomorphism, friendly design, applicability of locomotion, behavior within the human living environments. The more humanoid robots are expected to perform several application tasks in an actual human living environment (Kaneko et al. 2002).

A key factor for the successful co-existence of the humanoid robots with humans lies in their capacity to withstand unexpected perturbations without the loss of balance (Goswami 2005).

In papers (Gini et al. 2007; Federico et al. 2010) the authors present a human-oriented approach to the study of the biped gait for a humanoid robot. Starting from the analysis of the human lower-limbs, they figured out which features of the human legs are fundamental for a correct walking motion and can be adopted in the mechanical design of a humanoid robot. In particular they focused on the knee, designed as a compliant human-like knee instead of a classical pin-joint.

The method is used for future developments of LARP, the biped of Politecnico di Milano, but it can produce valid results for any robot, in evaluating design choices for future humanoid robots (Gini et al. 2007; Federico Moro et al. 2010).

Human knee joint is one of the most complex joints in the human body, taking into account the number of its components, their spatial geometry and their mechanical properties, the contacts between elements and the pressures acting on them.

Virtual modeling of human knee joint has been addressed in several articles (Bae 2012; Fening 2005; Bahraminasaba 2011; Sandholm 2011; Mohammad 2011; Kazemi 2011; Kubicek 2009; Hartley 2009; Harrysson 2007). Virtual models were analyzed with FEM, after performing a finite element model with tetrahedral type (Vidal 2008), hexahedral, or using automatic meshing methods. The articles have used an algorithm for meshing with hexahedrons and bricks in order to analyze with a much better approximation for the tibio–femoral contact area (Fening 2005; Mohammad 2011; Kazemi 2011; Kubicek 2009). Musculoskeletal disorders are the most frequent causes for long-lasting or chronic pain and for restrictions on mobility and physical performance; they can lead, in the extreme case, to an increased morbidity; they affect hundreds of millions of people worldwide with dramatic increases expected due to a doubling in the number of people over 50 years by 2020 (http://www.bme.master.unibe.ch/unibe/medizin/bioeng/content/e818/e820/e1697/e2045/FAMusculoskeletal_eng.pdf).

The knee osteoarthritis is one of the major chronic diseases usually found in people of middle age and old age and also mainly causes various disabilities. Osteoarthritis (OA) is the fourth most frequent cause of health problems in women and the eighth most frequent cause in men. About 40 % of all persons over the age of 70 are affected by osteoarthritis of the knee. About 80 % of persons with osteoarthritis suffer from limited mobility (http://www.bme.master.unibe.ch/unibe/medizin/bioeng/content/e818/e820/e1697/e2045/FAMusculoskeletal_eng.pdf). About 25 % of these OA persons can no longer perform the most important basic activities of daily life (http://www.bme.master.unibe.ch/unibe/medizin/bioeng/content/e818/e820/e1697/e2045/FAMusculoskeletal_eng.pdf). There are many causes of osteoarthritis like: deviation of the mechanical axis in the frontal plane, sagittal knee misalignment, overweight, excessive sport activities, trauma, biological, menisci lesion, instability due to the knee ligament injuries.

Knee osteoarthritis involves a degenerative process of cartilage in the knee joint leading to its loss (http://www.bme.master.unibe.ch/unibe/medizin/bioeng/content/e818/e820/e1697/e2045/FAMusculoskeletal_eng.pdf). It can also affect any or both compartments of the knee joint (Checa 2008). This degenerative process can be generally caused by obesity (Yang 2007), by excessive physical activity, by joint trauma, immobilization and hypermobility (Chantarapanich 2009). Knee misalignment is considered one of the biomechanical key factors, factors that influence the progression of the knee osteoarthritis (Yang 2009).

2 Method

To obtain the geometric model of the healthy knee joint, CT images were processed using SpaceClaim integrated application and to obtain the 3D virtual model the integrated application Design Modeler was used (Fig. 1). The CT images were obtained using a CT scanner. More than 500 images were obtained. To achieve bone contours we used SpaceClaim application, which is integrated in the ANSYS Workbench package. This application is a pre-processor for direct modeling. The CT files were imported in SpaceClaim as .jpg files, where contour lines were created. For each bone, the sections were imported one-by-one in Design-Modeler parallel sketches. The software allows the generation of the parametrical tridimensional models which can be modified, edited and exported in kinematical or FEA software.

The virtual biomechanical system of the human knee contains femur, tibia and fibula bones, medial and lateral ligaments, medial and lateral menisci, femoral and tibial cartilages (Catana and Tarnita 2012). Based on the modelled geometry of the bones, the ligaments, the cartilages and the menisci were created (Fig. 2).

The components were placed in a global system XYZ. Nonlinear structural analysis is static; non-linearity is done by the existence of the nonlinear contacts between the cartilages and menisci. Changes and proper positioning of the components was done using the package ANSYS Workbench 14.5, CAE software which allows rapid modeling of a proper record and control of the geometric problems arising in the contact zone. The correct position requires a real placement of components, a proper distance between them and correct geometric structure.

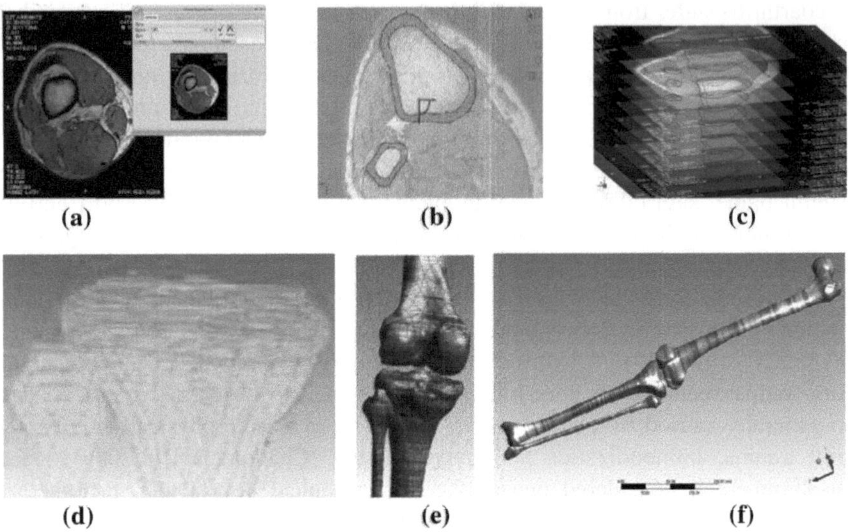

Fig. 1 **a** CT Images of the femur. **b** CT imported and prepared in SpaceClaim application. **c** Positioning of CT images in the same coordinate system XYZ. **d** Contour lines for distal head of tibia and peroneu. **e** Solid definition of the contour lines. **f** Solid geometry of bones: femur, tibia and peroneu

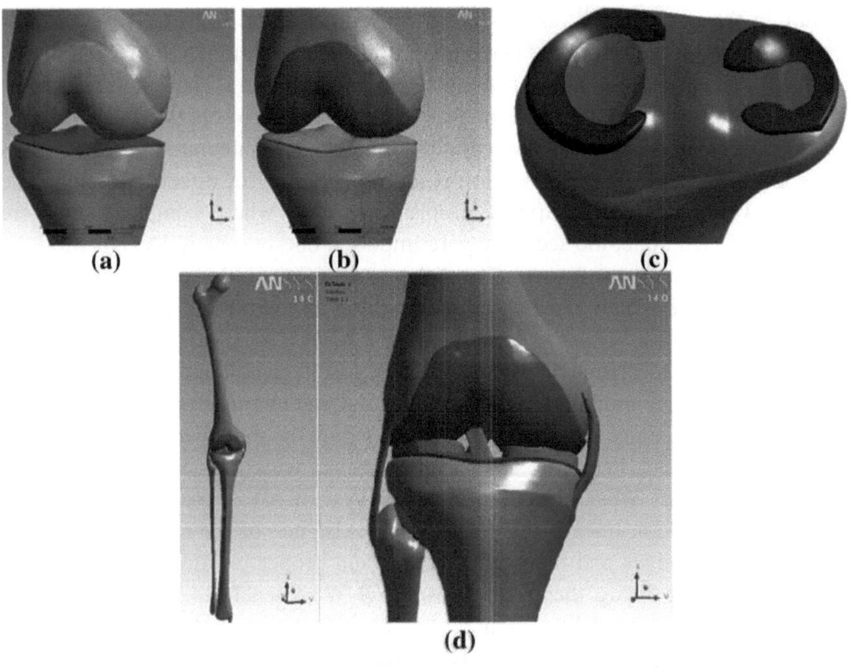

Fig. 2 Anterior views for: **a** Femoral articular cartilage. **b** Tibial articular cartilage. **c** 3D model of distal head of tibia with menisci. **d** Complex knee joint model in the normal position

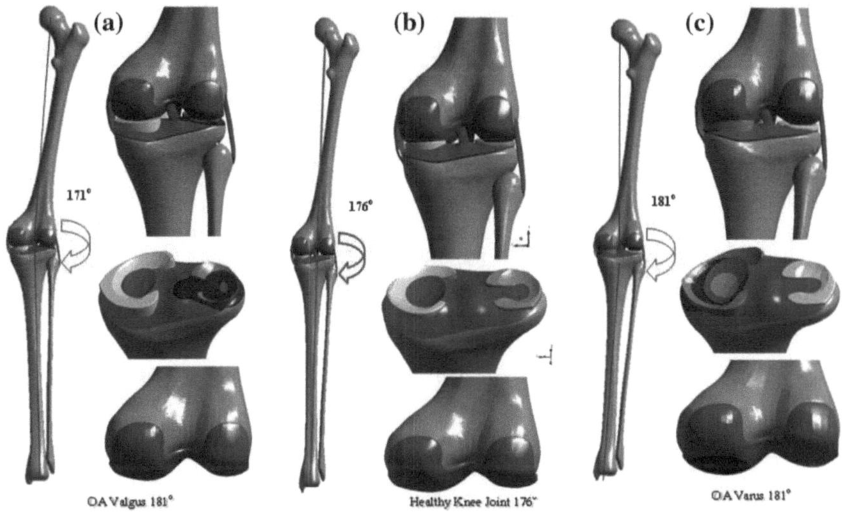

Fig. 3 Virtual 3D models for different cases: **a** OA valgus knee joint. **b** Healthy knee joint. **c** OA valgus knee joint

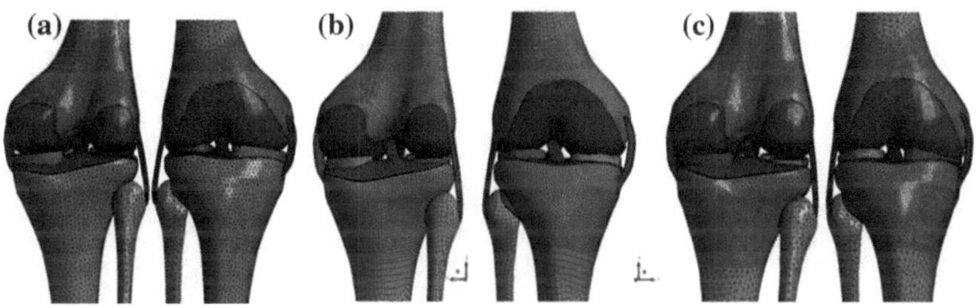

Fig. 4 The network nodes and elements for: **a** Healthy knee. **b** OA knee joint of knee varus inclination of 5°. **c** OA knee joint of knee valgus inclination of 5°

The healthy joint is featured by a 176° angle between femur and tibia, while, for he joint affected by osteoarthritis the analyzed geometry presented in this chapter, has an inclination of 171° for valgus and 181° for varus (Fig. 3).

For geometric discretization into nodes and elements, the Solid 186 and Solid 187 tetrahedron elements, which are defined by 20 nodes, and respectively by 10 nodes, having three degrees of freedom per node: translations in the nodal x, y, and z directions, are used. Advanced discretization methods such as "Sweep", "Hex Dominant" and "Patch Conforming" were used (Fig. 4).

The elements dimension for the areas of interest is 1 mm and for the rest of the structure, a global size of 4 mm was used. The transition between two regions

Table 1 Number of nodes and elements for all components of the healthy virtual knee

Component	Number of nodes	Number of elements
Femur	185,402	58,604
Femoral cartilage	80,036	22,061
Tibia	127,919	38,401
Tibial cartilage	33,787	8,795
Medial menisci	8,182	2,596
Lateral menisci	7,965	2,519
Peroneu	39,118	12,876
Peroneu–tibia cartilage	6,678	2,365
LCM	6,449	2,223
LCL	7,876	2,747
LIA	1,660	620
LIP	1,885	679
Total	488,092	148,397

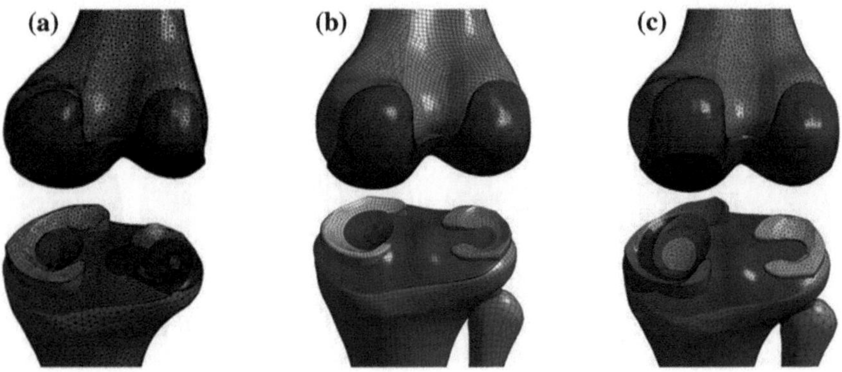

Fig. 5 The network nodes and elements for: **a** OA knee joint of knee varus inclination of 5°. **b** Healthy knee. **c** OA knee joint of knee varus inclination of 5°

(1–4 mm) was solved by the software, using a growth rate of 1.33. Taking into account the large number of nodes and elements, but also the presence of nonlinear contacts, for solving it is necessary to implement a "smaller steps" system; solver was set as Preconditioned Conjugate Gradient level 2 iterative types.

For each studied case, the virtual model is discretized individually, the contact areas are readjusted and the analysis is run (Fig. 5). In Table 1 the number of nodes and elements for all components of the healthy virtual knee are presented.

Table 2 Material properties used for knee geometric components (Lyu et al. 2012; Yang 2007; Chantarapanich 2009)

Geometry	Young's modulus (MPa)	Poisson's ratio
Cortical—femur bone	18,600	0.3
Cortical—tibia bone	12,500	0.3
Trabecular bone	500	0.3
Cartilage	12	0.475
Menisci	59	0.49
LCM—LCL	10	0.49
LIA—LIP	1	0.49

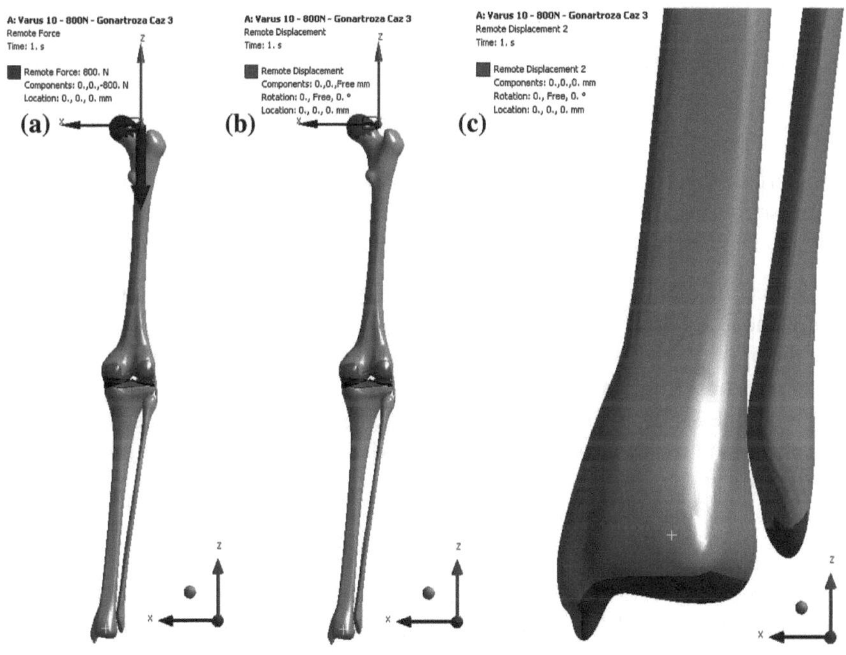

Fig. 6 Boundary conditions for the analyses

During the progressive stages of the osteoarthritis, the menisci and the cartilage change their structures and their material properties. For an accurate virtual simulation of the process, the settings take into account these aspects, by reducing with 50 % the elasticity of the menisci and cartilage.

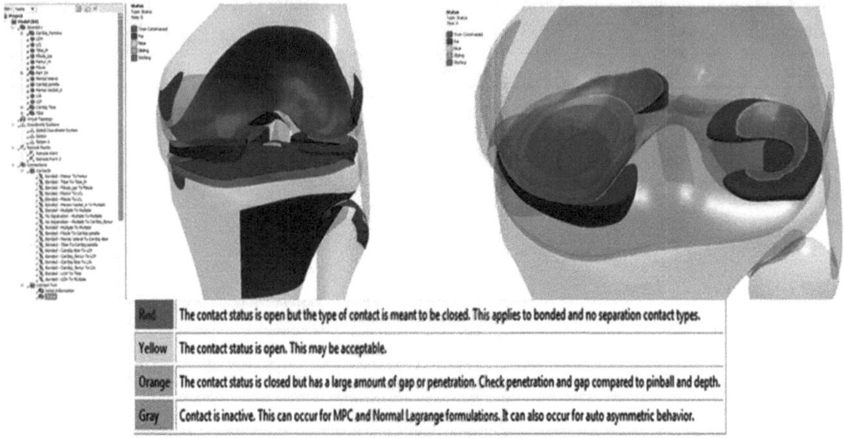

Fig. 7 The contacts status

Material properties of knee geometric components are presented in Table 2. The settings and the conditions (Fig. 6) for the analysis are:

- taking into account the large number of nodes and elements but, also, the presence of nonlinear contacts, for solving the analysis it is necessary to implement a "smaller steps" system;
- on the proximal head of the femur bone there is applied a 800 N force in the—Z axis direction (Fig. 6a);
- on the same location, the "Remote Displacement" is applied; this setting allows Z offset and RotY around the femur, which allows movement of the hip (Fig. 6b);
- on the tibia distal head the "Remote Displacement" is applied; this setting allows RotY (movement of the ankle around the tibia).

Contact stiffness was also adjusted for the time of settlement. If the difficulties arise, the stiffness will be reduced automatically. A setting called NSF analysis ("Normal Stiffness Factor"), a normal multiplication factor used to calculate the stiffness of the code, was introduced.

It is also possible to check the status for contacts participating in the analysis (Fig. 7). To better simulate the nonlinear contacts, "Bonded" and "No Separation" contacts type and "Augmented Lagrange" calculation algorithm were used. For a more efficient mathematical representation of these contact areas, the option "Pindball Region" with a radius of 0.1 mm was used. The program has the opportunity to establish automatically contacts.

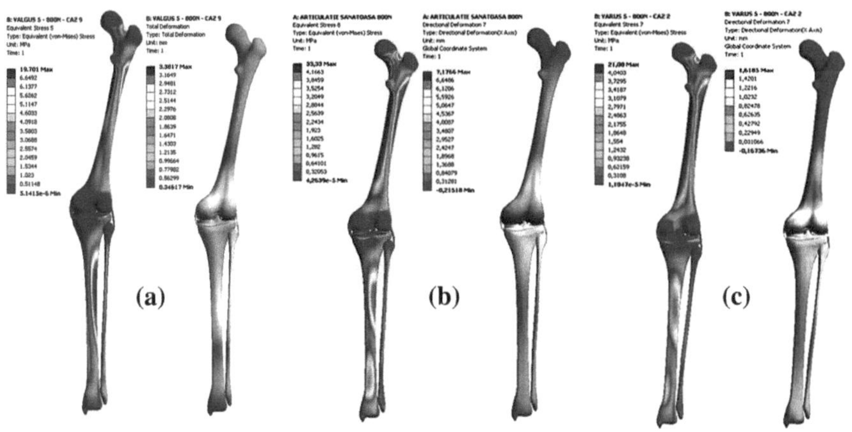

Fig. 8 von Mises stress and lateral displacement for **a** OA valgus knee. **b** Healthy knee. **c** OA varus knee

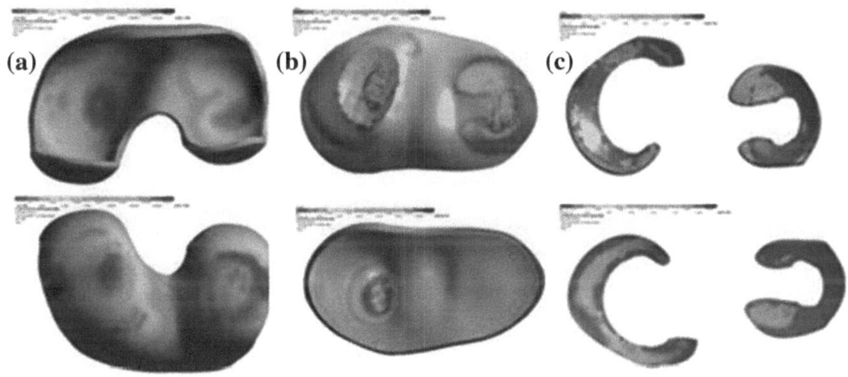

Fig. 9 Healthy Knee—von Mises stress for: **a** Femoral cartilage. **b** Tibial cartilage. **c** Menisci; *First line*—Top view; *Second line*—Bottom view

3 Results

To investigate the role of the articular cartilage in the developing of the osteoarthritis, and to analyze and simulate the biomechanical behavior of the knee joint, a non-linear analysis with finite element method was performed. The non-linearities are due to the presence of the contact elements modeled between components surfaces. For each analysis the maximum values of the von Mises stress and of the lateral displacements for entire assembly were extracted (Fig. 8). The maps of the von Mises stress for the femoral cartilage, for the tibial cartilage and for the menisci are presented: healthy knee joint (Fig. 9), OA varus knee (Fig. 10),

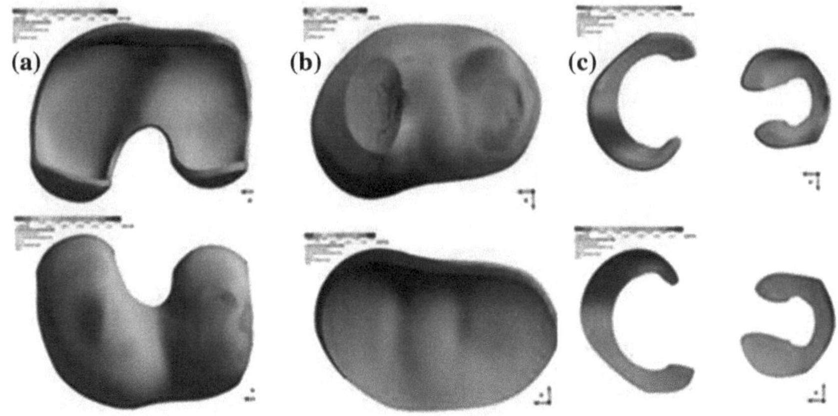

Fig. 10 Healthy knee—lateral displacement for **a** Femoral cartilage. **b** Tibial cartilage. **c** Menisci; *First line*—Top view; *Second line*—Bottom view

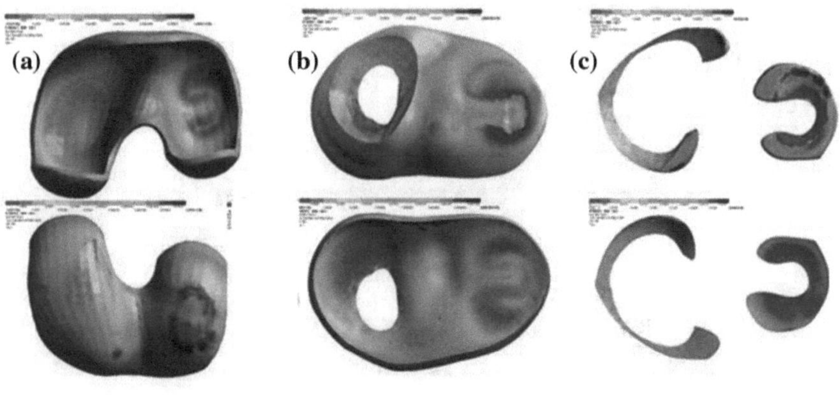

Fig. 11 OA varus knee—von Mises stress for **a** Femoral cartilage. **b** Tibial cartilage. **c** Menisci; *First line*—Top view; *Second line*—Bottom view

OA valgus knee (Fig. 11). The maps of the lateral displacements are presented for: healthy knee joint (Fig. 12), OA varus knee (Fig. 13), OA valgus knee (Fig. 14).

The maximum values resulted from this analysis are presented in Table 3. We can observe an increase of the stress values in the cartilages from healthy knee to OA knee joint cases.

The results show that the misalignment leads to an increase of stress value and this determines the damage of the articular cartilage and, finally, an augmenting of the osteoarthritis phenomenon (Fig. 15). The values obtained in this study are similar with those obtained by other authors: Haut et al. (2002), Riegger et al. (1998), Ihn et al. (1993), Thambyah et al. (2005).

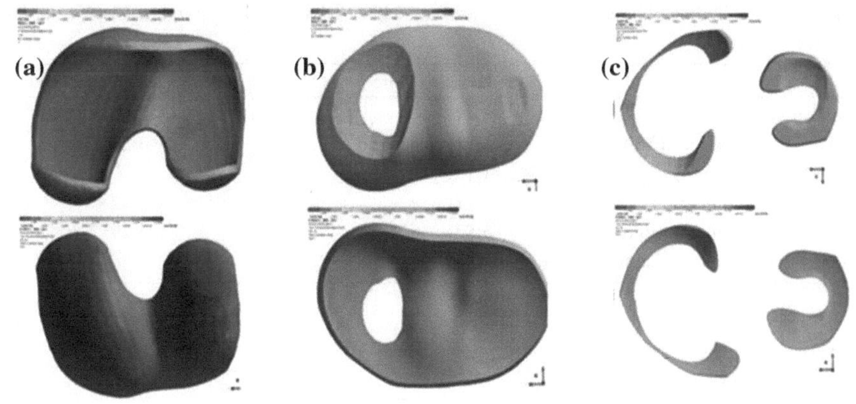

Fig. 12 OA varus Knee—Lateral Displacement for **a** Femoral cartilage. **b** Tibial cartilage. **c** Menisci; *First line*—Top view; *Second line*—Bottom view

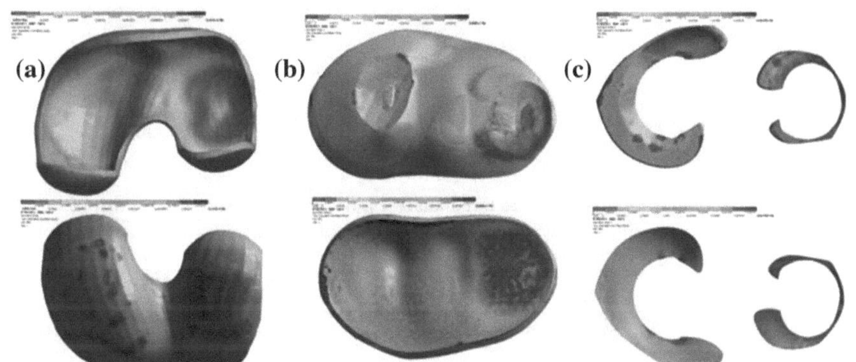

Fig. 13 OA valgus Knee—von Mises stress for cartilage **a** Femur cartilage. **b** Tibia cartilage. **c** Menisci; *First line*—Top view; *Second line*—Bottom view

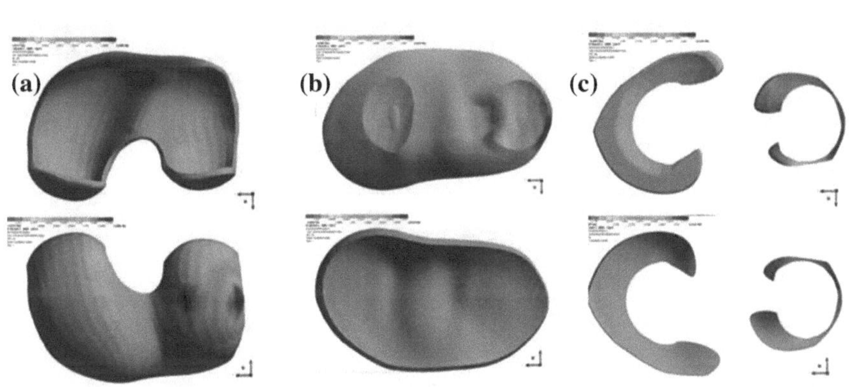

Fig. 14 OA valgus knee—lateral displacement for **a** Femur cartilage. **b** Tibia cartilage. **c** Menisci;; *First line*—Top view; *Second line*—Bottom view

Table 3 The results obtained for the analyses: von Mises stress (MPa) and lateral displacements (mm)

Component	Healthy knee	OA varus knee	OA valgus knee
Femoral cartilage stress (MPa)	2.41	3.42	2.65
Tibial cartilage stress (MPa)	1.71	2.08	3.89
Menisci stress (MPa)	1.12	1.54	2.87
Lateral displacements femur (mm)	7.17	1.61	3.32
Lateral displacements tibia (mm)	5.88	1.43	3.29
Lateral displacements menisci (mm)	6.05	1.52	3.24

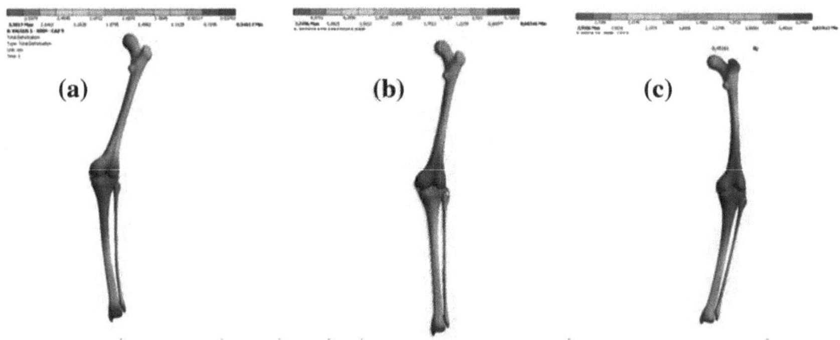

Fig. 15 Misalignments obtained for the three analyses: **a** OA valgus knee lateral displacement; **b** Healthy human knee joint; **c** OA vargus knee lateral displacement

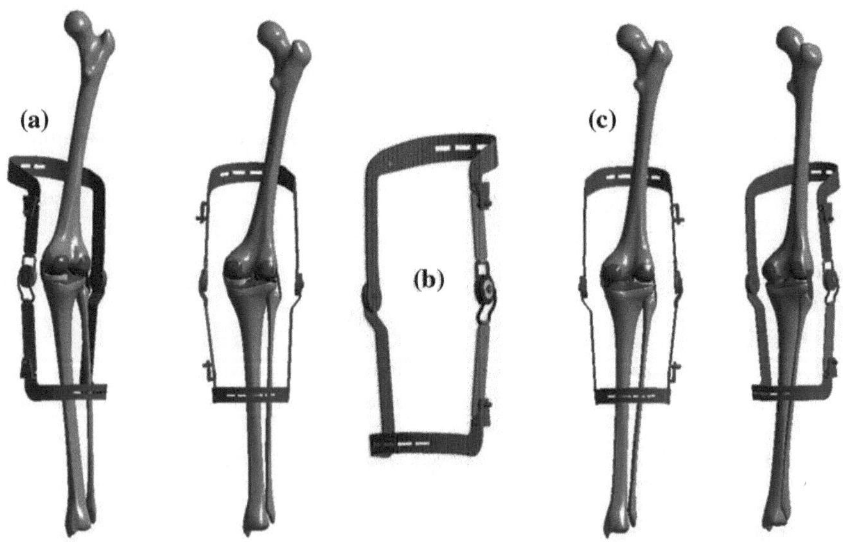

Fig. 16 **a** Knee joint *valgus* 5° with orthotic device; **b** Orthotic device; **c** Knee joint *varus* 5° with orthotic device

4 Conclusions

The biomechanical behavior of human knee cartilages is important in order to understand the OA phenomenon due to the mechanical factors. The advantage of the numerical simulations consists in the fact they can be done in advance in order to evaluate the osteoarthritic process without an invasive intervention. A standard finite element model of the knee model will help surgeons and biomechanical researchers to develop improved implants and treatment method for patients suffering bone loss and diseases.

The Finite Element Method Analysis is a modern and very power full method, useful for understanding the biomechanical behavior of human joints (normal and pathological). The results of our study show that the contact areas of initial cartilage damage are changing the misalignment, determining the increase of the stress magnitude. The damage magnitude could determine progressive cartilage erosion, and, finally, an augmenting of the osteoarthritis phenomenon. The values obtained in this study are similar with those obtained by other authors and similar with clinical observations. These conclusions confirm the fidelity and the accuracy of the knee virtual model and of the numerical simulations. A standard finite element model of the knee model will help surgeons and biomechanical researchers to develop improved implants and treatment method for patients suffering bone loss and diseases. Additionally, the finite element model used in the present study, characterized by a solid hexahedral element mesh, was able to analyze the stress and displacements in the human knee joint.

The results could be important for the future design of the knee joint used in the humanoid robots that are able to walk in an unstructured environment like home, where movements are based on the human kinematic abilities. The similarity between the behavior of human walking and of the humanoid robots can be exploited to promote a further research comparing the bipedal behavior with human gait.

The virtual model, patterned after human anatomy, can be a good base for future research:

- Improving the 3D virtual model of the human knee joint;
- The kinematical and dynamical simulations and analysis using FEA method for the knee joint in different normal or pathological situations;
- Virtual and experimental studies for orthotic and prosthetic devices design and their optimization for improving the knee mobility performances. In Fig. 16 the virtual model of an orthotic device designed for the osteoarthritic knee is presented. This device will be used to rehabilitate the knee movements and to ameliorate the pain caused by osteoarthritis disease.

Acknowledgments This work was supported by the strategic grant POSDRU/CPP107/DMI1.5/S/78421, Project ID78421 (2010), co-financed by the European Social Fund within the SO Program Human Resources Development 2007–2013.

References

Bae, Y.J.: Biomechanical analysis of the effects of medial meniscectomy on degenerative osteoarthritis, Med Biol Eng Comput, Springer, 50, 2012.

Bahraminasaba, M.: Finite Element Analysis of the Effect of Shape Memory Alloy on the Stress Distribution and Contact Pressure in Total Knee Replacement, Trends Biomater. Artif. Organs. 25, 3, 2011.

Catana, M., Tarnita, D.: The three-dimensional modeling of the complex virtual human knee joint, Bulletin of the Polytechnic Institute of Iasi, Tom LVIII (LXII) Fasc.3, 303–308, 2012.

Chantarapanich, N.: A finite element study of stress distributions in normal and osteoarthritic knee joints, J Med Assoc Thai. 92, 2009.

Checa, S., Influence of an interpositional spacer on the behaviour of the tibio-femoral joint: A finite element study. In: Clinical Biomechanics 23, 2008.

Federico Moro, F., Gini, G., Zefran, M., Rodic, A.: Simulation for the Optimal Design of a Biped Robot: Analysis of Energy Consumption, Proceeding SIMPAR'10, Proceedings of the Second international conference on Simulation, modeling, and programming for autonomous robots. Pages 449-460, Springer-Verlag Berlin, Heidelberg ©2010.

Fening, D.S.: The effects of meniscal sizing on the knee using finite element methods, College of Engineering and Technology of Ohio University. 2005.

Gini. G., Scarfogliero, U., Folgheraiter, M.: Human-Oriented Biped Robot Design: Insights into the Development of a truly Anthropomorphic Leg, 2007 IEEE International Conference on Robotics and Automation Roma, Italy. pp. 2910–2915, 2007.

Goswami, M.A.A.: A Biomechanically Motivated Two-Phase Strategy for Biped Upright Balance Control, Proceedings of the 2005 IEEE International Conference on Robotics and Automation, Barcelona, Spain. pp 2008–2013, 2005.

Harrysson, O.L.: Custom-designed orthopedic implants evaluated using finite element analysis of patient-specific computed tomography data: femoral-component case study, BMC Musculoskeletal Disorders, 2007.

Hartley, Y.N.: The effect of the frontal plane tibiofemoral angle on the contact stress and strain at the knee joint, Mechanical Engineering Dissertations, Department of Mechanical and Industrial Engineering, Northeastern University, 2009.

Haut, T.L., Hull, M.L., Rashid, M.M., Jacobs, C.R.: A finite element model of the human knee joint for the study of tibio-femoral contact, Journal of Biomechanical Engineering. 124, 273–280, 2002.

Ihn, J.C., Kim, S.J., Park, I.H.: In vivo study of contact area and pressure distribution in the human knee after partial and total meniscectomy, Int. Orthop. 17, 214–218, 1993.

Kaneko, M.K, Kajita, S., Kanehiro, F., Yokoi, K., Fujiwara, K., Hirukawa, H., Kawasaki, T., Hirata, M., Isozumi, T.: Design of Advanced Leg Module for Humanoid Robotics Project, Proceedings of the 2002 International Conference on Robotics & Automation, Washington. pp. 38–45, 2002.

Kazemi, M.: Creep Behavior of the Intact and Meniscectomy Knee Joints, Journal of the Mechanical Behavior of Biomedical Materials, 2011.

Kubicek, M.: Stress strain analysis of knee joint, Engineering Mechanics, 16, 5, 2009.

Lyu, S., Liu, D., Tseng, C., Wang, H., Chau, L.: Knee health promotion option for osteoarthritic knee: Cartilage regeneration is possible. In: Osteoarthritis - Diagnosis, Treatment and Surgery, ISBN 978-953-51-0168-0, 2012.

Mohammad, K.: A musculoskeletal model of a subject specific knee joint with menisci during the stance phase of a walk cycle, Dissertation in engineering and mathematics, University of Missouri-Kansas City, 2011.

Riegger, K.C., Gerhart, T.N., Power, W.R., Hayes, W.C.: Tibiofemoral contact pressures in degenerative joint disease, Clin. Orthop. 348, 233–245, 1998.

Sandholm, A.: Evaluation of a geometry-based knee joint compared to a planar knee joint, Virtual Reality Lab., École Polytechnique Fédérale de Lausanne, Lausanne, 2011.

Thambyah, A., Goh, J.C.H., De, S.D.: Contact stresses in the knee joint in deep flexion. Medical Engineering & Physics. 27, 329–335, 2005.

Vidal, A.: Analysis, simulation and prediction of contact stresses in articular cartilage of knee joint, Department of Mechanical Engineering, Instituto Tecnologico de Celaya, Mexico, International Conference Ansys, 2008.

Yang, N.: Effect of frontal plane tibio-femoral angle on the stress and strain at the knee cartilage during the stance phase of gait, Published online in Wiley Inter Science, 2009.

Yang, N.: The effects of tibio-femural angle and body weight on the stress field in the knee joint, International Mechanical Engineering Congress and Exposition, Seattle, 2007.

How to Control Anthropomimetic Robot: Engineering and Cognitive Approach

V. Potkonjak, K. Jovanovic and P. Milosavljevic

Abstract The anthropomimetics represents a relatively new discipline in the field of robotics that tends to go one step further than copying human shape and functionality. In order to fully transfer certain human behavior patterns to the robots working in a human adapted environment, it is necessary to fully copy human body and structure. However, the emerging issue in this field is how to control such a mechanism. This chapter presents some concepts related to the control of human- like drives. The first one is the biologically inspired and energy efficient puller-follower control concept for the antagonistically coupled compliant drives. Although the concept follows its biological paragon, it is still realizable in a conventional engineering way. Apart from the antagonistically coupled muscles, it is required to deal with the control of muscles crossing several joints (poly-articular muscles) or even multi-DOF joints, where conventional control techniques can hardly offer any solution. The second part of this chapter suggests possible approaches to dealing with these issues, by exploiting cognition and heuristics. The control algorithm involves two levels: feedforward (FF) and feedback (FB), both relying on the experience. Based on the prior knowledge of human-like motions, FF control is obtained using neural networks or heuristic approach. Regardless of the antagonistic drive structure, both methods are applicable to a wider class of robots. This chapter advocates these methods as an efficient tool to evade the exact mathematical modeling and conventional control of the nonlinear and redundant mechanical system. For fine movements, the FB

V. Potkonjak (✉) · K. Jovanovic
ETF Robotics Laboratory, School of Electrical Engineering,
University of Belgrade, Belgrade, Serbia
e-mail: potkonjak@yahoo.com

K. Jovanovic
e-mail: kosta.jovanovic@etf.bg.ac.rs

P. Milosavljevic
Automatic Control Laboratory, Swiss Federal Institute
of Technology Lausanne (EPFL), Lausanne, Switzerland
e-mail: predrag.milosavljevic@epfl.ch

A. Rodić et al. (eds.), *New Trends in Medical and Service Robots*,
Mechanisms and Machine Science 20, DOI: 10.1007/978-3-319-05431-5_20,

control is introduced through fuzzy logic. It presents a novel solution to issues emerging as a result of combining the experience-based learning and the "black-box" model of the system. Finally, we have compared and contrasted engineering and cognitive approaches, thus drawing attention to their advantages and disadvantages, as well as their possible applications.

Keywords Bio-inspired robotics · Musculoskeletal robot · Puller-follower control · Experience based control · Neural-fuzzy control

1 Introduction

Contemporary humanoid robots are built with the aim to achieve significant level of maneuverability and fit well within human centered environment. This further leads to distinguished human shape robots but also the robots of human size and proportion. Moreover, to act in a safe manner, significant level of intrinsic compliance must be embedded to them. Also, it is necessary to create robots whose mechanical structure resembles human anatomy so as to enable full transfer of some human behavior patterns to robots. This new direction in robotics is also known as anthropomimetic robotics (Holland and Knight 2006), and it already has numerous followers among distinguished research groups and project consortiums. Some of those include the University of Tokyo—robot Kenshiro (Asano et al. 2012), The Robot Studio—Eccerobot (Wittmeier et al. 2013), University of Osaka (Ikemoto et al. 2012), etc. Fig. 1.

Although novel materials and technology enable copying human form very successfully (Diamond et al. 2012), there is still some way to go in control of such mechanisms. This chapter presents some achievements in the field of anthropomimetic robot control from the conventional engineering standpoint, moving towards cognitive, learning and artificial intelligence perspective. In Sect. 2, feedback linearization is used as an efficient tool for controlling antagonistically coupled compliant drives. In order to compensate for the lack of model, bi-directional muscles, multi degree of freedom (DoF) joints, the solution in a form of experience exploitation, neural networks and fuzzy control is proposed in Sect. 3. Both FF and FB control levels are taken into consideration. The results of the proposed methodologies are reported in Sect. 4. Some advantages and drawbacks of the given approaches, limitations, as well as directions for future work are pointed out in Sect. 5.

2 Engineering Approach

Although human body and therefore anthropomimetic robots are not shaped in agreement with any engineering principle, some assumptions can be made for the purpose of gaining better understanding of the overall human behavior. Most

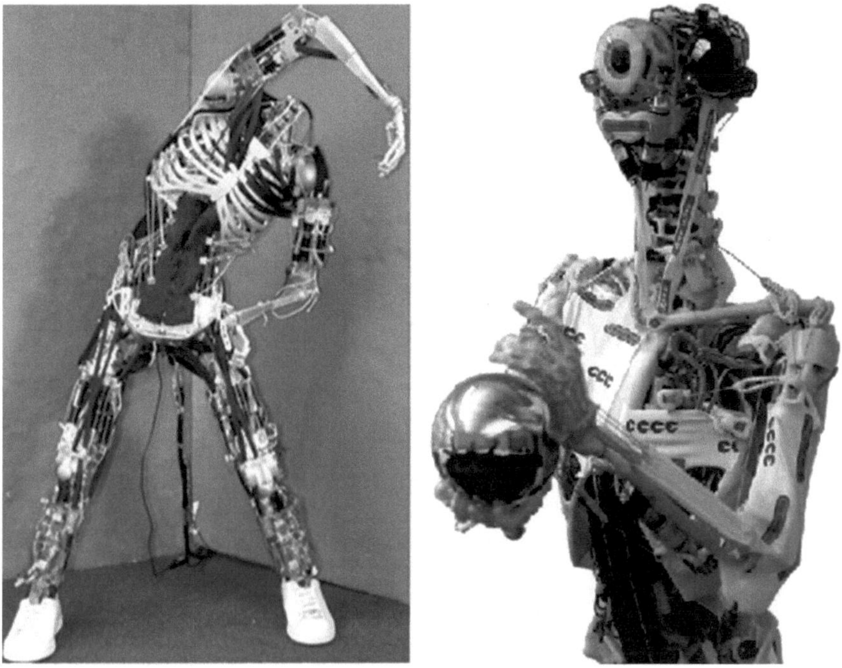

Fig. 1 Anthropomimetic robots—University of Tokyo JSK Laboratory's robot Kenshiro (on the *left*), The Robot studio and European Universities Consortium's Eccerobot (on the *right*)

human muscles are antagonistically coupled and using their co-contraction, movement is achieved. Considerable effort has already been put into optimizing muscle activities (Bortoletto et al. 2012; Oh et al. 2011). Even though they do not offer any finite solution, they all agree that the two basic principles are followed by different cost estimation: minimal energy consumption and accuracy of motion.

Barely any results have been presented with the aim to suggest the control of the antagonistically coupled compliant human-like drives (Wimbock et al. 2010; Potkonjak et al. 2011). Palli et al. (2008) used feedback linearization to achieve simultaneous control of the position and stiffness of antagonistic robot joints. However, this theory is not applicable if the elastic element is linear (as is the case in the operating range of human muscles), and it does not consider pulling limitation of muscle force and its representatives in technical implementation (tension in tendons must always be positive as human muscles can only pull and not push). Bearing in mind the above-mentioned restrictions and muscle-like features, we suggest novel control approach of antagonistic compliant joint—puller-follower control. It is inspired by electromyography signal patterns measured in antagonistically coupled human muscles (Hannaford and Stark 1985). The puller-follower approach uses feedback linearization to independently control joint position and pretension in the "following" tendon. While the "puller" controls joint positions,

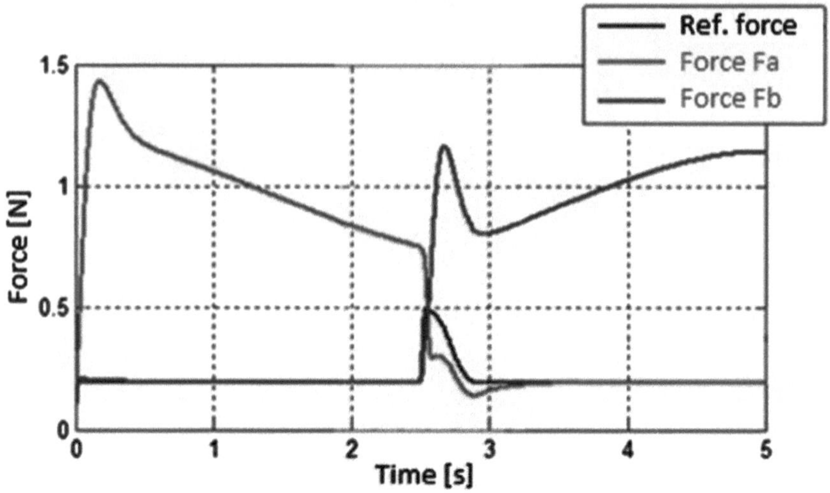

Fig. 2 Puller-follower principle. Due to energy efficiency, the reference tension force is kept on some low level, while during switching the adaptive reference force is increased to disable oscillation and slackening of the tendons

"follower" co-contracts the tendon to some prescribed tension level, which has to be low due to energy efficiency, but sufficiently high to prevent the slacking of the tendons. Of course, owing to the acceleration and deceleration phases and link movement in both directions, puller and follower need to occasionally change roles. This switching is followed by oscillations in tendon forces (switching shock), which can cause slackening. An optimal (relatively high) level of the follower tension that minimizes such shock has been proved in (Potkonjak et al. 2012). Therefore, in order to achieve energy efficiency as well as prevent tendon slackening during the switching, an adaptive reference tension has been proposed. It is low during regular motion and increases during the periods of switching (Fig. 2).

Puller-follower principle is demonstrated on a simple robotic joint driven by antagonistically coupled tendons with linear springs as a source of compliance (Fig. 3).

The dynamics of the antagonistic joint model is given in Eqs. (1–5) and finally in state space form (6) which considers joint and motor position and velocities $\mathbf{x} = [x_1 x_2 x_3 x_4 x_5 x_6]^T = [\theta_A \dot{\theta}_A \theta_B \dot{\theta}_B q\, \dot{q}]^T$ as state variables and motor torques $\mathbf{u} = [\tau_m{}^A \tau_m{}^B]^T$ as inputs.

$$I_j \ddot{q} = \frac{r_j}{r_m}(\tau_A - \tau_B) \tag{1}$$

$$I_m{}^A \ddot{\theta}_A + B_m{}^A \dot{\theta}_A + \tau_A = \tau_{mA} \tag{2}$$

$$I_m{}^B \ddot{\theta}_B + B_m{}^B \dot{\theta}_B + \tau_B = \tau_{mB} \tag{3}$$

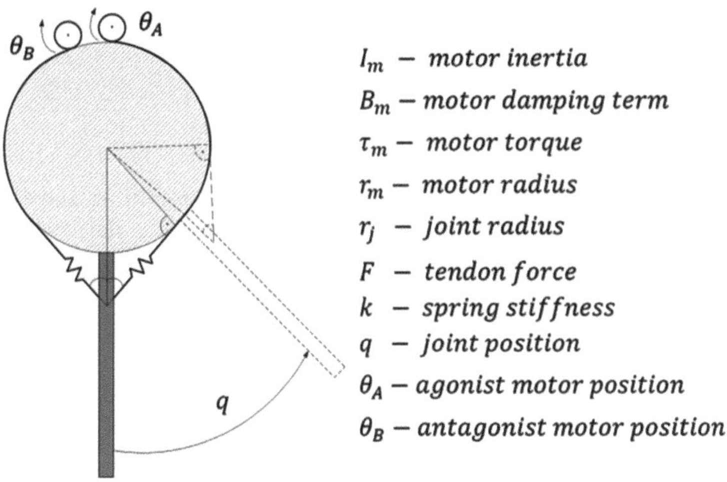

Fig. 3 Antagonistic robot joint and related parameters

$$\tau_A = F_{AG} r_m; F_{AG} = k\Delta l_A; \Delta l_A = -r_j q + r_m \theta_A \tag{4}$$

$$\tau_B = F_{ANT} r_m; F_{ANT} = k\Delta l_B; \Delta l_B = r_j q - r_m \theta_B \tag{5}$$

$$\dot{\mathbf{x}} = \mathrm{f}(\mathbf{x}) + \mathrm{g}(\mathbf{x})\mathbf{u} = \begin{bmatrix} \mathrm{x}_2 \\ \dot{\mathrm{x}}_2(\mathrm{x}_1, \mathrm{x}_2, \mathrm{x}_5, \mathrm{x}_6) \\ \mathrm{x}_4 \\ \dot{\mathrm{x}}_4(\mathrm{x}_3, \mathrm{x}_4, \mathrm{x}_5, \mathrm{x}_6) \\ \mathrm{x}_6 \\ \dot{\mathrm{x}}_6(\mathrm{x}_1, \mathrm{x}_2, \mathrm{x}_3, \mathrm{x}_4, \mathrm{x}_5, \mathrm{x}_6) \end{bmatrix} + \begin{bmatrix} 0 & 0 \\ 1/I_m{}^A & 0 \\ 0 & 0 \\ 0 & 1/I_m{}^B \\ 0 & 0 \\ 0 & 0 \end{bmatrix} \mathbf{u} \tag{6}$$

The idea of static feedback linearization is to decouple control of joint position and force in the antagonistic tendon, and transform system (6) into a new fully controllable and observable system. This could be accomplished if the sum of relative degrees of the outputs q and F_{ANT} is equal to the state dimension, and if the decoupling matrix of the system (6) is non-singular. Let us introduce $\mathbf{E}(\mathbf{x})$ as decoupling matrix, and $L_f h(\mathbf{x})$–Lie derivative of $h(\mathbf{x})$ along vector function $f(\mathbf{x})$. Then, by straightforward application of feedback linearization (Khalil 2002), we differentiate outputs q and F_{ANT} until linear relation to inputs $\tau_m{}^A$ and/or $\tau_m{}^B$ is given. To this end, output q is differentiated 4 times (7), while linear input/output relation for F_{ANT} is found in its second derivative (8). Therefore, relative degree of the outputs is $4 + 2 = 6$, which is equal to the system order. The second condition which must be fulfilled is non-singularity of decoupling matrix **E**. Decoupling matrix for the described system is diagonal and nonsingular (9).

$$q^{(4)} = L_f^4 h_q(x) + E_{11}\tau_m{}^A + E_{12}\tau_m{}^B \tag{7}$$

$$F_{ANT}{}^{(2)} = L_f^2 h_F(x) + E_{21}\tau_m{}^A + E_{22}\tau_m{}^B \tag{8}$$

$$\mathbf{E} = \begin{bmatrix} E_{11} & E_{12} \\ E_{21} & E_{22} \end{bmatrix} = \begin{bmatrix} \frac{kr_jr_m}{I_jI_m} & \frac{kr_jr_m}{I_jI_m} \\ 0 & -\frac{kr_m}{I_m} \end{bmatrix} \tag{9}$$

Therefore, input $\mathbf{u}$ can be transformed as it is done in (10), to achieve independent control of both joint position and antagonistic force via newly defined input $\mathbf{v} = \left[v_q v_F\right]^{\mathrm{T}}$. The novel state vector will be $\mathbf{z} = \left[q\dot{q}\,\ddot{q}\,q^{(3)}F_{ANT}\dot{F}_{ANT}\right]^{\mathrm{T}}$, and the complete state space model (11):

$$\mathbf{u} = \mathbf{E}^{-1}\left(-\begin{bmatrix} L_f^4 h_q(x) \\ L_f^2 h_F(x) \end{bmatrix} + \begin{bmatrix} v_q \\ v_F \end{bmatrix}\right) \tag{10}$$

$$\dot{\mathbf{z}} = \begin{bmatrix} 0 & 1 & 0 & 0 & 0 & 0 \\ 0 & 0 & 1 & 0 & 0 & 0 \\ 0 & 0 & 0 & 1 & 0 & 0 \\ 0 & 0 & 0 & 0 & 0 & 0 \\ 0 & 0 & 0 & 0 & 0 & 1 \\ 0 & 0 & 0 & 0 & 0 & 0 \end{bmatrix}\mathbf{z} + \begin{bmatrix} 0 & 0 \\ 0 & 0 \\ 0 & 0 \\ 1 & 0 \\ 0 & 0 \\ 0 & 1 \end{bmatrix}\mathbf{v} \tag{11}$$

Finally, to derive controllers and prove stability, it is necessary to note that $\left[q^{(4)}F_{ANT}{}^{(2)}\right]^{\mathrm{T}} = \left[v_q v_F\right]^{\mathrm{T}}$ stands from (7)–(11). Thus, if we chose q_d as a desired joint position and F_{ANT_d} as a desired pretension in antagonistic tendon, the simple control low (12) can be applied:

$$\begin{aligned} v_q &= q_d^{(4)} + K_{q3}\left(q_d^{(3)} - L_f^3 h_q(x)\right) + K_{q2}\left(\ddot{q}_d - L_f^2 h_q(x)\right) \\ &\quad + K_{q1}\left(\dot{q}_d - L_f h_q(x)\right) + K_{q0}\left(q_d - h_q(x)\right); \\ v_F &= \ddot{F}_{ANT\_d} + K_{F1}\left(\dot{F}_{ANT\_d} - L_f h_F(x)\right) + K_{F0}\left(F_{ANT\_d} - h_F(x)\right) \end{aligned} \tag{12}$$

Stability and convergence to zero tracking error are ensured for (12) if gains $K_{q0}, K_{q1}, K_{q2}, K_{q3}, K_{F0}, K_{F1}$ are chosen so the polynomials (13) are Hurwitz. If the desired joint positions are continuous up to the 4th order, and pretension is planned to be continuous up to the 2nd order, asymptotic trajectory/force tracking is achieved.

$$\begin{aligned} s^4 + K_{q3}s^3 + K_{q2}s^2 + K_{q1}s + K_{q0} &= 0; \\ s^2 + K_{F1}s + K_{F0} &= 0 \end{aligned} \tag{13}$$

One could note that puller-follower approach is strongly model dependent, as it is the case with all feedback linearization methods. To control multi-joint system, phenomena of dynamic coupling between joints, the variable effective joint inertia (depending on the entire distal mechanism position), and the influence of gravity should be faced. This is done in (Potkonjak et al. 2011) utilizing the H-infinity loop shaping method [a combination of loop shaping and robust stabilization proposed in (McFarlane and Glover 1992)] to achieve more robust controllers. However, application of puller-follower concept in musculoskeletal robots is still restricted by limitations in control of spherical joints or multi-articular muscles, besides precise system modeling. Therefore, we dealt with this problem through considering not only the conventional control techniques, but also experience exploitation and learning.

3 Cognitive Approaches

There is no doubt that control of anthropomimetic robots will rely solidly on experience and machine learning as is the case with humans. Furthermore, an accurate dynamic model can be hardly derived for a musculoskeletal robot. Therefore, a lack of mathematical modeling imposes the usage of algorithms for dealing with the black-box system. This section gives the procedure of biological pattern using computational intelligence and experience, neural networks and fuzzy logics. The following section shall propose few methods such as: heuristic methods of interpolation and neural network based FF, as well as the fuzzy logic approach to FB control.

3.1 "Nearest Neighbor" Feedforward Approach

In this subsection the interpolation of the control inputs for single-joint system is examined and later on expended to a multi-joint system. The pattern of the EMG activity in elbow flexors produced against small constant load (Tal'nov et al. 1999) is replicated and similar logic is used to control all joints of the robot (Fig. 4 Left). The figure demonstrates the input voltages of the joint agonist (AG) motor and its positions. By observing the input signal, one can distinguish two input voltage components: *the control signal burst* mainly responsible for the joint motion; and *the silent period* that maintains the steady state position.

Three motions of elbow joint with input voltages fed into AG and antagonist (AGN) actuators presented in three different colours individually can be seen in Fig. 4 (on the right). If the distance from p_1 to p_2 is considered as a region of potentially required final positions, the appropriate joint control would be interpolated. We define d_1 and d_2 as the distance from final position f_p to p_1 and p_2

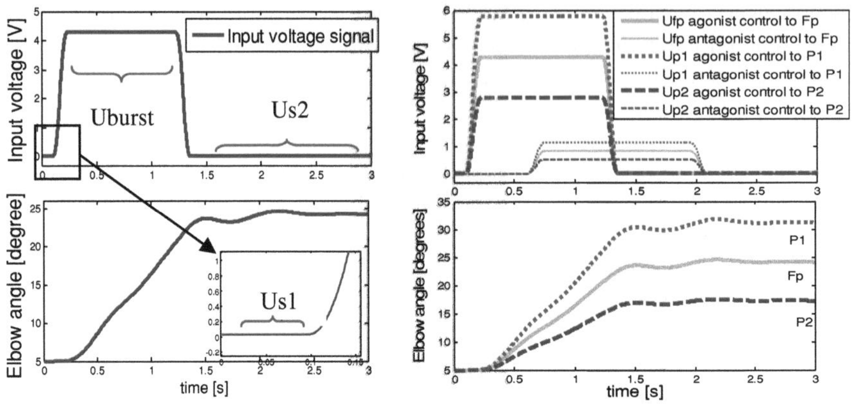

Fig. 4 (*Left top*) The control signal presented by: burst component before 1.5 s, silent period after 1.5 s and zoomed signal before the motion. (*Left bottom*) Elbow position as a result of the presented control; (*Right top*) agonist and antagonist input voltage control. (*Right bottom*) the elbow position p_1, p_2 and f_p as a result of presented control **Up1**, **Up2** and **Ufp,** respectively

respectively. The first row of U_{fp}, U_{p1} and U_{p2} matrixes is agonist, while the second row is antagonist voltage input, presented in (Fig. 4 Right).

$$\mathbf{U}_{fp}(t)_{2x1} = \frac{d_1\mathbf{U}_{p2}(t)_{2x1} + d_2\mathbf{U}_{p1}(t)_{2x1}}{d_1 + d_2} \tag{14}$$

This basic principle in controlling a single-joint is now generalized to the multi-joint robot arm. The given examples examine a fixed-base arm with seven single-degree-of-freedom joints moved by antagonistically coupled drives is considered. The experience acquiring is the set of motion experiments performed from a set of initial hand-tip positions X_s which define the initial region of 0.1 m radius, and ending in a region of final positions X_f (0.05 m radius). The initial and the final positions, together with the controls applied in these experiments are recorded and represent the system experience i.e. experience base. When performing a motion experiment, the joints are controlled by heuristically determined control voltages which follow the pattern presented in Fig. 4. The used pointing example does not specify the path, only the end point. In our example, for each initial position there are 90–130 final positions in the final sphere. The distances in the initial grid range between 2.5 and 3.5 cm and 2–2.5 cm in the final grid.

In exploitation phase, the robot is expected from the robot to reach a target point (F_0) that has not been previously reached in training, starting from a position (S_0) that has not been previously used. The interpolation and the calculation of the FF control are done before the robot moves, i.e. off-line.

Therefore, the first step of algorithm for FF calculation is sequential selection of the nearest four initial positions from data set X_s. Namely, the distance $d = \min(d_1 + d_2 + d_3 + d_4)$ is the minimum sum, where d_1, d_2, d_3, d_4 are the

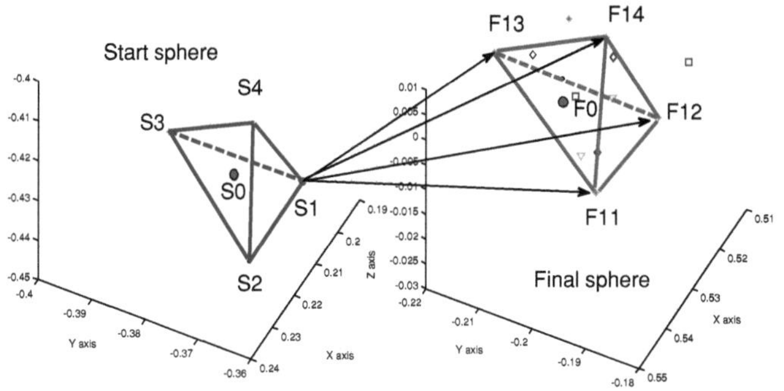

Fig. 5 *Left* Four initial positions with prescribed initial position S_0 is marked in the tetrahedron. *Right* The four final positions that derive from the initial position S_1

distances from the prescribed initial position S_0 (Fig. 5.), to first (S_1), second (S_2), third (S_3) and fourth (S_4) neighbour from data set X_s, respectively. S_0 must be inside the volume of the tetrahedron defined by S_1, S_2, S_3, and S_4.

The following step would be to declare useful final positions for each of the four initial neighbors. Firstly, we distinguish all final positions $X_{fi}, i \in (1,2,3,4)$, as the reached points of the robot arm, which derive from the initial position S_i. In order to estimate control sequence from S_i to F_0 (Fig. 5), we need to define four final positions F_{i1}, $F_{i2}\, F_{i3}$, F_{i4} from each distinguished data X_{fi}. Namely, the distance $d = \min(d_{i1} + d_{i2} + d_{i3} + d_{i4})$ is the minimum sum, where $i \in (1,2,3,4)$ and d_{i1}, d_{i2}, d_{i3}, d_{i4} are the distances from the prescribed final position (F_0) to first (F_{i1}), second (F_{i2}), third (F_{i3}) and fourth (F_{i4}) neighbour from distinguished data X_{fi}, respectively. F_0 must be inside the volume of the tetrahedron defined by F_{i1}, F_{i2}, F_{i3}, F_{i4}.

This way we found four tetrahedrons with the smallest volume, with F_0 inside them. Each tetrahedron is from distinguished data X_{fi}. Equation (14) gives an example for obtaining the control for problem in one dimension, when a convex interpolation between two neighbor vertexes is actually a line. In order to drive hand tip from S_0 to F_0 we need to deal with the problem of interpolation in 3D. The desired control is found as a linear combination of control signals in experience base that drive hand tip from S_i to F_{i1}, F_{i2}, F_{i3} and F_{i4}. Similar to Eq. (14), the final expression depend on distances from S_i to S_0 and distances form F_0 to F_{i1}, F_{i2}, F_{i3} and F_{i4}. This algorithm is discussed in details and experimentally verified in (Milosavljevic et al. 2012).

3.2 Neural Network Feedforward Approach

This section considers neural networks as another approach to calculating FF. The insufficient acquired data in the experience base with regard to the complexity of the antagonistically coupled system, suggest the usage of radial basis neural networks (RBN). Also, Gaussian RBN represents an efficient solution since it can smoothly approximate any function (Thrishantha Nanayakkara et al. 2001). By observing Fig. 4 (Left), one can distinguish three parameters that define input signal fed into actuator:

U_{s1} The value of control signal while the arm is in initial position
U_{s2} The value of the control signal during silent period after the arm motion
U_{burst} The dynamic component also know as the control signal burst

The shift of the joint depends on the integral of the control signal burst over time *T*. This parameter is calculated for the each motor from the antagonistic pair of the motors per joint. The motors are driven by DC motors with the maximum voltage supply of 12 V.

$$E = \int_0^T U_{burst}(t)dt \tag{15}$$

For the network input vector in (16), the initial and final positions of the hand tip presented in Cartesian space are used. The final outcome of this section should be the input control signal for each motor of the anthropomimetic robot arm, defined in (17). As previously mentioned, the joint position and its shift are defined by $U_{s1,}$ U_{s1} and parameter *E,* defined in (15). In order to derive the hand tip from S_0 to F_0, it is needed to estimate these parameters for all motors of the robot arm. Therefore, the network inputs and outputs are:

$$Input = \begin{bmatrix} x_{initial} & y_{initial} & z_{initial} & x_{final} & y_{final} & z_{final} \end{bmatrix} \tag{16}$$

$Output = [Output_i]_{1xn}$, where $Output_i$ is defined for each joint:

$$Output_i = \begin{bmatrix} U_{s1} & U_{s2} & E & w \end{bmatrix} \tag{17}$$

For a new initial (s_0) and final (F_0) position, the network will generate an output with the corresponding values for each motor: the value of control signal (U_{s1new}) during silent period of both drives in position S_0, as well as (U_{s2new}) in position F_0 and the value of the parameter E_{new}. The output *w*, shall determine if the motor in the joint is the puller. Considering this, there are four parameters for each of 14 motors which make 56 outputs of the network. The entire procedure and possibility of neural network control of antagonistic joint are reported in (Milosavljevic et al. 2012).

3.3 "Nearest Neighbor" Feedback Approach

This subsection presents FB control based on interpolation, and exploiting knowledge from the experience base, very similar to the approach used for reported FF in Sect. 3.1. FB component contributes to the final control signal and enables fine tuning of hand tip while FF provides hand tip to the prescribed vicinity of the final point F_0. In order to reduce the terminal error $\Delta X_f = X^* - X_f$, for each final point reached at the FF level, a new set of experiments is defined and conducted by making small shifts and relating them to the applied control inputs. Since we cannot determine which joint is responsible for the hand tip motion along x, y or z axis, we shall try to avoid this black-box disadvantage by carrying out a new set of experiments during the acquiring phase. After properly accomplished FF motion, we increase the puller input voltage up to U_{apm} and record the caused hand tip shift. This voltage increment would drive joint j and therefore the hand tip to the new steady state position $\mathbf{X}(t+T)$ with the new FF voltage $\mathbf{U_{FF}}(t+T)_{2nx1}$. We have applied this logic for each joint (n = 7) during jth simulation, $j \in (1, 2 \ldots n)$ and the following variables have been recorded:

$$\Delta\widehat{\mathbf{U}}_{j_{nx1}} = \mathbf{U_{FF}}(t+T)_{nx1} - \mathbf{U_{FF}}(t)_{nx1} = \begin{bmatrix} 0_{[j-1x1]} \\ dU_j \\ 0_{[n-jx1]} \end{bmatrix}_{nx1} \tag{18}$$

$$\Delta\widehat{\mathbf{X}}_{j_{3x1}} = \mathbf{X}(t+T)_{3x1} - \mathbf{X}(t)_{3x1} = \begin{bmatrix} dx_j \\ dy_j \\ dz_j \end{bmatrix}_{3x1} \quad ; j \in (1, 2 \ldots n) \tag{19}$$

$\Delta\widehat{\mathbf{U}}_{j_{nx1}}$ is matrix of n estimated values of agonist motors; dU_j is a voltage increment of *jth* joint from steady state moment (*t*) to steady state moment (*t* + *T*). After *nth* simulation we can define *input voltage increment matrix* $\Delta\widehat{\mathbf{U}}_{nxn}$ and *position increment matrix* $\Delta\widehat{\mathbf{X}}_{3xn}$. The diagonal matrix $\Delta\widehat{\mathbf{U}}_{nxn}$ have elements $u_{ij} = dU_j; i = j$ and $u_{ij} = 0; i \neq j;$, where $\Delta\widehat{\mathbf{X}}_{3xn} = \widehat{\mathbf{H}}_{3xn}\Delta\widehat{\mathbf{U}}_{nxn}$.

Since $\widehat{\boldsymbol{H}}_{3xn}$ is not a square matrix, modified pseudo inversion with weight matrix $\mathbf{W} = \mathbf{I}$ is applied. Solving this problem we calculate FB gain $\widehat{\mathbf{K}}_{nx3}$ for each final position:

$$\Delta\mathbf{U}_{nx1} = \mathbf{W}^{-1}\widehat{\mathbf{H}}^T\left(\widehat{\mathbf{H}}\mathbf{W}^{-1}\widehat{\mathbf{H}}^T\right)^{-1}\Delta\mathbf{X}_{3x1} \tag{20}$$

$$\widehat{\mathbf{K}}_{nx3} = \mathbf{W}^{-1}\widehat{\mathbf{H}}^T\left(\widehat{\mathbf{H}}\mathbf{W}^{-1}\widehat{\mathbf{H}}^T\right)^{-1} \tag{21}$$

After accomplished FF motion, in exploitation stage the robot will be asked to reach the target point that has no previously calculated $\mathbf{K}_{nx3}$. In such case, the interpolation of the FB gain neighbours presented in (21), would obtain new $\mathbf{K}_{nx3}$. The interpolation of $\widehat{\mathbf{K}}_{nx3}$ and $\Delta\widehat{\mathbf{U}}_{nxn}$ is done by the same algorithm described in Sect. 3.1. This algorithm is discussed in details and experimentally verified in (Milosavljevic et al. 2012). After this increment, position control is regulated on-line with proportional controller $\mathbf{K}_{nx3}$, based on actual sensory data.

3.4 Feedback Approach Based on Online Estimation of Kinematic Coefficients and Fuzzy Logic

The assumption that we lack any mathematical model of the robot kinematics or dynamics means that we are missing all relevant characteristics to use conventional tools to solve the point-to-point control problem in the global frame. This subsection proposes the approach that exploits experience base to calculate kinematic coefficient and exploit fuzzy logic with the aim to obtain fine tuning of the hand tip position. The most challenging and demanding task is how to determine the influence of each control input on the hand tip motion in the global frame. Once the FB exploitation starts, it is necessary to know how a particular input influences the Cartesian motion of the hand tip. In order to solve the problem, we have proposed the experience-based estimation algorithm for the so-called kinematic coefficients. Kinematic coefficients are defined as parameters which describe the relation between control inputs and the axes of the global frame. For each joint *i*, three normalized coefficients $nc_{x_i}, nc_{y_i}, nc_{z_i}$ are assigned for x, y and z axis respectively.

Suppose that pure FF brings the hand tip to point $\widehat{F}_0 = (\widehat{x}, \widehat{y}, \widehat{z})$. Coordinates of the points from the narrow environment (neighbors of $\widehat{F}_0$) are denoted as $S_j = (x_j, y_j, z_j), j = 1, 2, \ldots, N$ (*j*-neighbour number). The nearest neighboring points (neighbours) form the experience base to target motion, used for the calculation of coefficients, are chosen just like in Sect. 3.1.

An influence of each joint to hand tip movements along x, y and z axis is estimated using all available and measurable data—current and desired hand tip position, current joint angles (available from sensors); positions of chosen neighbours, and corresponding joint angles (available from experience base). Therefore, we estimate the contribution of each neighbour to desired position in Cartesian coordinates, as well as joint position and their configuration for each neighbour, to finally estimate dependence of joint movement and hand tip position in Cartesian space. The method of heuristic evaluation of normalized coefficients $nc_{x_i}, nc_{y_i}, nc_{z_i}$ is omitted here due to lack of space, but presented in details in (Jovanovic et al. 2013). The paper demonstrates reported logic where kinematic coefficients are presented for the example of 2 DOFs planar robot.

Once the kinematic coefficients are calculated to estimate contribution of each actuator to the hand tip position, the deviation of the achieved motion form desired motion should be estimated. Therefore a fuzzy controller is implemented. The detailed explanation can be seen in (Potkonjak et al. 2012). The paper proposes membership functions of fuzzy controller as well as defined two input variables (position error and derivative of position error) and one output variable (voltage) for each axis. The fuzzy controller provides voltages as outputs in each axis $U_{fuzzy}(x)$, $U_{fuzzy}(y)$, and $U_{fuzzy}(z)$. Together with kinematic coefficients, one can calculate FB voltage in each actuator separately for fine tuning of the hand tip position. Accordingly, the final equation for the control input during FF plus FB

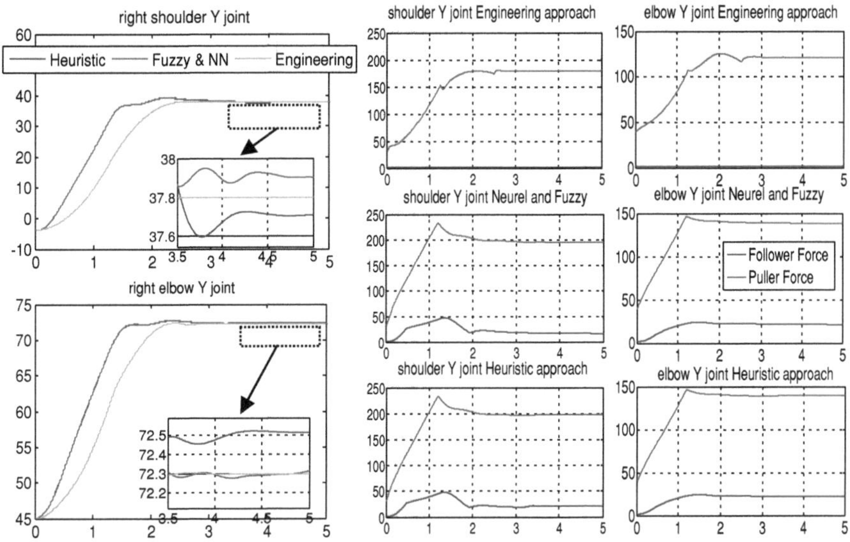

Fig. 6 Lifting the arm in vertical plane using engineering approach, and cognitive approaches based on nearest neighbour methods for both FF and FB as well as neural network based FB in combination with Fuzzy FB: (*Left*) Positions of the most representative joints during motion in vertical plane with zoomed position during FB phase; (*Right*) Tendon forces in antagonistic joints

phase is given in (22). The variable $U_{static}(i)$ is a static voltage of i—joint required to keep the joint in the prescribed position during steady state. The static voltage is estimated for the target position using feedforward algorithm (see Sect. 3.1).

$$U_i = U_{i,static} + n_{C_{x_i}} U_{fuzzy}(x) + n_{C_{y_i}} U_{fuzzy}(y) + n_{C_{z_i}} U_{fuzzy}(z) \quad (22)$$

4 Simulation Results and Comparative Analysis

The results of lifting the robot arm in vertical plane with control based on Engineering and Cognitive approach are presented in Fig. 6. To point out capabilities of all mentioned approaches, we present results for Puller-follower approach (Sect. 2) as an engineering control technique based on feedback linearization as well as combination of two cognitive approaches. The first one contains combination of Nearest neighbor approach based on interpolation for both FF (Sect. 3.1) and FF (Sect. 3.3), while the second one combines RBNN for FF (Sect. 3.2) and Fuzzy with kinematic coefficient estimation for FB (Sect. 3.4). The results of performance comparison for all three methodologies have been reported.

Numerous examples have proven that Puller-follower approach is preferable from the standpoint of energy efficiency (in Fig. 6 right, note that tendon forces are lower for engineering then cognitive approaches). The assumption that the model of robot dynamics is known, also speaks in favour of the Engineering method since the movement is faster and more accurate. This is obvious in zoomed FB phase in Fig. 6 (on the left). However, the feature that distinguishes Cognitive from Engineering approach is their use in cases when accurate model is not available, which is often case in anthropomimetic robots. Therefore, the applicability of cognitive approaches to a wider class of robots (containing bi-articular muscles and multi DOF joints beside intrinsic compliance) represents their major advantage, while their performance remains satisfactory as one can conclude from Fig. 6.

5 Conclusions

The future of service robotics will certainly be in human like compliant robots. Since our daily ambience is fully adapted to humans, the greatest challenge in robotics is how to build a robot capable of maneuverability and safe interaction in such environment. Anthropomimetic robots are being built with a lot of success but the control of such robots is still challenge. This chapter considered both conventional control techniques (puller-follower control based on feedback linearization) and control based on learning and experience exploitation (nearest neighbors control based on interpolation, neural networks and fuzzy control). We pointed out advantages and drawbacks of all developed methods as well as their possible application. The results presented unequivocally lead to conclusion that for successful control of such highly complex mechanical systems, it is necessary to exploit all benefits of the given methods. Therefore, once the final control scheme is solved, it should represent the mixture of all presented control techniques. The symbiosis of presented approaches will be the topic of our future research.

Acknowledgments The research work reported here was made possible by Grant No. 35003 and No. 44008 of Serbian Ministry of Science and Technological Development.

References

Asano, Y., Miyoguchi, H., Kozuki, T., Motegi, Y., Osada, M., Urata, J., Nakanishi, Y., Okada, K. and Inaba, M.: Lower Thigh Design of Detailed Musculoskeletal Humanoid – Kenshiro. In: Proc. of IEEE-RSJ International Conference on Intelligent Robots and Systems, Algarve, Portugal, 4367–4372 (2012)

Bortoletto, R., Sartori, M., He, F., and Pagello, E.: Modeling and Simulating Compliant Movements in a Musculoskeletal Bipedal Robot. Simulation, Modeling, and Programming for Autonomous Robots (Lecture Notes in Computer Science), 7628, 237–250 (2012)

Diamond, A. Knight, R., Devereux, D. and Holland, O.: Anthropomimetic Robots: Concept, Construction and Modelling. International Journal of Advanced Robotic Systems, 9, 1–14 (2012)

D.P. Thrishantha Nanayakkara, Keigo Watanabe, Kazuo Kiguchi, and Kiyotaka Izumi: Fuzzy Self-Adaptive Radial Basis Function Neural Network-Based Control of a Seven-Link Redundant Industrial Manipulator. Advanced Robotics, 15(1), 17–43 (2001)

Hannaford, B. and Stark, L.: Roles of the elements of the triphasic control signal. Experimental Neurology, 90(3), 619–634 (1985)

Holland, O. and Knight, R.: The Anthropomimetic Principle. In Burn, J. and Wilson, M. (eds.), In: Proceedings of the AISB06 Symposium on Biologically Inspired Robotics, (2006)

Ikemoto, S., Nishigori, Y. and Hosoda, K.: Advances of flexible musculoskeletal robot structure in sensory acquisition. Artificial Life Robotics, 17, 63–69 (2012)

Jovanovic, K., Milosavljevic, P. and Potkonjak, V.: Fuzzy Feedback Control Based on On-line Estimated Kinematic Coefficients. Submitted to Transactions on Computational Collective Intelligence (date of submission: September 2013)

Khalil, H. K.: Nonlinear Systems (3rd ed.). Upper Saddle River, Prentice Hall (2002)

McFarlane D. and Glover, K.: A loop-shaping design procedure using $H\infty$synthesis. IEEE Transactions on Automatic Control, 37(6), 759–769 (1992)

Milosavljevic, P., Bascarevic, N., Jovanovic, K. and Kvascev, G.: Neural networks in feedforward control of a robot arm driven by antagonistically coupled drives. In: Proceedings of the 11th Symposium on Neural Networks Applications in Electrical Engineering (NEUREL 2012), Belgrade, Serbia, 77–80 (2012)

Milosavljevic, P., Jovanovic, K., Bascarevic, N., Potkonjak, V. and Holland, O.: Heuristic Machine-Learning Approach to the Control of an Anthropomimetic Robot Arm. In: Proceedings of 10th IFAC Symposium on Robot Control, Dubrovnik, Croatia, 301–306 (2012)

Oh, S., Salvucci, V. and Hori, Y.: Development of Simplified Statics of Robot Manipulator and Optimized Muscle Torque Distribution based on the Statics. In: Proceedings of American Control Conference, 4099–4104 (2011)

Palli, G., Melchiorri, C. and De Luca, A.: On the feedback linearization of robots with variable joint stiffness. In: Proceedings of IEEE International Conference on Robotics and Automation (ICRA 2008), 1753–1759 (2008)

Potkonjak, V., Bascarevic, N., Milosavljevic, P., Jovanovic, K. and Holland, O.: Experience-Based Fuzzy Control of an Anthropomimetic Robot. In: Proceedings of International Joint Conference on Computational Intelligence, Barcelona, Spain, 389–394 (2012)

Potkonjak, V., Jovanovic, K., Milosavljevic, P., Bascarevic, N. and Holland, O.: The Puller-Follower Control Concept For The Multi-Joint Robot With Antagonistically Coupled Compliant Drives. In: Proceedings of 2nd IASTED Intl. Conf. on Robotics (Robo2011), Pittsburgh, USA, 375–381 (2011)

Potkonjak, V., Svetozarevic, B., Jovanovic, K. and Holland, O.: Anthropomimetic Robot with Passive Compliance – Contact Dynamics and Control, In: Proceedings of 19th IEEE Mediterranean Conference on Control and Automation, Corfu, Greece, 1059–1064 (2011)

Potkonjak, V., Svetozarevic, B., Jovanovic, K. and Holland, O.: The puller-follower control of compliant and noncompliant antagonistic tendon drives in robotic systems. International Journal of Advanced Robotic Systems, 8(5), 143–155 (2012)

Tal'nov, A., Serenko, S., Strafun, S., Kostyukov, A.: Analysis of the electromyographic activity of human elbow joint muscles during slow linear flexion movements in isotorque conditions. Neuroscience, 90, 1123–1136 (1999)

Wimbock, T., Ott, C. and Hirzinger, G.: Immersion and Invariance Control for an Antagonistic Joint with Nonlinear Mechanical Stiffness. In: Proceedings of IEEE Conference on Decision and Control, Atlanta, GA, USA, 1128–1135; (2010)

Wittmeier, S., Alessandro, C., Bascarevic, N., Dalamagkidis, K., Diamond, A., Jeantsch, M., Jovanovic, K., Knight, R., Marques, H.G., Milosavljevic, P., Svetozarevic, B., Potkonjak, V., Pfeifer, R., Knoll, A. and Holland, O.: Toward Anthropomimetic Robotics: Development, Simulation, and Control of a Musculoskeletal Torso. Artificial Life, 19(1), 171–193, (2013)

Kinematic and Dynamic Modeling of a Parallel Manipulator with Eight Actuation Modes

Stéphane Caro, Damien Chablat, Philippe Wenger and Xianwen Kong

Abstract Kinematic and dynamic performances of parallel manipulators are usually not homogeneous throughout their operational workspace. This problem is usually solved by introducing actuation redundancy, which involves force control algorithms. Another approach is the selection of the best actuation modes along a trajectory to be followed with regard to the kinetostatic, elastostatic and dynamic performances of the parallel manipulator. Accordingly, this chapter introduces a novel three degree-of-freedom planar parallel manipulator with variable actuation modes, named NAVARO. NAVARO stands for NAntes Variable Actuation RObot and has eight actuation modes. First, the prototype of the manipulator is presented. Then, its transmission systems are presented. Finally, the kinematic and dynamic models of the NAVARO are developed.

1 Introduction

A drawback of serial and parallel mechanisms is the inhomogeneity of the kinetostatic performance within their workspace. For instance, dexterity, accuracy and stiffness are usually bad in the neighbourhood of singularities that can appear in

S. Caro (✉) · D. Chablat · P. Wenger
Institut de Recherche en Communications et Cybernétique de Nantes,
Nantes, France
e-mail: stephane.caro@irccyn.ec-nantes.fr

D. Chablat
e-mail: damien.chablat@irccyn.ec-nantes.fr

P. Wenger
e-mail: philippe.wenger@irccyn.ec-nantes.fr

X. Kong
School of Engineering and Physical Sciences, Heriot-Watt University,
Edinburgh EH14 4AS, UK
e-mail: X.Kong@hw.ac.uk

A. Rodić et al. (eds.), *New Trends in Medical and Service Robots*,
Mechanisms and Machine Science 20, DOI: 10.1007/978-3-319-05431-5_21,

the workspace of such mechanisms. As far as the parallel mechanisms are concerned, their inverse kinematics problem (IKP) has usually many solutions, which correspond to the *working modes* of the mechanism (Chablat and Wenger 1998; Chablat et al. 2002). Nevertheless, it is difficult to come up with a large operational workspace free of singularity with a given working mode. Consequently, a trajectory planning may require a change of the working mode by means of an alternative trajectory in order to avoid singular configurations. In such a case, the initial trajectory would not be followed. The common approach to solve this problem is to introduce actuation redundancy, that involves force control algorithms (Alba-Gomez et al. 2005). Another approach is to use the concept of joint-coupling as proposed by Chen et al. (2007) or to select the actuated joint in each limb with regard to the pose of the moving-platform, (Arakelian et al. 2007).

In this chapter, a three degree-of-freedom planar parallel manipulator with variable actuation modes, named NAVARO, is introduced. NAVARO stands for NAntes Variable Actuation RObot and has eight actuation modes. First, the prototype of the manipulator is presented. Then, its transmission systems are presented. Finally, the kinematic and dynamic models of the NAVARO are developed.

2 Mechanism Architecture

The concept of *variable actuated mechanism* (VAM) was introduced in (Arakelian et al. 2007; Chen et al. 2007). Indeed, they derived a VAM from the architecture of the 3-RPR planar parallel manipulator (PPM) by actuating either the first revolute joint or the prismatic joint of its limbs.

This chapter deals with the study of a VAM introduced in Rakotomanga et al. (2008) and illustrated in Fig. 1. This mechanism is derived from the architecture of the 3-RRR PPM. The first link of each limb of the conventional 3-$\underline{R}$RR manipulator is replaced by parallelogram $A_iB_iD_iE_i$ to come up with the mechanism at hand. Accordingly, links A_iB_i and B_iC_i can be driven independently, i.e., angles α_i and δ_i are actuated and uncoupled, by means of an actuator and a transmission system, mounted to the base and located in point A_i, $i = 1, 2, 3$.

It turns out that the VAM has eight *actuating modes* as shown in Table 1. Indeed, the actuating mode of the mechanism depends on its actuated joints. For instance, the first actuating mode corresponds to the 3-$\underline{R}$RR mechanism, also called $\underline{R}RR_1-\underline{R}RR_2-\underline{R}RR_3$ mechanism in the scope of this chapter, as the first revolute joints (located at point A_i) of its limbs are actuated. Likewise, the eighth actuating mode corresponds to the 3-R$\underline{R}$R manipulator, also called $\underline{R}RR_1-\underline{R}RR_2-\underline{R}RR_3$ mechanism, as the second revolute joints (located at point B_i) of its limbs are actuated.

The moving platform pose of the VAM is determined by means of the Cartesian coordinates (x, y) of operation point P expressed in the base frame $\mathscr{F}_b$ and angle ϕ, namely, the angle between frames $\mathscr{F}_b$ and $\mathscr{F}_p$. Moreover, the passive and actuated joints do not have any stop. Points A_1, A_2 and A_3 (C_1, C_2 and C_3, respectively) lie at the corners of an equilateral triangle, of which the geometric center is point O (point P, resp.).

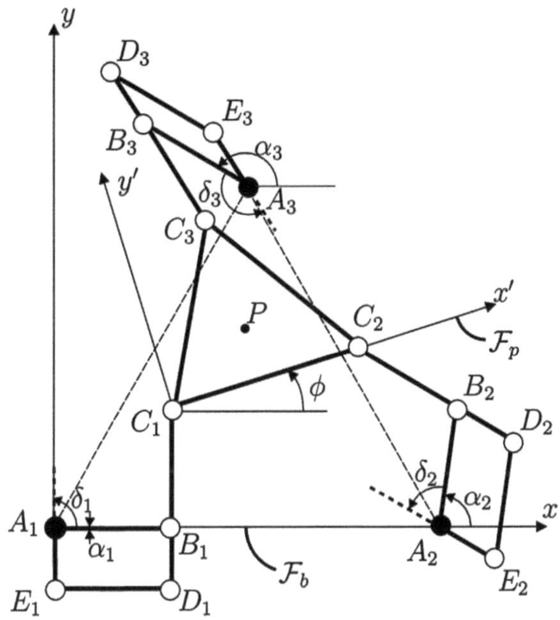

Fig. 1 3-RRR PPM with variable actuation

Table 1 The eight actuating modes of the NAVARO

Actuating mode number		Driven links	Active angles
1	$\underline{R}RR_1-\underline{R}RR_2-\underline{R}RR_3$	A_1B_1, A_2B_2, A_3B_3	α_1, α_2, α_3
2	$\underline{R}RR_1-\underline{R}RR_2-R\underline{R}R_3$	A_1B_1, A_2B_2, A_3E_3	α_1, α_2, δ_3
3	$\underline{R}RR_1-R\underline{R}R_2-\underline{R}RR_3$	A_1B_1, A_2E_2, A_3B_3	α_1, δ_2, α_3
4	$R\underline{R}R_1-\underline{R}RR_2-\underline{R}RR_3$	A_1E_1, A_2B_2, A_3B_3	δ_1, α_2, α_3
5	$\underline{R}RR_1-R\underline{R}R_2-R\underline{R}R_3$	A_1B_1, A_2E_2, A_3E_3	α_1, δ_2, δ_3
6	$R\underline{R}R_1-R\underline{R}R_2-\underline{R}RR_3$	A_1E_1, A_2E_2, A_3B_3	δ_1, δ_2, α_3
7	$R\underline{R}R_1-\underline{R}RR_2-R\underline{R}R_3$	A_1E_1, A_2B_2, A_3E_3	δ_1, α_2, δ_3
8	$R\underline{R}R_1-R\underline{R}R_2-R\underline{R}R_3$	A_1E_1, A_2E_2, A_3E_3	δ_1, δ_2, δ_3

Figure 2 shows the prototype of the NAVARO, which has been developed at IRCCyN.[1]

3 Transmission System

A transmission system has been developed and mounted in each leg of the NAVARO in order for the manipulator to be able to switch smoothly from one actuation mode to another along a prescribed trajectory. Figure 3 illustrates a CAD

[1] IRCCyN: Institut de Recherche en Communications et Cybernétique de Nantes.

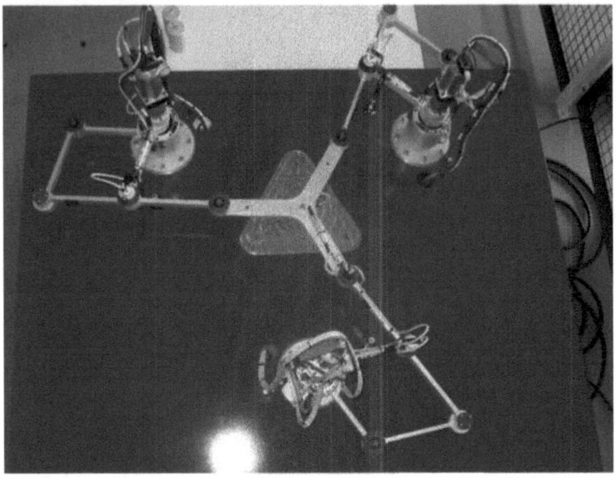

Fig. 2 The NAVARO prototype

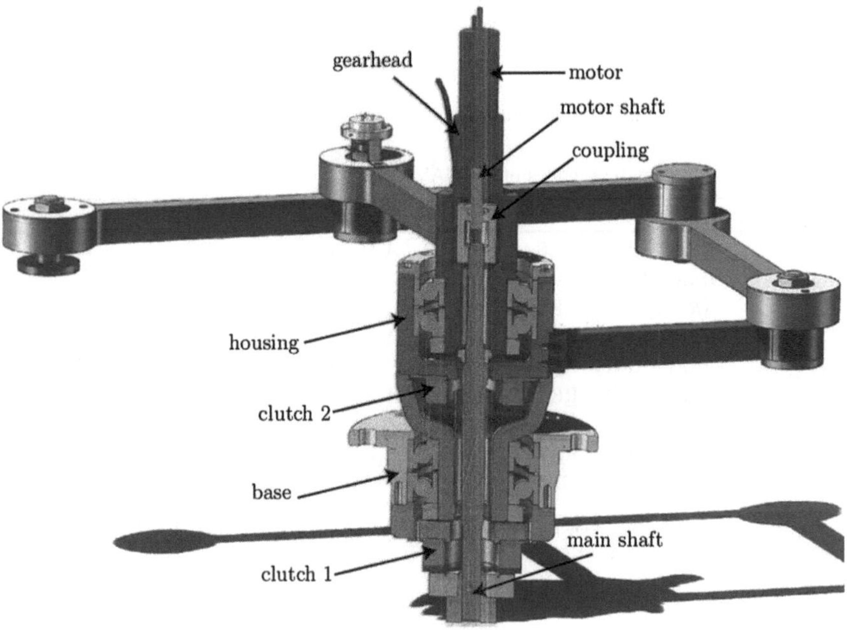

Fig. 3 The NAVARO transmission system

modeling of the transmission system of the NAVARO. This system can be seen as a double clutch system and contains: (1) a motor, (2) a gearhead, (3) a motor shaft, (4) a main shaft (in cyan), (5) a base (in yellow), (6) a housing (in purple) and (7) two clutches (in brown). As a matter of fact, the two clutches 1 and 2 are electromagnetic brakes.

Each transmission system has four actuation schemes that are defined thereafter:

1. **None of clutches 1 and 2 are active**: The main shaft is free to move with respect to the housing and the base. In that case, none of the first two revolute joints of the corresponding legs are actuated, namely, angles α_i and δ_i are passive, $i = 1, 2, 3$.
2. **Clutch 1 is active while Clutch 2 is not**: The main shaft is fixed with respect to the base, i.e., the link A_iB_i is driven thanks to the rotation of the motor shaft. In that case, angle α_i is active and angle δ_i is passive, $i = 1, 2, 3$.
3. **Clutch 2 is active while Clutch 1 is not**: The main shaft is attached to the housing, but is free to move with respect to the base. In that case, angle α_i is passive and angle δ_i is active, $i = 1, 2, 3$.
4. **Both clutches 1 and 2**: The blue shaft is attached to both the base and the housing. It means that the housing cannot move and link A_iE_i is fixed. In that case, link C_iD_i performs a circular translation with respect to point A_i, $i = 1, 2, 3$. This actuation scheme amounts to an actuated Π joint.[2]

Only the second and third actuation schemes of each transmission system are used in the NAVARO prototype in order to keep the three degrees of freedom motion of the moving-platform and to avoid any actuation redundancy and under-actuation. However, it is noteworthy that the NAVARO behaves like a five-bar mechanism when the fourth actuation scheme of the transmission system is used in one leg, the second or the third actuation scheme is used in one of the other two legs two and the first actuation scheme is used in the third leg.

4 Kinematic Analysis of the NAVARO

4.1 Kinematic Modeling

The velocity $\dot{\mathbf{p}}$ of point P can be obtained in three different forms, depending on which leg is traversed, namely,

$$\dot{\mathbf{p}} = \dot{\alpha}_1\mathbf{E}(\mathbf{c}_1 - \mathbf{a}_1) + \dot{\delta}_1\mathbf{E}(\mathbf{c}_1 - \mathbf{b}_1) + \dot{\phi}\mathbf{E}(\mathbf{p} - \mathbf{c}_1) \tag{1}$$

$$\dot{\mathbf{p}} = \dot{\alpha}_2\mathbf{E}(\mathbf{c}_2 - \mathbf{a}_2) + \dot{\delta}_2\mathbf{E}(\mathbf{c}_2 - \mathbf{b}_2) + \dot{\phi}\mathbf{E}(\mathbf{p} - \mathbf{c}_2) \tag{2}$$

$$\dot{\mathbf{p}} = \dot{\alpha}_3\mathbf{E}(\mathbf{c}_3 - \mathbf{a}_3) + \dot{\delta}_3\mathbf{E}(\mathbf{c}_3 - \mathbf{b}_3) + \dot{\phi}\mathbf{E}(\mathbf{p} - \mathbf{c}_3) \tag{3}$$

[2] A Π joint is also called parallelogram joint (Caro et al. 2010).

with matrix $\mathbf{E}$ defined as

$$\mathbf{E} = \begin{bmatrix} 0 & -1 \\ 1 & 0 \end{bmatrix}$$

$\mathbf{a}_i$, $\mathbf{b}_i$ and $\mathbf{c}_i$ are the position vectors of points A_i, B_i and C_i, respectively. $\dot{\alpha}_i$, $\dot{\delta}_i$ and $\dot{\phi}$ are the rates of angles α_i, δ_i and ϕ depicted in Fig. 1, i = 1, 2, 3.

The kinematic model of the VAM under study can be obtained from Eq. (1)c by eliminating the idle joint rates. However, the latter depend on the actuating mode of the mechanism. For instance, $\dot{\delta}_1, \dot{\delta}_2$, and $\dot{\delta}_3$ are idle with the first actuating mode and the corresponding kinematic model is obtained by dot-multiplying Eqs. (1)–(3) with $(\mathbf{c}_i - \mathbf{b}_i)^T$, i = 1, 2, 3. Likewise, $\dot{\delta}_1, \dot{\delta}_2$ and $\dot{\delta}_3$ are idle with the second actuating mode and the corresponding kinematic model is obtained by dot-multiplying Eqs. ~(1)–(2) with $(\mathbf{c}_i - \mathbf{b}_i)^T$, i = 1, 2, and Eq. (3) with $(\mathbf{c}_3 - \mathbf{a}_3)^T$.

The kinematic model of the VAM can now be cast in vector form, namely,

$$At = B\dot{\mathbf{q}} \quad \text{with} \quad t = [\dot{p}\,\dot{\phi}]^T \quad \text{and} \quad \dot{q} = [\dot{q}_1\,\dot{q}_2\,\dot{q}_3]^T \tag{4}$$

with $\dot{\mathbf{q}}$ thus being the vector of actuated joint rates. $\dot{q}_i = \dot{\alpha}_i$ when link A_iB_i is driven and $\dot{q}_i = \dot{\delta}_i$ when link A_iE_i is driven, i = 1, 2, 3. $\mathbf{A}$ and $\mathbf{B}$ are respectively, the direct and the inverse Jacobian matrices of the mechanism, defined as

$$\mathbf{A} = \begin{bmatrix} (\mathbf{c}_1 - \mathbf{h}_1)^T & -(\mathbf{c}_1 - \mathbf{h}_1)^T\mathbf{E}(\mathbf{p} - \mathbf{c}_1) \\ (\mathbf{c}_2 - \mathbf{h}_2)^T & -(\mathbf{c}_2 - \mathbf{h}_2)^T\mathbf{E}(\mathbf{p} - \mathbf{c}_2) \\ (\mathbf{c}_3 - \mathbf{h}_3)^T & -(\mathbf{c}_3 - \mathbf{h}_3)^T\mathbf{E}(\mathbf{p} - \mathbf{c}_3) \end{bmatrix} \tag{5}$$

$$\mathbf{B} = \text{diag}\left[(\mathbf{c}_i - \mathbf{b}_i)^T\mathbf{E}(\mathbf{b}_i - \mathbf{a}_i)\right], \quad i = 1, 2, 3 \tag{6}$$

where $\mathbf{h}_i = \mathbf{b}_i$ when link A_iB_i is driven and $\mathbf{h}_i = \mathbf{a}_i$ when link B_iC_i is driven, i = 1, 2, 3.

When $\mathbf{A}$ is non singular, we obtain the relation

$$\mathbf{t} = \mathbf{J}_p\dot{\mathbf{q}} \quad \text{with} \quad \mathbf{J}_p = \mathbf{A}^{-1}\mathbf{B} \tag{7}$$

Likewise, we obtain

$$\dot{\mathbf{q}} = \mathbf{K}_p\mathbf{t} \tag{8}$$

when $\mathbf{B}$ is non singular with $\mathbf{K}_p$ denoting the inverse of $\mathbf{J}_p$.

4.2 Singularity Analysis

The singular configurations associated with the direct-kinematic matrix of PPMs are well known (Merlet 2006). For the 3-RRR PPM, such configurations are reached whenever lines (B_1C_1), (B_2C_2) and (B_3C_3) intersect (possibly at infinity). For the 3-R$\underline{R}$R PPM, such configurations are reached whenever lines (A_1C_1), (A_2C_2) and (A_3C_3) intersect. Consequently, the singular configurations associated with the direct-kinematic matrix of the NAVARO are reached whenever lines (H_1C_1), (H_2C_2) and (H_3C_3) intersect where H_i stands for B_i (A_i, resp.) when link A_iB_i (B_iC_i, resp.) is driven, $i = 1, 2, 3$.

From Eq. (6), the singular configurations associated with the inverse-kinematics of the NAVARO are reached whenever points A_i, B_i, and C_i are aligned.

5 Dynamic Modeling of the NAVARO

The inverse dynamic model of a robot provides its joint torques and forces as a function of the joint positions and its time derivatives. The direct dynamic model gives the joint accelerations as a function of joint positions, velocities and torques. Different approaches such as virtual work principle, Lagrange formalism and Newton Euler equations have been adopted in the literature (Merlet 2006). Here the method developed in Khalil and Ibrahim (2007) is used to derive the dynamic model of the NAVARO. In Khalil and Ibrahim (2007), the dynamic models of the legs are obtained with classical methods used for serial robots, while the dynamic model of the platform is obtained with Newton-Euler equations. Then, they are projected onto the actuated joint axes by means of Jacobian matrices. It is noteworthy that the legs of the NAVARO contain some closed loop chains contrary to the legs of the parallel manipulators analyzed in Khalil and Ibrahim (2007). As a consequence, the methodology presented in Khalil and Ibrahim (2007) used to express the dynamic modeling of parallel manipulators is improved in this chapter in order to be suitable for the dynamic modeling of the NAVARO. One difficulty lies in the choice of the joint to be cut to come up with an appropriate tree structure of the NAVARO for its dynamic modeling as explained thereafter.

5.1 Inverse Dynamic Model

To project the dynamics of the legs onto the active joint space, the Jacobian between the two spaces is used. The projection of the platform dynamics is performed by multiplying the expression with the transpose of the kinematic Jacobian matrix:

$$\Gamma = \mathbf{J}_p^T \mathbf{F}_p + \sum_{i=1}^{m} \left(\frac{\partial \dot{\mathbf{q}}_i}{\partial \dot{\mathbf{q}}_a} \right)^T \mathbf{H}_i \tag{9}$$

where $\mathbf{J}_p$ is the kinematic Jacobian matrix of the robot defined by Eq. (7), $\mathbf{F}_p$ contains the total forces and moments applied on the platform, $\dot{\mathbf{q}}_a$ is the vector of active joint velocities and $\mathbf{H}_i$ is the inverse dynamic model of the ith leg.

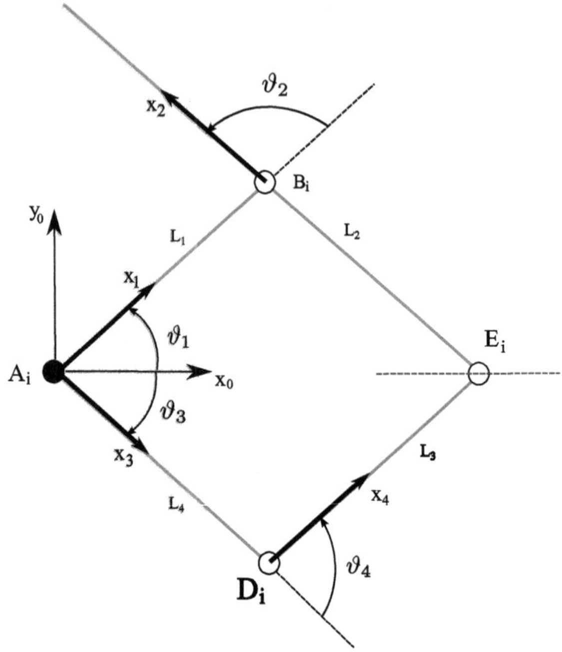

Fig. 4 Geometric model of the equivalent tree structure of the leg of the NAVARO

The following relationship holds:

$$\left(\frac{\partial \dot{\mathbf{q}}_i}{\partial \dot{\mathbf{q}}_a}\right) = \mathbf{J}_i^{-1}\mathbf{J}_{vi}\mathbf{J}_p \tag{10}$$

Matrix $\mathbf{J}_i$ is the Jacobian matrix of leg i ($i = 1, \ldots, m$, being m the number of legs), $\mathbf{J}_{vi}$ is the matrix that maps the velocity $\mathbf{v}_i$ of the ith leg into the moving platform twist $\mathbf{t}_p$:

$$\mathbf{v}_i = \mathbf{J}_i\dot{\mathbf{q}}_i \tag{11}$$

$$\mathbf{v}_i = \mathbf{J}_{vi}\mathbf{t}_p \tag{12}$$

As the active joint variables are independent, Eq. (9) is rewritten as:

$$\Gamma = \mathbf{H}^a + \mathbf{J}_p^T\left(\mathbf{F}_p + \sum_{i=1}^{m}\mathbf{J}_{vi}^T\mathbf{J}_i^{-T}(:,p_i)\mathbf{H}_i^p\right) \tag{13}$$

where $\mathbf{H}^a$ is the vector of active torques of the legs and index p_i of matrix $\mathbf{J}_i^{-T}$ refers to the passive joint variable number.

Each leg of the NAVARO contains a parallelogram closed loop and its dynamics should be first computed. Accordingly, the loop is opened and its

Table 2 Modified Denavit-Hartenberg parameters of the equivalent tree structure of one leg of the NAVARO

j	$a(j)$	σ_j	γ_j	b_j	α_j	d_j	ϑ_j	r_j
1	0	0	0	0	0	0	ϑ_1	0
2	1	0	0	0	0	L_1	ϑ_2	0
3	0	0	0	0	0	0	ϑ_3	0
4	3	0	0	0	0	L_4	ϑ_4	0

equivalent tree structure is analyzed. The open loop is described using the Modified Denavit Hartenberg parameters (Khalil and Dombre 2004) as illustrated in Fig. 4, where the cut joint is located at point E_i and highlighted by the red dotted line. The parameters are given in Table 2.

The dynamic model of the equivalent tree structure is defined as:

$$\Gamma_{tr,i} = \mathbf{A}_{tr,i}\ddot{\mathbf{q}}_i + \mathbf{h}_{tr,i} = \begin{bmatrix} \Gamma_{i1} \\ \Gamma_{i2} \\ \Gamma_{i3} \\ \Gamma_{i4} \end{bmatrix} \tag{14}$$

with

$$\ddot{\mathbf{q}}_i = \begin{bmatrix} \ddot{q}_{i1} \\ \ddot{q}_{i2} \\ \ddot{q}_{i3} \\ \ddot{q}_{i4} \end{bmatrix} \tag{15}$$

Once the dynamic model of the open loop is computed, it is projected onto the closed loop in order to obtain the torques $\mathbf{H}_i$ of the ith leg:

$$\mathbf{H}_i = P^T \Gamma_{tr,i} = \left(\frac{\partial \mathbf{q}_i}{\partial \mathbf{q}_{ai}}\right)^T \Gamma_{tr,i} = \begin{bmatrix} H_{i1} \\ H_{i2} \end{bmatrix} \tag{16}$$

The joint angle vector is expressed as:

$$\mathbf{q}_i = \begin{bmatrix} q_{i1} \\ q_{i2} \\ q_{i3} \\ q_{i4} \end{bmatrix} = \begin{bmatrix} \vartheta_1 \\ \vartheta_2 \\ \vartheta_3 \\ \vartheta_4 \end{bmatrix} \tag{17}$$

The passive joint angles ϑ_3 and ϑ_4 are defined as a function of angles ϑ_1 and ϑ_2 as follows:

$$\begin{aligned} \vartheta_3 &= -\pi + \vartheta_1 + \vartheta_2 \\ \vartheta_4 &= \pi - \vartheta_2 \end{aligned} \tag{18}$$

Therefore, the projection matrix **P** is defined as:

$$\mathbf{P} = \left(\frac{\partial \mathbf{q}_i}{\partial \mathbf{q}_{ai}}\right) = \begin{bmatrix} 1 & 0 \\ 0 & 1 \\ 1 & 1 \\ 0 & -1 \end{bmatrix} \tag{19}$$

The platform dynamics is calculated following the Newton-Euler equations and is defined for the general case as:

$$\mathbf{F}_p = \mathbb{J}_p \begin{bmatrix} \dot{\mathbf{v}}_P - \mathbf{g} \\ \dot{\omega}_p \end{bmatrix} + \begin{bmatrix} \omega_p \times (\omega_p \times \mathbf{MS}_p) \\ \omega_p \times (\mathbf{I}_p \quad \omega_p) \end{bmatrix} \tag{20}$$

where $\mathbf{MS}_p$ is the vector of first moments of the platform around the origin of the platform frame:

$$\mathbf{MS}_p = \begin{bmatrix} MX_p & MY_p & MZ_p \end{bmatrix}^T \tag{21}$$

$\mathbb{J}_p$ is the spatial inertia matrix of the platform:

$$\mathbb{J}_p = \begin{bmatrix} M_p \mathbf{I}_3 & -\hat{\mathbf{MS}}_p \\ \hat{\mathbf{MS}}_p & \mathbf{I}_p \end{bmatrix} \tag{22}$$

$\mathbf{I}_p$ is the inertia matrix of the platform:

$$\mathbf{I}_p = \begin{bmatrix} XX_p & XY_p & XZ_p \\ YX_p & YY_p & YZ_p \\ ZX_p & ZY_p & ZZ_p \end{bmatrix} \tag{23}$$

$\hat{\mathbf{MS}}_p$ is the skew matrix associated with the vector $\mathbf{MS}_p$:

$$\hat{\mathbf{MS}}_p = \begin{bmatrix} 0 & -MZ_p & MY_p \\ MZ_p & 0 & -MX_p \\ -MY_p & MX_p & 0 \end{bmatrix} \tag{24}$$

Since the moving-platform of the NAVARO performs a planar motion, vector $\mathbf{MS}_p$ takes the form:

$$\mathbf{MS}_p = \begin{bmatrix} MX_p & MY_p & 0 \end{bmatrix}^T \tag{25}$$

and

$$\mathbf{I}_p = \begin{bmatrix} 0 & 0 & 0 \\ 0 & 0 & 0 \\ 0 & 0 & ZZ_p \end{bmatrix} \tag{26}$$

Therefore, Eq. (9) becomes:

$$\Gamma = \mathbf{J}_r^T \mathbf{S}^T \mathbf{F}_p + \sum_{i=1}^{m} \left(\mathbf{J}_i^{-1} \mathbf{J}_{vi} \mathbf{S} \mathbf{J}_r \right)^T \mathbf{H}_i \tag{27}$$

5.2 Direct Dynamic Model

The direct dynamic model (DDyM) gives the platform Cartesian accelerations as a function of the Cartesian position and velocity of the platform and the motorized joint torques. In (Khalil and Ibrahim 2007) it is shown that the direct dynamic model can be computed with the following general form:

$$\dot{\mathbf{t}}_r = \mathbf{A}_{robot}^{-1} \left(\mathbf{J}_r^{-T} \Gamma - \mathbf{h}_{robot} \right) \tag{28}$$

where $\mathbf{A}_{robot}$ is the total inertia matrix of the robot with respect to the Cartesian space, $\mathbf{h}_{robot}$ is a term that includes the Coriolis, centrifugal and gravity forces.

The inverse dynamic model of the ith leg is formulated as:

$$\mathbf{H}_i(\mathbf{q}_i, \dot{\mathbf{q}}_i, \ddot{\mathbf{q}}_i) = \mathbf{A}_i \ddot{\mathbf{q}}_i + \mathbf{h}_i(\mathbf{q}_i, \dot{\mathbf{q}}_i) \tag{29}$$

Upon differentiation of Eqs. (11) and (12) we obtain:

$$\dot{\mathbf{v}}_i = \mathbf{J}_i \ddot{\mathbf{q}}_i + \dot{\mathbf{J}}_i \dot{\mathbf{q}}_i \tag{30}$$

$$\dot{\mathbf{v}}_i = \dot{\mathbf{J}}_{vi} \mathbf{t}_p + \mathbf{J}_{vi} \dot{\mathbf{t}}_p \tag{31}$$

The joint accelerations in Eq. (29) are then substituted with:

$$\ddot{\mathbf{q}}_i = \mathbf{J}_i^{-1} \left(\dot{\mathbf{J}}_{vi} \mathbf{t}_p + \mathbf{J}_{vi} \dot{\mathbf{t}}_p - \dot{\mathbf{J}}_i \dot{\mathbf{q}}_\mathbf{i} \right) \tag{32}$$

For the NAVARO the leg inertia matrix $\mathbf{A}_{it}$ and the Coriolis, centrifugal and gravity torques $\mathbf{h}_{it}$ were first computed for the equivalent tree structure with

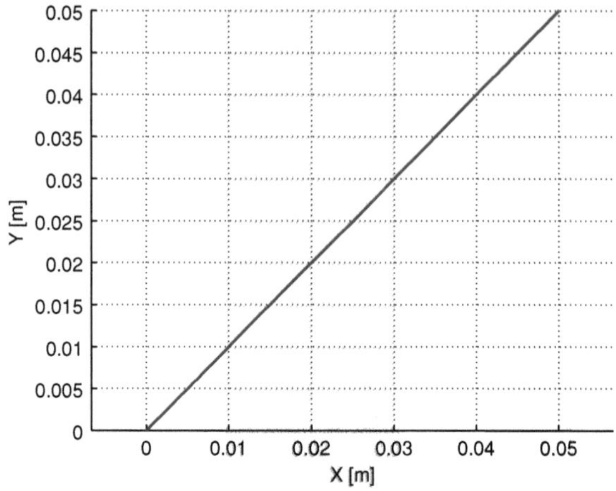

Fig. 5 Path of the test trajectory in the Cartesian space

SYMORO+ (Khalil and Creusot 1997), then projected onto closed loop by means of the projection matrix P defined by Eq. (19) to obtain $\mathbf{A}_i$ and $\mathbf{h}_i$:

$$\mathbf{A}_i = \mathbf{P}^T \mathbf{A}_{it} \mathbf{P} \tag{33}$$

$$\mathbf{h}_i = \mathbf{P}^T \mathbf{h}_{it} \tag{34}$$

Having all these elements, the robot platform acceleration is computed with Eq. (28).

5.3 Validation of the Dynamic Model

Both inverse and direct dynamic models of the NAVARO were implemented in Matlab. A model was realized in Simulink to simulate the behaviour of the dynamic model of the NAVARO in response to a test trajectory. The actuation mode is specified in the definition of the trajectory in order to select the appropriate robot Jacobian during the computation of both inverse and direct dynamic models.

Figure 5 illustrates the path of the test trajectory in the Cartesian space. Figure 6 shows the velocity and acceleration profiles of the test trajectory. Figure 7 provides the required motor torques computed with the dynamic model of the NAVARO written in Matlab to follow the test trajectory with the first actuation mode of the NAVARO. Figure 8 depicts the position and linear acceleration errors

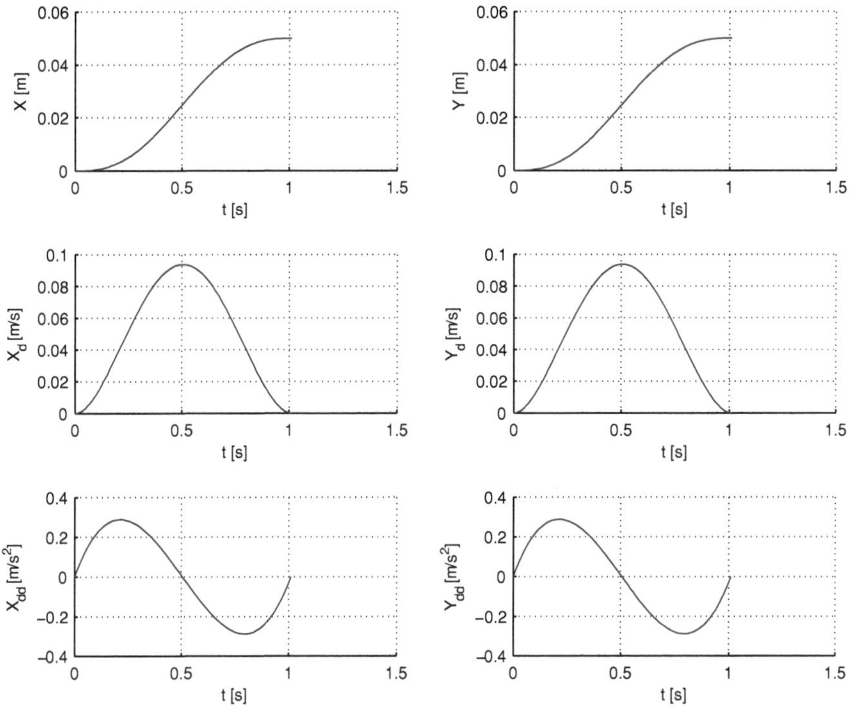

Fig. 6 Velocity and acceleration profiles of the test trajectory

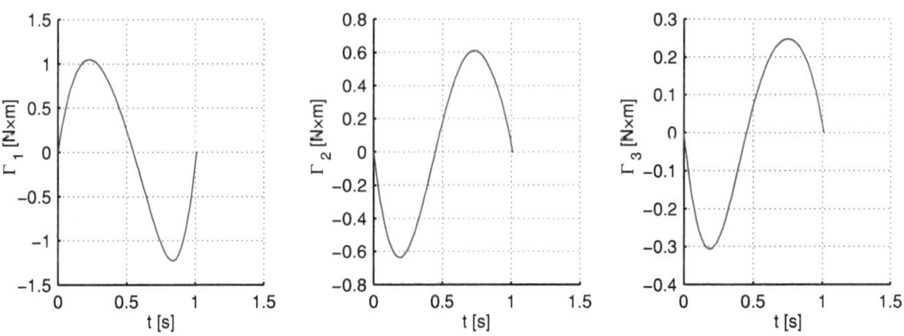

Fig. 7 Required motor torques to follow the test trajectory with the 1st actuation mode

of the moving platform along the test trajectory. The acceleration errors are of order 10^{-16}. The position errors are instead of order 10^{-4}. Considering that there are possible integration errors, those errors are acceptable. Finally, those results were also compared with those obtained with MapleSIM software and the correlation turned to be good.

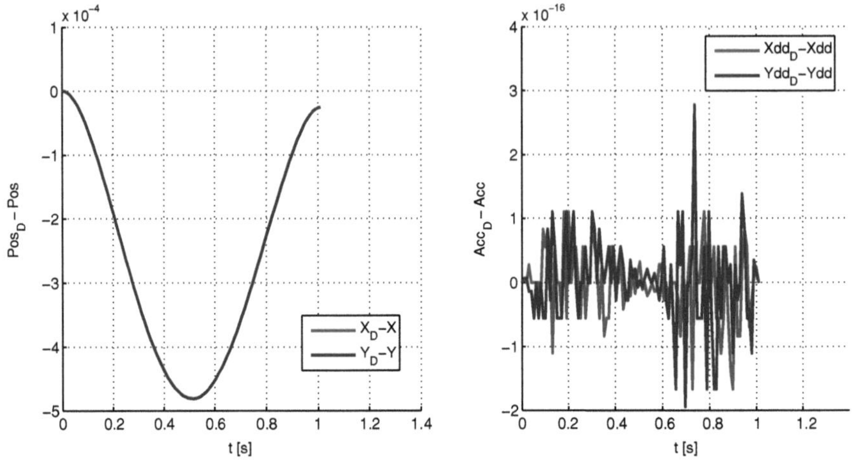

Fig. 8 Position and linear acceleration errors of the moving platform along the test trajectory

6 Conclusions

In this chapter, a three degree-of-freedom planar parallel manipulator with variable actuation modes, named NAVARO, was introduced. NAVARO stands for NAntes Variable Actuation RObot and has eight actuation modes. First, the prototype of the manipulator was presented. Then, its transmission systems were described. The kinematic and dynamic models of the NAVARO have also been developed. It is noteworthy that the legs of the NAVARO contain some closed loop chains contrary to the legs of the parallel manipulators analyzed in Khalil and Ibrahim (2007). As a consequence, the methodology presented in Khalil and Ibrahim (2007) used to express the dynamic modeling of parallel manipulators has been improved to be suitable for the dynamic modeling of the NAVARO. The development of an algorithm to deal with the actuation mode changing of the NAVARO and optimal path placement will be part of the future work. The kinematic and dynamic models will be also validated experimentally.

Acknowledgements The first three authors would like to acknowledge the financial support of the French "Agence Nationale de la Recherche" (Project "SiRoPa", SIngularités des RObots PArallèles). The four authors would like to thank the Royal Society, United Kingdom, through an International Joint Project No. JP100715. M. Iván Sáinz and Prof. Wisama Khalil are also acknowledged for their great help during the design of the double clutch system and the dynamic modeling of the NAVARO, respectively.

References

Alba-Gomez, O., Wenger, P. and Pamanes, A. (2005), Consistent Kinetostatic Indices for Planar 3-DOF Parallel Manipulators, Application to the Optimal Kinematic Inversion, *Proceedings of the ASME 2005 IDETC/CIE Conference*.

Arakelian, V., Briot, S. and Glazunov, V. (2007). Increase of Singularity-Free Zones in the Workspace of Parallel Manipulators Using Mechanisms of Variable Structure. *Mech. Mach. Theory*, Available online at www.sciencedirect.com.

Caro, S., Khan, W.A., Pasini, D. and Angeles, J. (2010), The Rule-based Conceptual Design of the Architecture of Serial Schönflies-motion Generators *Mechanism and Machine Theory*, vol. 45, no. 2, pp. 251–260.

Chablat, D. and Wenger, P. (1998), Working Modes and Aspects in Fully-Parallel Manipulator, *Proceeding IEEE International Conference on Robotics and Automation*, pp. 1964–1969, May.

Chablat, D., Wenger, P., Caro, S. and Angeles, J. (2002), The Isoconditioning Loci of Planar Three-DOF Parallel Manipulators, *Proc. DETC ASME*, Montreal, Canada.

Khalil, W. and Creusot, D. (1997) SYMORO+: A system for the symbolic modelling of robots. *Robotica*, 15:153–161.

Khalil, W. and Dombre, E. (2004) *Modeling, Identification and Control Of Robots*. Elsevier Butterworth Heinemann.

Khalil, W. and Ibrahim, O. (2007) General solution for the dynamic modeling of parallel robots. *Journal of intelligent and robotic systems*, 49:19–37.

Merlet, J-P. (2006), *Parallel robots*, Springer.

Rakotomanga, N., Chablat, D. and Caro, S. (2008), Performance of a Planar Parallel Mechanism with Variable Actuation, *Advances in Robot Kinematics*, Batz-sur-Mer, France, June 22–26, pp. 311–320.

Theingin, Chen, I.-M., Angeles, J. and Li, C. (2007), Management of parallel-manipulator singularities using joint-coupling *Advanced Robotics*, vol. 21, no. 5–6, pp. 583–600.

Experiences on Service Robots at LARM in Cassino

Marco Ceccarelli and Giuseppe Carbone

Abstract Service robots are presented in this chapter from authors' perspective as based on experiences at LARM in Cassino. Peculiarities of service robots can be challenges for their wide diffusion in terms of low-cost user-oriented features both in design and operation. Comments on direct authors' experiences help to outline possibilities for developing service robots with low-cost user-oriented features with design activity without large resources.

Keywords Service robots · Design · Experimental robotics · Prototypes

1 Introduction

Service robots and their applications are new areas for Robotics and its future. Since more than one decade attention has been addressed to bring robots out of industrial frames in servicing in tasks with humans interaction. A considerable experience and corresponding literature are available to understand and outline peculiarities in service robots, mainly from those past successful applications, even in attempts at lab levels. A reader can refer to (Ceccarelli 2011; Robot Vision 2009; Siciliano and Khatib 2008) as sources for a better insight of this emerging field with already real positive achievements. Main characters of service robots can be recognized in multi-disciplinary aspects and human-machine interactions. Both require preliminary research activity and lab experimental testing. In this chapter challenges and trends with more developments of service robots are

M. Ceccarelli (✉) · G. Carbone
LARM, University of Cassino and South Latium, Cassino, Italy
e-mail: ceccarelli@unicas.it

G. Carbone
e-mail: Carbone@unicas.it

A. Rodić et al. (eds.), *New Trends in Medical and Service Robots*,
Mechanisms and Machine Science 20, DOI: 10.1007/978-3-319-05431-5_22,

outlined by looking at direct experiences at LARM in Cassino with a specific approach for low-cost user-oriented solutions. Those experiences can be considered illustrative examples of how approaching the field by a small team with interesting successful solutions for specific implementations.

2 Service Robots

Service robots give the possibility of new fields of applications for Robotics by wide spreading robots also into non technical areas. But new requirements and goals need to be carefully considered both in designing and operating specific solutions. In this chapter, main aspects and challenges are discussed both as problems and advantages in developing and using robots in service operations for new areas of applications, by taking particular attention to non engineering aspects that are deduced from new service areas. Key problems for developing service robots for a successful acceptance and use by even non technical users can be considered in terms of specific technical problems for low-cost user-oriented operation systems, but mainly in terms of implications for human-machine interactions.

In general challenges for service robots can be seen in:

- operating together with/or for human users, with suitable behaviours and careful users-friendly operation;
- operating service tasks with proper easy-operation modes at user-oriented cost.

One key point for service robots can be considered human-machine interaction and corresponding interfaces that can determine the success or failure of a service operation. Indeed, a mechanical design of human-machine interface is not very often considered as a critical issue, but it is often included as an issue part of the overall design of mechanical solutions within servo controlled operation and environment interaction. A second important issue is related with the acceptance of robotic systems and corresponding psychological aspects, when robots are proposed to operators and users in fields with very low level of technical means in current work practice.

Beside comfort issues, aspects involving users are the most challenging since they include issues of education, training, acceptance, and appreciation from users, who are in general common people. Thus, it can take time that a good service robot will achieve the success even if it is based on innovative technology developments. This is the case for example for home cleaning robots which, although conceived and developed more than ten years ago, only now are used successfully worldwide in house applications.

User-oriented operation requires developing a system having functional characteristics well suited to users' capabilities and requirements, mainly in term of technical understanding as pointed out in (Ceccarelli 2011, 2013). This aims not only at reducing the complexity of service robots, but also at promoting suitable education and training of potential users. Those problems bridge mechatronic design of service robots with adequate formation and continuous education of humans in an integrated framework which includes creators of service robots too.

3 Challenges and Trends

Challenges for service robots with new designs and new applications can be faced in two main frames, namely for new advances and for low-cost solutions. New advances are searched as per innovation and implementation of new technologies. They can be considered a necessary background for feasible implementations, although most of the times they are developed costly and in research labs. The natural evolution is in low-cost solutions at levels for market availability and users acceptance. Even low-cost solutions still require research and design activities both in design and operation aspects (Ceccarelli 2013). Indeed trends and challenges for practical use of service robots can be recognised mainly in the above-mentioned aspects, namely human-machine interfaces (not only for operability by non technical users) and users acceptance (with proper understanding and appreciation).

Low-cost solutions are characterized by design components from the market and operation features with user-oriented modes. Most of the challenges can be identified in problems that arise when advanced solutions are evolved in constructions and operations by market components and facilities. Nevertheless, trends are well indicated in the directions that service robots will have functionalities for well specified service tasks at operation complexity and system costs that are specified by capabilities of potential users.

4 Experiences at LARM in Cassino

At LARM, Fig. 1, research activity is carried out in the following specific subjects of Robotics and Mechatronics regarding with Mechanics, Design, and Experimental Validation: serial and parallel manipulators; grippers and hands; walking machines and humanoid robots; electro-pneumatic systems; dynamics of mechanical systems for automation; robotised manipulations; low-cost robots; mechanical transmissions. Within LARM activity a specific attention has been addressed to development of service systems for specific tasks mainly by looking at technological solutions that could give low-cost solutions both in design and operation. Main achievements are reported in the following with the aim both of presenting LARM contributions and discussing developments for low-cost solutions with limited resources as those available at LARM.

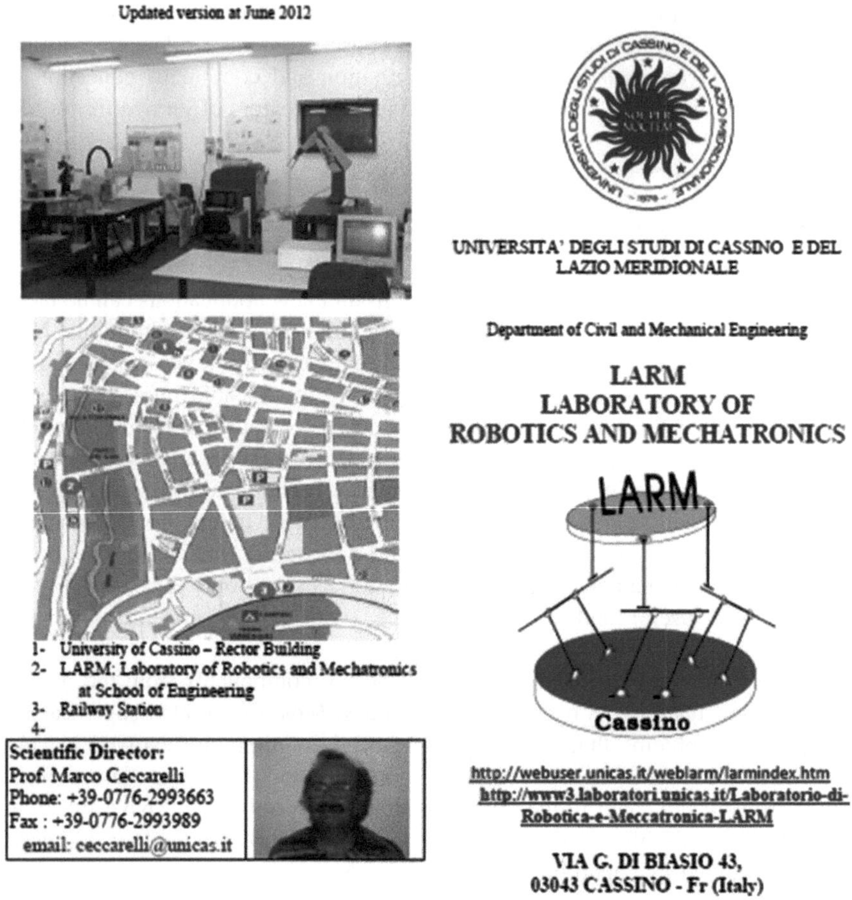

Fig. 1 Current flyer of LARM

4.1 An Account of History of LARM

LARM history can be outlined shortly as in (Ceccarelli 2012) by reporting main achievements during the several phases of development with different capabilities, namely 1990–1995: early days just after the foundation; 1996–2001: full establishment; 2002–2009: inter-nationalization of the activities; 2010-present towards the future. The laboratory started as LARI (Laboratory of Industrial Robotics) in 1990 as a first laboratory of the School of Engineering in Cassino and in 1996 when prof. Papa for health reasons passed leadership to prof. Ceccarelli it was decided to update name and field of interest with the current name of LARM.

Main developments are illustrated as referring to figures in the chapter. In particular, the historical evolution has been characterized by the main following aspects during the above-mentioned phases. In early days the activities were

Table 1 Chronicle of main achievements on service robots at LARM

Year	Event
1995	Design and construction of CaTraSys (Cassino Tracking System)
1996	Design and construction of a prototype of CaPaMan (Cassino Parallel Manipulator)
1998	Design and construction of a micro-gripper
1999	Earthquake simulation by CaPaMan
2001	Design and construction of LARM Hand
2003	Design and construction of Cassino leg mechanism for Biped robots and Cassino Rickshaw robot
2004	Design and construction of CaLoWi (Cassino Low-Cost Wire Parallel Manipulator)
2005	Design and construction of Cassino Hexapod
2006	Design and construction of LARM Hand Vers IV
2007	Application of CaTraSys for human gait analysis
2009	Design and construction of LARM Clutched Arm
2010	Application of CaLoWi for human limb exercise
2010	Design of LARM finger exoskeleton for finger exercising
2012	Design and construction of BaPaMan II (Binary Parallel Manipulator)

mainly carried out with computer-oriented work; experiences were initiated with the equipment that was little by little installed in the laboratory space. In the period of full establishment the laboratory was properly located with space that permitted also to acquire more equipment, to run continuously experimental activities and to build first constructions of devices and prototypes, also thanks to the increased number of staff members. In the internationalization period the activities were fully developed with relevant collaborations within international research projects and student exchange programs. Since 2010 the activities have been oriented to well-focused subjects to service robot applications also because of the reduction of staff members and limits in budget resources (due reforming plans at national and local levels). The history of LARM development is summarized in the chronicle of Table 1 with indication of main events as related to service robots. More information and full list of publications as well as summaries of activities are reported in LARM webpage (2013).

4.2 Developments for an Earthquake Simulator

A first service task was attached by applying CaPaMan (Cassino Parallel Manipulator) prototype to earthquake experimental simulations. The seismic motions were modelled for a proper reproduction in the motions of CaPaMan platform through a suitable path planning in 1999 (Carvalho and Ceccarelli 2002). Planar seismic motions were reproduced in a sensored mobile platform for prescribed displacements and acceleration. Later in 2003 3D seismic motions were analyzed and reproduced by a sensored CaPaMan that was settled up as an

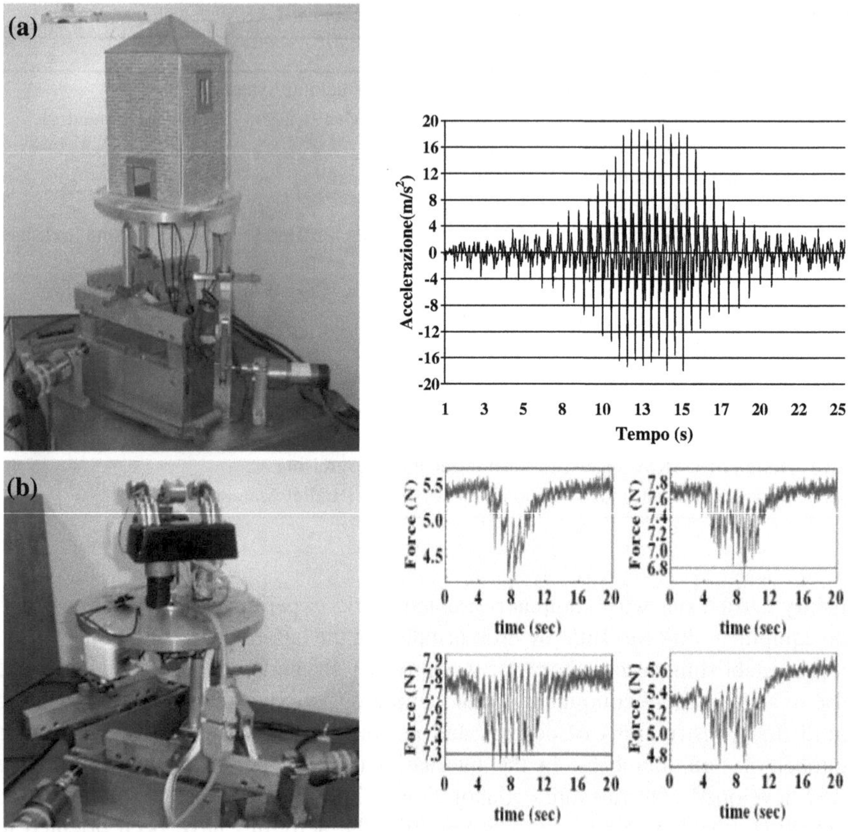

Fig. 2 Service experiences with CaPaMan as earthquake simulator; **a** with civil structures in 1999; **b** for characterization of seismic effects on machine operation since 2010

earthquake simulator (Ceccarelli et al. 2002; Ottaviano and Ceccarelli 2006). The mobile platform under seismic motion is used as a test-bed to study effects of earthquake on scaled systems. Thus, experiences were worked out not only on structures of civil engineering, Fig. 2a but even to investigate on robustness of robotic systems and machinery in general under shaking disturb dynamics, Fig. 2b.

Recently, tests have been applied to characterize experimentally the effects of seismic disturbances on machine operation (Sula et al. 2011). Examples have been tested with scaled set up of linkages, driving mechanisms, and robotic structures. Service features have been implemented by adjusting CaPaMan operation as earthquake simulator through suitable user-oriented earthquake programming and proper test area on the mobile platform with monitoring sensors.

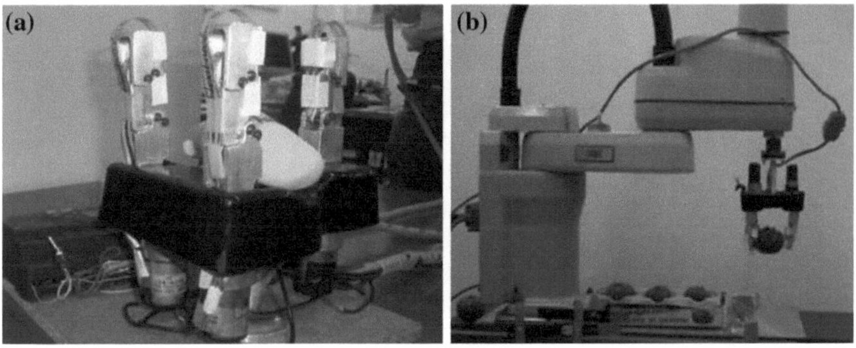

Fig. 3 Service experiences with LARM Hand: **a** Vers III for teaching; **b** in tomato packaging application

4.3 Developments for an Artificial Hand

LARM hand was conceived as robotic grasping device for application on robots even with humanoid solutions since 2000, as outlined in Carbone and Ceccarelli (2008). However, since the beginning the overall design was developed with low-cost features that made possible service applications, like tomato packaging and prosthesis designs, mainly with students' thesis works. In particular, a version was developed with fairly simple sensor and programming units, with the aim to join the fairly simple linkage design which is the driving mechanism of each finger.

The LARM finger mechanism has been designed with a linkage structure for 1 DOF actuation and a kinematic solution to insure proper human-like motion of the linkage within a finger body. As depending of planned services, solutions have been developed with control systems of different levels of performance as function of service tasks, namely from a threshold force signal binary regulation up to a servo control with advanced actuators. Further activities are planned to develop a LARM finger mechanism that can adapt to the object shapes with an underactuation design (Ceccarelli et al. 2012).

Grasping service has been thought for LARM hand not only in robots, and particularly humanoids, but even non technical applications, like prosthesis. In fact, a development has been conceived with finger structures as exoskeletons for exercising in finger rehabilitation.

LARM hand has been also used in teaching and training students and robot users in handling grasping issues and specifically a robotic hand. Indeed, teaching service is a common aspects in all LARM experiences as due to the formation mission of the academic institution within which LARM operates (Fig. 3).

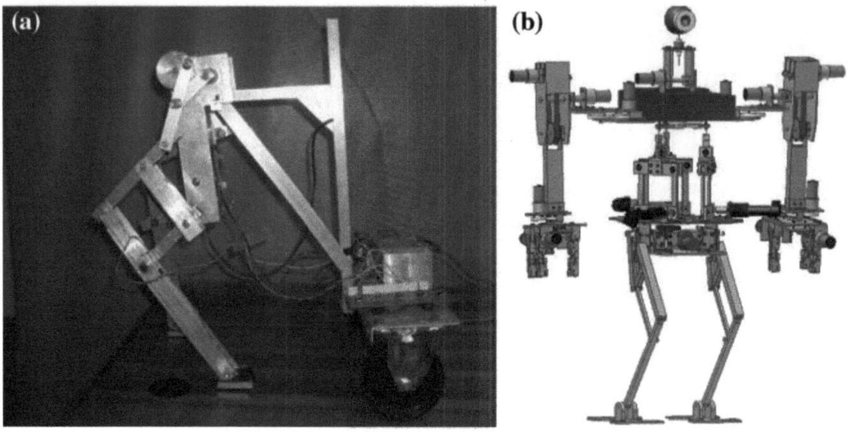

Fig. 4 Service applications of LARM leg mechanism: **a** in a rickshaw robot; **b** in a humanoid robot design

4.4 Developments for Legged Robots

Legged robots have been developed at LARM for biped solutions and hexapod mobile robots for different service applications. Biped leg mechanisms have been designed with a robust linkage structure based on Chebyshev 4-bar mechanism as actuating mechanism of a pantograph leg. Different solutions have been investigated (Li and Ceccarelli 2012) and prototypes have been tested for payload transportation in rickshaw solutions (Li and Ceccarelli 2011), Fig. 4a. Implementations of designed leg mechanisms are planned also in a humanoid design (Nava Rodriguez et al. 2008), Fig. 4b, and multi-legged mobile robot platforms, with the specific characteristics of low-cost 1-DOF actuated leg. Also in this case, the robotic leg mechanism has been extrapolated into a leg exoskeleton that is underdevelopment for human walking rehabilitation (Copilusi et al. 2012).

A specific activity for a service goal has been worked out to develop a hexapod robot for survey and restoration services in interventions in archaeological sites, Fig. 5 (Ceccarelli and Cigola 2012). The robot structure and its operation have been conceived for operators in Cultural Heritage activities with robust modular design and fairly simple control in order to achieve a user-oriented operation with a structure whose maintenance and reparation is possible on field. Hexapod architecture has been designed to ensure a tripod gait that permits the robot platform body available in stable posture for data acquisition procedures (Carbone and Ceccarelli 2008). Wheeled foot is added to each leg both to move in wheeled mode but to have the possibility to regulate the contact force with the ground.

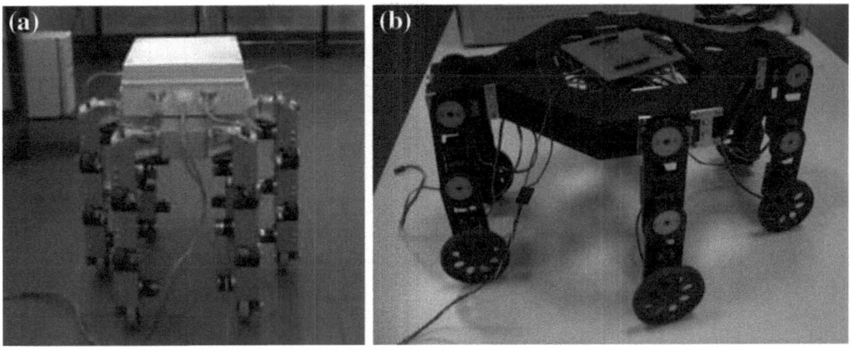

Fig. 5 Prototype of Cassino hexapod for survey service in restoration: **a** 2003 solution; **b** scaled design in 2013

4.5 Developments for Cable-Based Parallel Manipulators

Catrasys (Cassino Tracking System) and CaLoWi (Cassino low-Cost Wire manipulator) are cable-based manipulators that have been developed at LARM for technical issues as results of expertise in kinematics of parallel manipulators, but soon after they have been implemented in service applications.

CoTraSys has been successfully developed in service tasks to monitor motion of human limbs for experimental characterization towards diagnosis procedures (Ceccarelli 2012), Fig. 6. Its main features are easy transportation thanks to the sensor platform, comfortable application thanks to strand attaching connectors, and fairly easy on-line computation thanks to closed form kinematics and commercial equipment.

The connector design as human-machine interface has been a crucial point both for operation efficiency and users acceptance. This is still an open issue for CaLoWi use in applications for limb exercising, as point out in (Ceccarelli and Romdhane 2010).

CaLoWi has been attempted in guiding human limb motions for rehabilitation exercises, after its design for disaster rescue application (Ottaviano et al. 2005), Fig. 7. An open frame structure with parallel architecture can be suitable also for active guidance of a connected limb with proper indications that need supervision and strategy by doctors and nurses.

At LARM, although medical operators have been attracted by the capabilities of CaTraSys and CaLoWi, it is not yet possible to implement the above service applications in medical frames for hospital or home use, also for constrains in medical protocols. Such an implementation will require additional developments both to adjust the design and its component to medical environment constraints and to optimize the operation and its flexibility to patient's therapy.

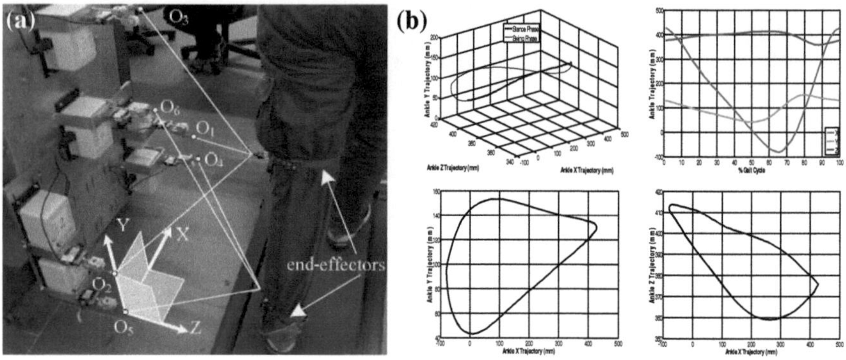

Fig. 6 CaTraSys as diagnostic device for human limb motion: **a** an experimental setup; **b** numerical outputs for ankle point trajectory

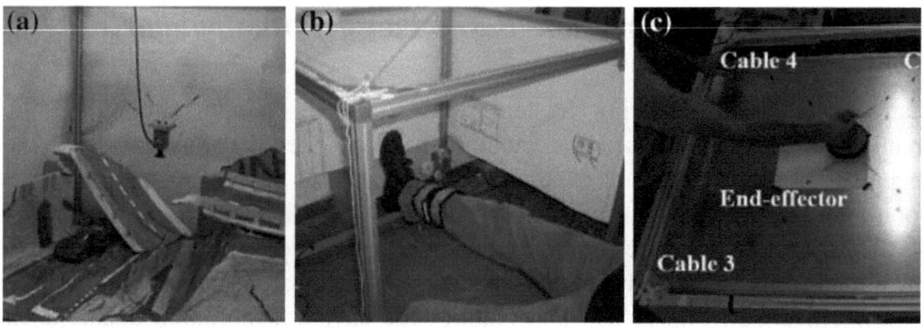

Fig. 7 CaLoWi as service robots in: **a** disaster rescue lab design; **b** medical assisting device in human leg exercise; **c** medical assisting device in human arm exercise

4.6 Developments for a Clutched Arm

LARM clutched arm has been development for investigating a manipulator arm with a reduced number of actuators that could be useful in humanoid robots, space robots, or in assisting robots for disabled people.

The conceived design has been developed in a prototype (Gu et al. 2010), Fig. 8, with market components that suggests an implementation as support arm in a wheel chair of disabled people. The operation has been planned with a light structure of the arm by concentrating the bulk system in a shoulder box with only one motor for the 3 anthropomorphic DOFs (Gu and Ceccarelli 2012).

Interfaces are needed for a specific human-machine interaction in specific service tasks as well as for operation control and command by disabled people users. The prototype solution has been successfully tested in operation efficiency through lab experiments, but open issues are related to light mechanical design, proper size and equipment for well identified service tasks.

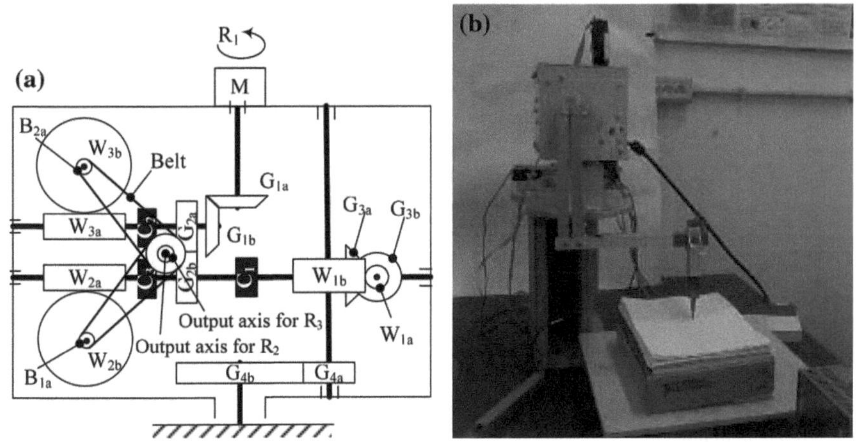

Fig. 8 Experience with LARM clutched arm: **a** a built prototype; **b** test for writing service

4.7 Development of Micro Scaled Devices

Micro-scaled systems have been experienced at LARM for specific manipulation tasks of small objects with the aim of not only developing solutions for attached problems but even for investigating expertise transfer to applications of micro-scale.

A micro-gripper was developed in 1998 (Carbone et al. 2001), Fig. 9a, by using the technology of flexural joints and SMA cable actuation as to implement two-finger grasping through planar mechanisms of proper structure. The micro-gripper overall size was achieved in 2 × 2 cm and objects of 0.1 mm were grasped as a possibility for micro-manufacturing.

In Fig. 9b a micromanipulator prototype is shown as a result of a design purpose for a multi-module structure that is based on micro parallel manipulators with flexural joints (Borchert et al. 2013).

Main constrains for a micro-manipulation design can be considered its dimensions, accuracy, displacement and force capability. In micro-scale service tasks are characterized and indeed constrained by micro-movements and additional force phenomena, like adhesive actions (gluing, capillarity, Van der Walls, electrostatic) with considerable influence of friction effects. The required accuracy can be considered inversely proportional to the geometric dimensions since smaller objects require greater positioning accuracy. The displacement and force capability are directly proportional to the geometric dimensions since bigger objects require larger displacements of fingers and greater grasping force. For these reasons in micro-manipulative tasks the needed accuracy is high while displacement and force capability are of small magnitude in agreement with the dimensions of the handled objects. For example, grasping an object of 1 mm and 0.1 N weight can require an accuracy of 0.1 mm, a grasping force of 1 N and a finger opening

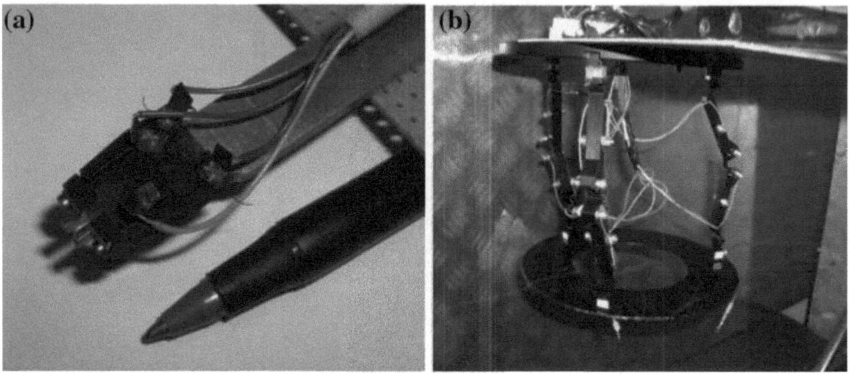

Fig. 9 LARM micro-mechanisms for service tasks: **a** a microgripper; **b** BaPaMan (Binary Barallel Manipulator

displacement of 0.5 mm. Therefore, high accuracy is required in tasks like micro-assembly and microsurgery, which are typical field of application of micromanipulators and microgrippers.

5 Conclusions

This chapter is aimed to discuss the possibility to develop service robots with low-cost user-oriented features with design activity without large resources. Main problems for a successful design can be recognized in full understanding of potential users' acceptance both in terms of operation benefits and personal satisfaction. Thus, technical aspects must be completed with non-engineering requirements in order to obtain a feasible solution. Simplicity of the design can be a key issue both for users' understanding and implementation of other nature features. Direct experiences of the authors are reported to show successfully activity with the above-mentioned approach in developing LARM prototypes.

References

Borchert G., Löchte C., Carbone G., Raatz A., A modular design kit for task-adaptable low-cost robots based on BaPaMan design, Frontiers of Mechanical Engineering, March 2013, Volume 8, Issue 1, pp 33–41 (2013)

Carbone G., Ceccarelli M., Design of LARM Hand: Problems and Solutions, Journal of Control Engineering and Applied Informatics, Vol.10, n.2, pp. 39–46 (2008)

Carbone G., Ceccarelli M., A Low-Cost Easy-Operation Hexapod Walking Machine, International Journal of Advanced Robotic Systems, Vol.5, n.2, pp.161–166 (2008)

Carbone G., Ceccarelli M., Kerle H., Raatz A.,Design and Experimental Validation of a Microgripper, Fuji International Journal of Robotics and Mechatronics, Vol.13, No.3, pp.319–325 (2001)

Carvalho J.C.M., Ceccarelli M., Seismic Motion Simulation Based on Cassino Parallel Manipulator, Journal of the Brazilian Society of Mechanical Sciences, Vol.25, n.3, July pp.213–219 (2002)

Ceccarelli M., Problems and issues for service robots in new applications, International Journal of Social Robotics: Volume 3, Issue 3, p. 299–312 (2011)

Ceccarelli M., An Illustrated History of LARM in Cassino, Proceedings of RAAD 2012 international Workshop on Robotics in Ale-Adria-Danube Region, Napoli, Edizioni Scientifiche e Artistiche,pp. 35–42 (2012)

Ceccarelli M., The Historical Development of Catrasys - a Cable System; In: Explorations in the History of Machines and Mechanisms, Book series on History of Machines and Machine Science, Vol.15, Springer, Dordrecht, pp.365–379 (2012)

Ceccarelli M., Problems and Experiences on Cable-Based Service Robots for Physiotherapy Applications, in: New Trends in Medical and Service Robots, Pisla D. (Ed), Springer Book series on MMS, Dordrecht, pp.27–42 (2013).

Ceccarelli M., and Cigola M., Service Robots for Restoration of Goods of Cultural Heritage, Chapter 12 in: Service Robots and Robotics: Design and Application, Engineering Science Reference (IGI Global), Hershey, pp.213–228 (2012).

Ceccarelli M., Romdhane L., Design issues for human-machine platform interface in cable-based parallel manipulators for physiotherapy applications, Journal of Zhejiang University SCIENCE A, Vol.11 No.4 p.231–239 (2010)

Ceccarelli M., Ottaviano E., Galvagno M., "A 3-DOF Parallel Manipulator as Earthquake Motion Simulator", Proceedings of the 7th International Conference on Control, Automation, Robotics and Vision ICARCV 2002, Singapore, paper P1534 (2002)

Ceccarelli M., Yao S., Carbone G., Zhan Q., Lu Z., "Analysis and optimal design of an underactuated finger mechanism for robotic fingers", Proceedings of the Institution of Mechanical Engineers, Part C, Journal of Mechanical Engineering Science, Volume 226 Issue 1, pp. 242–256 (2012)

Copilusi C., Ceccarelli M., Dumitru, N. Carbone G., Design and Simulation of a Leg Exoskeleton Linkage for a Human Rehabilitation System, The 11th IFToMM International Symposium on Science of Mechanisms and Machines SYROM'13, Springer, Dordrecht pp.117–125 (2012)

EUROP, Robot Vision – to 2020 and Beyond, the Strategic Research Agenda for European Robotics, Brussels (2009)

Gu H., Ceccarelli M., Carbone G., Design and Simulation of a 1-DOF Anthropomorphic Clutched Arm for Robots International Journal of Humanoid Robotics, Vol. 7, No. 1 157–182 (2010)

Gu H., Ceccarelli M., A Multi-objective Optimal Path Planning for a 1-DOF Clutched ARM, Mechanics Based Design of Structures and Machines, 40:1, 109–121 (2012)

LARM webpage, http://webuser.unicas.it/weblarm/ larmindex.htm, (2013)

Li T., Ceccarelli M., A Method for Topological Design of Mechanism, CD Proceedings of MEDER2012, the IFToMM Symposium on Mechanism Design for Robotics, Beijing, 12–14 October 2012, paper n. 1 (2012)

Li T., Ceccarelli M., An Experimental Characterization of a Rickshaw Prototype, Proceedings of MeTrApp 2011 Mechanism, Transmissions, Applications Workshop, Springer, Dordrecht, pp. 205–216 (2011)

Nava Rodriguez N.E., Carbone G., Ceccarelli M., Simulation results for design and operation of CALUMA, a new low-cost humanoid robot, Robotica, volume 26, pp. 601–618. Cambridge University Press (2008)

Ottaviano E., Ceccarelli M., An Application of a 3-DOF Parallel Manipulator for Earthquake Simulations, IEEE Transactions on Mechatronics, Vol. 11, No. 2, pp. 140–146, (2006)

Siciliano B., Khatib O. (Eds.), Springer Handbook of Robotics, Part F: Field and Service Robotics (Alexander Zelinsky), Springer (2008)

Sula S., Ceccarelli M., Pîslă D., An Experimental Evaluation of Earthquake Effects on Mechanism Operation, International Journal of Mechanics and Control, JoMaC Special issue for RAAD10, pp.91–98, Vol.12, no.2 (2011).

Moving From 'How to go There?' to 'Where to go?': Towards Increased Autonomy of Mobile Robots

Francesco Amigoni, Nicola Basilico and Alberto Quattrini Li

Abstract Autonomous mobile robots have seen a widespread development in recent years, due to their possible applications (e.g., surveillance and search and rescue). Several techniques have been proposed for solving the path planning problem, in which a user specifies spatial targets and the robots autonomously decide how to go there. In contrast, the problem of where to go next, in which the targets themselves are autonomously decided by the robots, is largely unexplored and lacking an assessed theoretical basis. In this work, we make a step towards a framework for casting and addressing this problem. The framework includes the following dimensions: the amount of knowledge about the environment the robots have, the kind of that knowledge, the criteria used to evaluate the success of the decisions, the number of decision makers, and the possible adversarial nature of the settings. We focus on applications relative to exploration and patrolling.

Keywords Navigation strategies · Autonomous mobile robots · Exploration · Patrolling

1 Introduction

It is widely recognized that autonomous mobile robots will be increasingly employed in tasks that are difficult, dangerous, or simply boring for humans. Several steps have been made towards this goal. For example, most mobile robots

F. Amigoni (✉) · A. Quattrini Li
Politecnico di Milano, Milan, Italy
e-mail: francesco.amigoni@polimi.it

A. Quattrini Li
e-mail: alberto.quattrini@polimi.it

N. Basilico
University of Milan, Milan, Italy
e-mail: nicola.basilico@unimi.it

A. Rodić et al. (eds.), *New Trends in Medical and Service Robots*, Mechanisms and Machine Science 20, DOI: 10.1007/978-3-319-05431-5_23, deployed in service applications are currently able to plan a path between their current pose and a target pose, exploiting a plethora of algorithms that have been developed over the years. Indeed, *path planning* has been one of the long-standing topics of mobile robotics and, although some extensions and variants are still actively investigated (e.g., multirobot path planning), has a solid and relatively stable set of pivotal techniques (Latombe 1991; LaValle 2006). A naïve path planning problem formulation involves: a starting pose s for the robot, a target pose t for the robot, some knowledge about the environment, and a criterion O to measure path quality. The outcome is a feasible and safe path that connects s to t satisfying O (at least to some degree) and that, basically, answers the question: 'how to go there?'

Comparatively much less effort has been devoted to investigate the techniques that allow a mobile robot to autonomously determine the target poses t. In some applications, the target pose is provided by the user or imposed by the task (e.g., reach a screw to turn it). However, in many applications of service robots, the target pose is not known in advance but largely depends on the current history of interactions between robots and environments and on the goal of the robots. In such situations, the robots themselves have to autonomously decide where to go, and usually they need to do so at runtime while performing a task.

In this chapter, we address the problem of making such decisions, which we call the problem of developing *navigation strategies* for autonomous mobile robots. Navigation strategies answer the question: 'where to go?'. The main contribution of this work is the proposal of a framework for casting and addressing the issues related to the development of effective navigation strategies and, as such, it is more a conceptual, rather than a technical, contribution. With this work we provide some insights in addressing the problems about navigation strategies, without claiming to entirely solve the problem.

This chapter is structured as follows. The next section analyses some examples of navigation strategies with the aim of both surveying some significant areas in which they are employed and showing that each area is currently using its own techniques and methods for defining them. Section 3 introduces our framework for navigation strategies, which attempts at representing a common ground independent of any specific application. The framework is then applied in practice to suggest new research directions for developing better navigation strategies in Sect. 4. Finally, Sect. 5 concludes the chapter.

2 Navigation Strategies

As motivated in the previous section, the development of fully autonomous mobile robots requires the development of adequate navigation strategies that allow the robots themselves to select the next locations to visit, according to the specific application. In this section, we discuss some examples of navigation strategies, with the aim of introducing the general idea and not of providing an exhaustive survey of the works presented in the literature.

To better focus the situations we address, we provide a very general abstract model of the behavior of a fully autonomous mobile robot while executing a generic task:

(a) perform some action in the current location,
(b) decide a location of the environment where to move,
(c) reach the selected location,
(d) return to Step (a).

Although over-simplified, the above model evidences some interesting issues. Step (c) involves low-level planning (e.g., path planning and localization), while Step (a) relates to actions specific to the task that the robot executes at the reached location (e.g., acquire sensorial data or move some object). The navigation strategy is involved in Step (b) and, as already said, we will refer to it as the set of techniques that allow an autonomous mobile robot to answer the question 'where to go next?', given the knowledge it possesses so far.

In general, a navigation strategy significantly impacts on the task execution's performance. Therefore, the problem is to define *good* navigation strategies, i.e., strategies that allow the robot to perform its task maximizing some performance metric or criterion.

The major challenges related to this problem mainly derive from two issues. The first one is that the definition of a navigation strategy strongly depends on the robot's particular task. Compare, for example, a robot employed for exploration of unknown environments with another robot that has to patrol an environment to prevent intrusions (these two cases are discussed in detail below). In the first case, the robot should select the locations to reach such that it can obtain good views of the surroundings to be integrated in its current knowledge of the environment. In the second case, the robot has to account also for tactical issues such as preventing an intruder to predict its movements and elude it. As this example suggests, completely different navigation strategies could be developed for different tasks.

The second issue is related to the goodness of a navigation strategy. Sometimes this concept is intuitively easy to define. For example, in the case of the patrolling robot, one could define the optimal strategy as the one that minimizes the probability for an intruder to break in without being detected. However, in other situations the goodness of a navigation strategy is harder to capture. In the exploration example, different criteria contribute to the goodness of a strategy, e.g., the amount of mapped area in a given time, the total traveled distance, the quality of the obtained map, the time spent to map a given area, and many others. In general, searching for the best strategy according to some metric increases the problem's difficulty with respect to the case in which a sub-optimal strategy is employed.

Although these application-dependent specific issues, in the next section we will attempt to define a general framework for developing navigation strategies. In the remaining of this section, we discuss more deeply two specific examples of navigation strategies. They have been selected only based on the expertise of the authors and are not intended to endorse any claim of generality or importance. Other examples include continuous monitoring of temporal-spatial phenomena in partially known environments [e.g., ocean monitoring (Smith et al. 2011)], olfactory exploration (Marjovi and Marques 2013), tactile exploration of object properties (Pezzementi et al. 2011), information gathering (Singh et al. 2009), and pursuit/evasion (Durham et al. 2012).

2.1 Exploration of Unknown Environments

Consider the following problem: an autonomous mobile robot is deployed in an initially unknown (static) environment with the aim of discovering its physical structure, namely of building its map (Thrun 2002). A map of an environment represents the location of the obstacles and of the free space. The robot is equipped with sensors (e.g., laser range scanners) that allow it to acquire spatial data in its surroundings. It moves, repeatedly sensing different portions of the environment, and builds a corresponding map. This exploration problem (and its immediate variants, also including multiple robots) is fundamental for several applications, ranging from classical map building, to search and rescue (Tadokoro 2010), and to coverage (Choset 2001).

One of the main challenges of exploration of unknown environments is related to the navigation strategy, namely where to move to perform the next sensing action in partially-known environment? Consider, as an example, the situation represented in Fig. 1.

The mainstream approach to define navigation strategies for exploration is to pick, from a set of candidate locations (usually obtained by sampling the frontier between known and unknown space, as shown in Fig. 1), the best one that maximizes an utility function that combines different evaluation criteria. This selection is performed at each step of the exploration process, within the so-called *next-best-view* approach.

Several proposals have been made for evaluation criteria and utility functions. For example, the work in (Gonzáles-Baños and Latombe 2002) proposes the following utility function to evaluate a candidate location p:

$$A(p)\exp(-\lambda d(p)) \tag{1}$$

where $A(p)$ is the expected information gain that the robot can get in p (measured as the maximum amount of unknown area visible from p), $d(p)$ is the distance between the current position of the robot and p, and λ is a parameter that weights the two criteria.

The system proposed in (Visser and Slamet 2008) uses the following utility function:

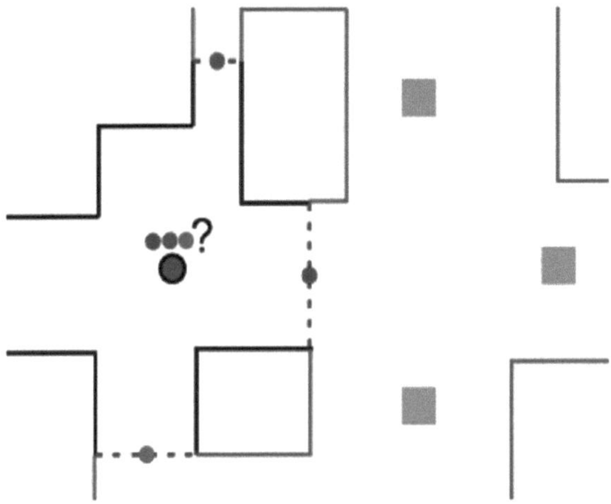

Fig. 1 A partially explored environment. *Black line* segments are the known part of the environment, while the *grey* ones are still unknown to the robot (*red dot*). *Dotted red lines* are the frontiers between known and unknown portions of the environment. The robot has to decide which location it should reach for performing the next perception among the three available possibilities (*green*, *blue*, and *orange dots*)

$$\frac{A(p)P(p)}{d(p)} \tag{2}$$

that considers also the estimated probability $P(p)$ of a successful communication between the robot (once at p) and a fixed base station.

Burgard et al. (2005) use the following linear utility function:

$$U_{t'} - \beta \cdot V_{t'}^{i'} \tag{3}$$

where $U_{t'}$ and $V_{t'}^{i'}$ are similar to the expected information gain and travelled distance, respectively, used by the works presented above, and β is the relative weight of benefit versus cost of candidate location t' for robot i'.

Tovar et al. (2006) use an utility function that evaluates a sequence of m candidate locations (poses) with the following multiplicative function:

$$\sum_{i=1}^{m}\left(\exp(lv_i - sv_i)\prod_{j=1}^{q_i}\left(\frac{\exp(-|\theta_j|)}{\sqrt{s_j}+1}\right) \times \left(\frac{1}{n_i}\sum_{k=1}^{n_i} p_k + Ne_i\right) fmin_i(d_l)\right) \tag{4}$$

where q_i is the total number of robot stops to reach location i, lv_i is the length of the closest frontier edge at i, s_j is the distance from the robot to the next possible location j, sv_i is the distance from the next possible location i to the closest frontier edge, θ_j is the orientation change to reach the next configuration j, p_k identifies the probability of viewing landmark k at i, n_i and Ne_i are the number of landmarks and of corners inside a visibility region at i, and $fmin_i$ is a function that penalizes i when it is too close to an obstacle, according to distance d_l.

While all the above navigation strategies (and most of others proposed in the literature) are rather *ad hoc*, we recently developed a more general and flexible approach based on Multi-Criteria Decision Making (MCDM) that provides a solid approach, grounded in decision-theoretical field, for selecting the next candidate location in exploration (Basilico and Amigoni 2011).

2.2 Patrolling Environments to Prevent Intrusions

A patrolling problem involves a robot that is deployed in a (usually known) environment with the objective of protecting it from intrusions. Intruders can come from outside the environment (e.g., a building). The robot is equipped with sensors (e.g., cameras) that allow it to detect the presence of a possible intruder. It moves, repeatedly monitoring different portions of the environment. The problem of patrolling environments with autonomous mobile robots has attracted the attention of many researchers both within the Autonomous Robotics and the Multiagent Systems communities (Agmon et al. 2011; Fang et al. 2013). It can be considered as an instance of a general class of problems related to surveillance and security (Jain et al. 2012) and can be generalized from detecting intruders to detecting any kind of threats.

The challenge of finding the navigation strategy that maximizes the protection level of a given environment has been mainly tackled adopting an explicit model of the intruder (its preferences over the possible targets, its knowledge on the patroller's strategy). Note that, the stance that is often taken is relative to a worst-case scenario, in which the intruder knows the strategy of the patroller (but not its actual actions, since the strategy is usually randomized).

Given this model, a game theoretical perspective is adopted (Jain et al. 2012): the patroller (i.e., the autonomous mobile robot) and the intruder are considered to play a strategic game that develops along a discrete timespan. At each time step, one of the two players performs an action (for the patroller, moving from one location of the environment to another location; for the intruder, entering or not the environment) and the combination of their actions determines the final outcome of the game (e.g., the intruder has been detected or the intruder successfully entered the environment). It can be shown that the optimal navigation strategy for the patroller (namely, the navigation strategy that minimizes the probability of an intruder to break in) is equivalent to a particular equilibrium, called *leader-follower*, of such game (Paruchuri et al. 2007).

In this context, we recently provided an approach that calculates deterministic and randomized strategies in environments with any topology, allowing the adversary to always know the current position of the patroller. A set of heuristic techniques were also defined with the objective of reducing the computational effort in settings of realistic size (Basilico et al. 2012).

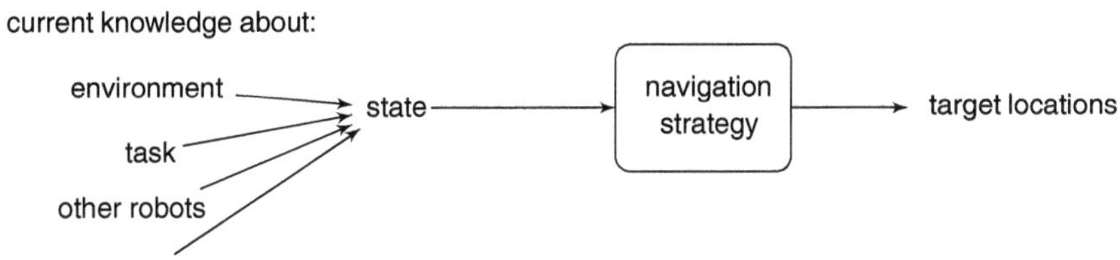

Fig. 2 The intuitive idea of navigation strategy

3 Towards a Framework for Navigation Strategies

In this section, we introduce a framework in the attempt to capture the main issues of navigation strategies in a way that is independent of the specific applications. In general, a robot needs a navigation strategy to select its target locations using its current knowledge about its environment and task (Fig. 2). Almost all navigation strategies take as input a *state* enclosing task-related information about the environment (e.g., in exploration usually it is a map of the currently explored space and the current position of the robot) and provide the locations to reach as output.

As the examples of Sect. 2 partially show, several techniques have been proposed to tackle the problem of the definition of good navigation strategies, including decision-theoretical techniques (PO)MDPs, game-theoretical techniques, and many others, but no general framework for the navigation strategy problem has been proposed so far.

Navigation strategies can be characterized along many dimensions, here we discuss some of those, being aware that the list is far from being definitive and complete.

- Offline versus online strategies.
- Global versus partial knowledge of the environment.
- Kind of knowledge used to make decisions.
- Optimality criterion.
- Number of decision makers.
- Adversarial versus non-adversarial scenario.

A first distinction can be done between *offline* and *online* strategies. In the first case, the locations to reach are computed for every possible input state before the robot actually executes the task, i.e., before the robot actually employs the strategy. With an online strategy, instead, the decision is computed during the task execution for the different situations the robot encounters.

This distinction can also be described with respect to another dimension, namely the amount of available information about the environment. If the environment (or, more precisely, all the information needed for making decisions) is fully known in advance, the robot has a *global knowledge*. Conversely, if only partial or no environment's information is initially available, the robot has a *partial knowledge* and should increase its knowledge to make more informed decisions. The availability of global knowledge results in the possibility of computing the strategy offline and, possibly, searching for an optimal solution. On the other hand, a partial knowledge is typically associated with the use of an online navigation strategy where sub-optimal algorithms are employed. As an example, consider the two common tasks of coverage and exploration. In coverage (Choset 2001), the environment is known in advance and the robot should cover (possibly, under some constraints) all the free area with the footprint of its sensors. In exploration, the environment is unknown at the beginning and the robot has to "discover" it. The first case is characterized by a global knowledge and the optimal strategy, e.g., the shortest route, can be computed offline. The second case is an example of partial knowledge situation for which decisions have to be made online, due to the impossibility to predict the states that the robot will face. The optimal strategy cannot be found in general and sub-optimal greedy algorithms (e.g., next-best-view approaches) must be employed. Note that in both cases the optimal strategy can be the one that minimizes the travelled distance.

The *kind of knowledge* used by the robot to make decisions can be of different natures. A specific kind of knowledge induces how decisions are made. For example, in exploration, criteria used in the utility function usually derive from the robot's knowledge about the spatial features that has been collected in the map built so far. However, in principle, there are other types of knowledge that can be used, like high-level information coming from human users.

The *optimality criterion* is a crucial dimension for the design of a navigation strategy, which is evaluated according to the selected optimality criterion. It is strongly dependent on the task the robot should perform, but also on the robot capabilities. Sometimes, this concept is easy to define, like in the patrolling case, in which the optimal solution is the one that minimizes the probability for an intruder to break in. However, in some applications, like search and rescue, it is hard to define which optimality criterion should be selected to measure the performance of the system, because there are more criteria that should be optimized. They are sometimes conflicting, as some measure the benefits obtained, while others measure costs to perform the assigned task (e.g., explored area vs. robot's battery and travelled distance). In such a case, a trade-off between benefits and costs should be addressed. Furthermore, in other cases the optimality criterion is not naturally evident. For example, in a pursuit/evasion scenario, there is not any main optimality criterion, but only feasibility (i.e., either the evader is caught or not caught).

The *number of decision makers* (robots) is another dimension. The presence of multiple agents can pose significant difficulties. Determining a navigation strategy for a team of robots has to deal with the exponential growth (in the number of robots) of the number of possible actions, and usually involves a task-assignment problem (Gerkey and Mataric 2004), where the task is a location to be reached by a robot. Multiple robots can cooperate to make a globally optimal decision or can compete to make individually optimal decisions.

The presence of multiple agents introduces another dimension represented by the *adversarial nature* of the setting, which is related to the possible presence of adversaries. An adversary can be defined as a rational agent acting against the robot's objectives, and whose interaction has to be considered when computing the navigation strategy. Intuitive examples of these last two dimensions can be found in patrolling. An adversary, i.e., a possible intruder, can be considered by the patrolling robot in deciding where to move for protecting the environment. In this case, a competitive interacting scenario emerges and game theoretical techniques are employed to find navigation strategies (see Sect. 2.2).

Let us apply the general framework just defined to the two examples of Sects. 2.1 and 2.2. In the case of exploration, the navigation strategy is online and based on a partial knowledge of the environment. Decisions are made from knowledge embedded in a metric map of the environment (consisting of obstacles, free space, distances,…) and the optimality criteria considered include travelled distance or number of perceptions to fully explore the environment, area discovered in a given time interval,…. In most of the examples presented in Sect. 2.1, there is a single decision-maker, but there can be several ones, and the scenario is clearly non-adversarial.

In the case of patrolling, the navigation strategy is calculated offline based on the global knowledge of the environment. Decisions are made from knowledge of the environment and of the adversary and the optimality criteria adopted are related to the probability of an intruder to break in the locations of interest of the protected environment. There is a single decision-maker that operates in an adversarial scenario.

4 Generating Novel Research Directions

The framework proposed in the previous section can stimulate novel ideas and research directions for enhancing the development of navigation strategies by facilitating the identification of significant open issues.

For example, according to what we discussed above, in developing navigation strategies for exploring initially unknown environments, the decision about the next destination location is usually based only on the information provided by a *metric map* of the environment. A metric map represents the geometrical and spatial features of an environment, like the position of obstacles. All the works presented in Sect. 2.1 use a metric map to extract the values for criteria they use in the utility function, like the expected information gain or the distance between a robot and a candidate location. One interesting, and potentially effective, extension can be to consider also information contained in *semantic maps* of environment. A semantic map associates spatial concepts to spatial entities. For example, a room identified in the metric map can be labeled as 'kitchen' or as 'bathroom' using one of the several methods that have been proposed (e.g., Mozos et al. 2005; Wolf and Sukhatme 2008). Moreover, a priori information about the task can be provided by the user and usually biases the behavior of the robot. For example, in a search and rescue operation, such information can be used to prefer the selection of candidate locations in offices if a disaster happened during working hours, because the user thinks that it is more likely to find victims there than in other places (e.g., in a canteen). Combining high-level knowledge of places in buildings (provided by semantic maps) and information coming from users for developing better exploring robots proves to be an interesting and largely uninvestigated research line, which we have preliminarily tackled in (Cipolleschi et al. 2013).

Another research direction stimulated by the framework is about experimental methodologies. A lively debate on good experimental methodologies is currently ongoing in the autonomous robotics community, which has recognized that the lack of sound procedures, globally accepted benchmarks, and well-established metrics for autonomous robotic systems slow down research and make the transfer of existing research results to market products rather difficult (Amigoni et al. 2009; Amigoni and Schiaffonati 2014). For example, experimental evaluation of navigation strategies for exploration is problematic (Basilico and Amigoni 2008). One relevant question is about which data should be used for evaluation. In real environments, evaluation can be clearly performed only *ex post*, once the environment has been completely mapped. Data sets acquired by real robots [like those on Rawseeds (Ceriani et al. 2009) and Radish (Howard and Roy 2003)] are usually not so dense to cover every perception in every pose of the environment and cannot be used to evaluate navigation strategies for exploration. Simulation is sometimes the only viable solution (Amigoni and Schiaffonati 2010). Another question is about which metric should be used for evaluation. This is related to the difficulty of establishing an optimality criterion that we evidenced for the corresponding dimension of our framework. The number of sensing actions performed by the robot and the total amount of distance travelled to completely explore an environment are two common metrics, but there currently is no agreement on this (Basilico and Amigoni 2008). Another important issue, which has been largely overlooked so far, is the availability of a reference (optimal) performance for conducting the experimental evaluation. Without such a reference performance, navigation strategies for exploration can be compared only in a relative way, against each other, and not in an absolute way, according to their distance from optimum. An initial attempt to overcome this problem has been presented in (Quattrini Li et al. 2012).

Other possible research directions that are expected to help developing better navigation strategies include the integration of human decisions within the framework, leading to mixed-initiative systems (Horvitz 2007). For example, in a search and rescue scenario, a robotic system could exchange knowledge and cooperate with human rescuers to more effectively find victims in a collapsed building; while, in exploration, a human operator can remotely bias the behavior of a team of robots by dynamically assigning priorities to portions of the environment (see above). Some of the challenges holding in these scenarios involve the design of human-robot interaction frameworks as well as the definition of mixed decision-theoretic layers, where human decisions could be combined with those made by robots in an effective way (Adams et al. 2004).

5 Conclusions

In this work, we proposed a general abstract framework to coherently address the analysis and the development of navigation strategies, which allow mobile robots to autonomously decide target poses. The framework has been defined and shown useful to stimulate new research directions, towards better navigation strategies.

The proposed framework will be further enhanced, especially providing a more formal decision-theoretical definition of its basic elements in order to pave the way towards the easy development and the theoretical and experimental assessment of good navigation strategies that make mobile robots more autonomous.

References

Adams, J., Rani, P., Sarkar, N.: Mixed initiative interaction and robotic systems. In: AAAI Workshop on Supervisory Control of Learning and Adaptive Systems (2004)

Agmon, N., Kaminka, G., Kraus, S.: Multi-robot adversarial patrolling: facing a full-knowledge opponent. J Artif Intell Res **42**(1), 887–916 (2011)

Amigoni, F., Reggiani, M., Schiaffonati, V.: An insightful comparison between experiments in mobile robotics and in science. Auton Robot **27**(4), 313–325 (2009)

Amigoni, F., Schiaffonati, V.: Autonomous mobile robots as technical artifacts: A discussion of experimental issues. In: L. Magnani (ed.) Model-Based Reasoning in Science and Technology, *Studies in Applied Philosophy, Epistemology and Rational Ethics*, vol. 8, pp. 527–542. Springer (2014)

Amigoni, F., Schiaffonati, V.: Good experimental methodologies and simulation in autonomous mobile robotics. In: L. Magnani, W. Carnielli, C. Pizzi (eds.) Model-Based Reasoning in Science and Technology, *Studies in Computational Intelligence*, vol. 314, pp. 315–332. Springer (2010)

Basilico, N., Amigoni, F.: Exploration strategies based on multi-criteria decision making for searching environments in rescue operations. Auton Robot **31**(4), 401–417 (2011)

Basilico, N., Amigoni, F.: On evaluating performance of exploration strategies for an autonomous mobile robot. In: IROS Workshop on Performance Evaluation and Benchmarking for Intelligent Robots and Systems (2008)

Basilico, N., Gatti, N., Amigoni, F.: Patrolling security games: Definition and algorithms for solving large instances with single patroller and single intruder. Artif Intell **184–185**, 78–123 (2012)

Burgard, W., Moors, M., Stachniss, C., Schneider, F.: Coordinated multi-robot exploration. IEEE T Robot **21**(3), 376–386 (2005)

Ceriani, S., Fontana, G., Giusti, A., Marzorati, D., Matteucci, M., Migliore, D., Rizzi, D., Sorrenti, D., Taddei, P.: Rawseeds ground truth collection systems for indoor self-localization and mapping. Auton Robot **27**(4), 353–371 (2009)

Choset, H.: Coverage for robotics: A survey of recent results. Ann Math Artif Intel **31**(1–4), 113–126 (2001)

Cipolleschi, R., Giusto, M., Quattrini Li, A., Amigoni, F.: Semantically-informed coordinated multirobot exploration of relevant areas in search and rescue settings. In: Proc. ECMR, pp. 216–221 (2013)

Durham, J., Franchi, A., Bullo, F.: Distributed pursuit-evasion without mapping or global localization via local frontiers. Auton Robot **32**(1), 81–95 (2012)

Fang, F., Jiang, A., Tambe, M.: Optimal patrol strategy for protecting moving targets with multiple mobile resources. In: Proc. AAMAS, pp. 957–964 (2013)
Gerkey, B., Mataric, M.: A formal analysis and taxonomy of task allocation in multi-robot systems. Int J Robot Res **23**, 939–954 (2004)
Gonzáles-Baños, H., Latombe, J.C.: Navigation strategies for exploring indoor environments. Int J Robot Res **21**(10-11), 829–848 (2002)
Horvitz, E.: Reflections on challenges and promises of mixed-initiative interaction. AI Mag **28**(2), 3 (2007)
Howard, A., Roy, N.: The robotics data set repository (Radish). http://radish.sourceforge.net/ (2003)
Jain, M., An, B., Tambe, M.: An overview of recent application trends at the AAMAS conference: Security, sustainability and safety. AI Mag **33**(3), 14–28 (2012)
Latombe, J.C.: Robot Motion Planning. Kluwer Academic Publishers (1991)
LaValle, S.: Planning Algorithms. Cambridge University Press (2006)
Marjovi, A., Marques, L.: Multi-robot topological exploration using olfactory cues. In: Proc. DARS, pp. 47–60 (2013)
Mozos, O., Stachniss, C., Burgard, W.: Supervised learning of places from range data using AdaBoost. In: Proc. ICRA, pp. 1742–1747 (2005)
Paruchuri, P., Pearce, J., Tambe, M., Ordonez, F., Kraus, S.: An efficient heuristic approach for security against multiple adversaries. In: Proc. AAMAS, pp. 311–318 (2007)
Pezzementi, Z., Plaku, E., Reyda, C., Hager, G.: Tactile-object recognition from appearance information. IEEE T Robot **27**(3), 473–487 (2011)
Quattrini Li, A., Amigoni, F., Basilico, N.: Searching for optimal off-line exploration paths in grid environments for a robot with limited visibility. In: Proc. AAAI, pp. 2060–2066 (2012)
Singh, A., Krause, A., Guestrin, C., Kaiser, W.: Efficient informative sensing using multiple robots. J Artif Intell Res **34**(1), 707–755 (2009)
Smith, R., Schwager, M., Smith, S., Rus, D., Sukhatme, G.: Persistent ocean monitoring with underwater gliders: Towards accurate reconstruction of dynamic ocean processes. In: Proc. ICRA, pp. 1517–1524 (2011)
Tadokoro, S.: Rescue Robotics. Springer-Verlag (2010)
Thrun, S.: Robotic mapping: A survey. In: Exploring Artificial Intelligence in the New Millenium, pp. 1–35. Morgan Kaufmann (2002)
Tovar, B., Munoz, L., Murrieta-Cid, R., Alencastre, M., Monroy, R., Hutchinson, S.: Planning exploration strategies for simultaneous localization and mapping. Robot Auton Syst **54**(4), 314–331 (2006)
Visser, A., Slamet, B.: Including communication success in the estimation of information gain for multi-robot exploration. In: Proc. WiOPT, pp. 680–687 (2008)
Wolf, D., Sukhatme, G.: Semantic mapping using mobile robots. IEEE T Robot **24**(2), 245–258 (2008)

Safety for an Autonomous Bucket Excavator During Typical Landscaping Tasks

Gregor Zolynski, Daniel Schmidt and Karsten Berns

Abstract The Robotics Research Lab in Kaiserserlautern, Germany, pursues the goal of automating a mobile bucket excavator for excavation and loading tasks. This document contains a short introduction to the autonomous bucket excavator THOR, a concept for low-level safety using laser scanners, and a high-level collision avoidance system using behavior-based control.

1 Introduction

Today's research in the domain of construction machines moves into the field of intelligent robotics. In the future fully autonomous machines will take over more and more complex construction tasks. To reach this goal, small steps need to be taken. The Robotics Research Lab in Kaiserserlautern, Germany, pursues the goal of automating a mobile bucket excavator for excavation and loading tasks. During this process many different problems need to be solved. One of these problems is the safety of the vehicle and of course the safety of humans. This document contains a short introduction to the autonomous bucket excavator THOR, a concept for low-level safety using laser scanners, and a high-level collision avoidance system using behavior-based control.

G. Zolynski (✉) · D. Schmidt · K. Berns
University of Kaiserslautern, Kaiserslautern, Germany
e-mail: zolynski@cs.uni-kl.de

D. Schmidt
e-mail: d_smith@cs.uni-kl.de

K. Berns
e-mail: berns@cs.uni-kl.de

A. Rodić et al. (eds.), *New Trends in Medical and Service Robots*,
Mechanisms and Machine Science 20, DOI: 10.1007/978-3-319-05431-5_24,

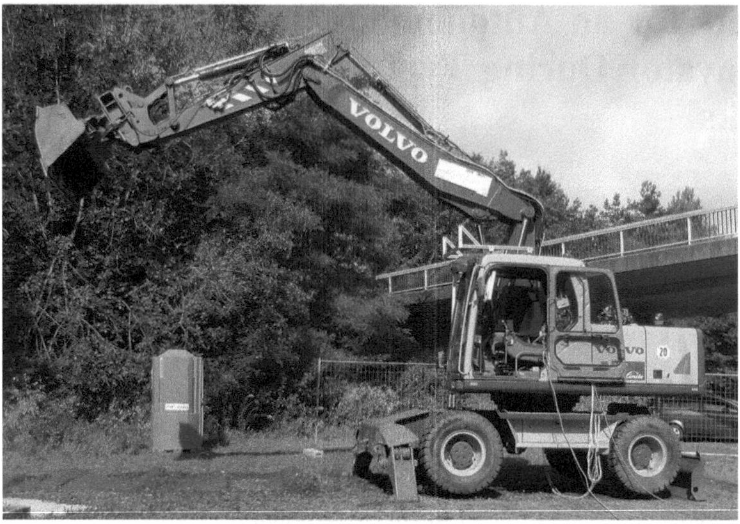

Fig. 1 The autonomous bucket excavator THOR (*Terraforming Heavy Outdoor Robot*)

2 Autonomous Bucket Excavator THOR

The test platform at the Robotics Research Lab is the robot THOR (*Terraforming Heavy Outdoor Robot*) which is based on a VOLVO EW 180B excavator (Fig. 1). The long-term goal of the project is to develop an excavator which is capable to perform material movement and landscaping tasks on a construction site in a fully autonomous manner.

Apart from developing the complex software control system which generates autonomous decisions to solve the problems, the standard human-driven 18 ton wheeled excavator had to be converted into a PC-controllable robot.

Therefore, electrohydraulic control valves (Fig. 2) for steering the machine, length measurement sensors (Fig. 3) for indirectly measuring the joint angles from cylinder lengths, angular joint encoders (Fig. 4) for measuring joint angles and velocities, electric circuit boards (Fig. 5) for closed-loop control of the joints and a powerful embedded PC (Fig. 6) were installed on the machine. For environment perception the machine uses multiple outdoor laser scanners from SICK (Fig. 7) which deliver precise distance data around the machine and can store multiple hardware safety fields for low-level safety (explained in Sect. 4).

As the decisions of the machine have to be taken in a highly dynamic environment full of disturbances no "classical" preliminary planning and trajectory generation system could be chosen.

Instead, a reactive behavior-based control approach was chosen which already proved to deliver good results for complex offroad-navigation in unstructured

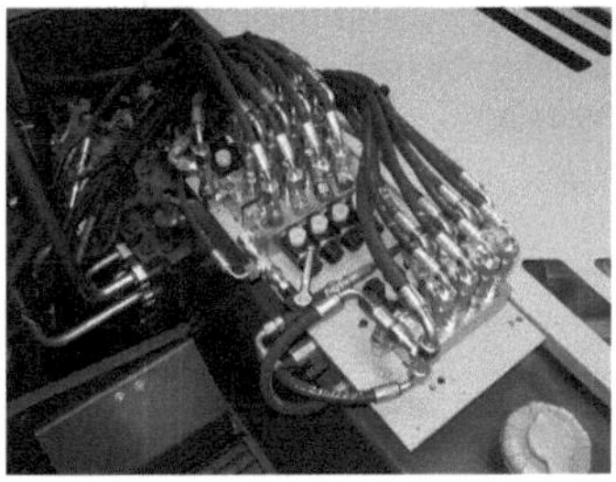

Fig. 2 Electrohydraulic control valves for steering the machine

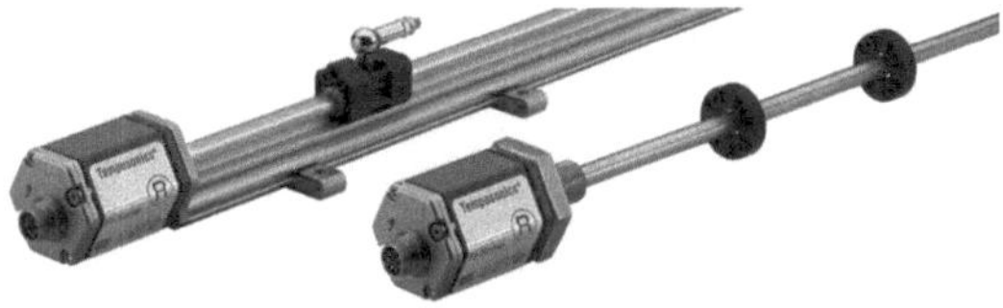

Fig. 3 Length measurement sensors for indirectly measuring the joint angles from cylinder lengths

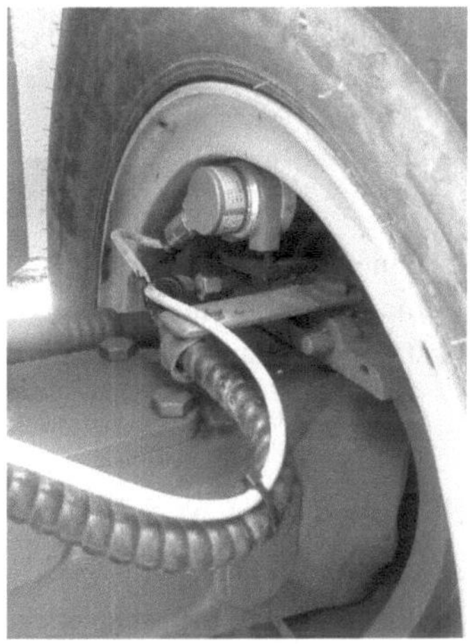

Fig. 4 Wheel encoders for measuring joint angles and velocities

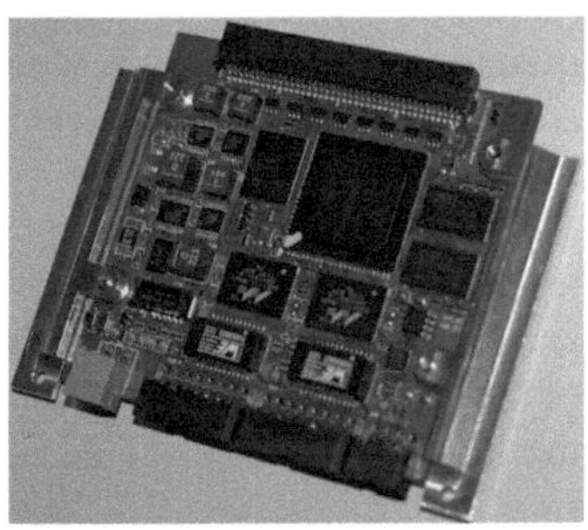

Fig. 5 Electronic circuit boards for closed-loop control of the joints

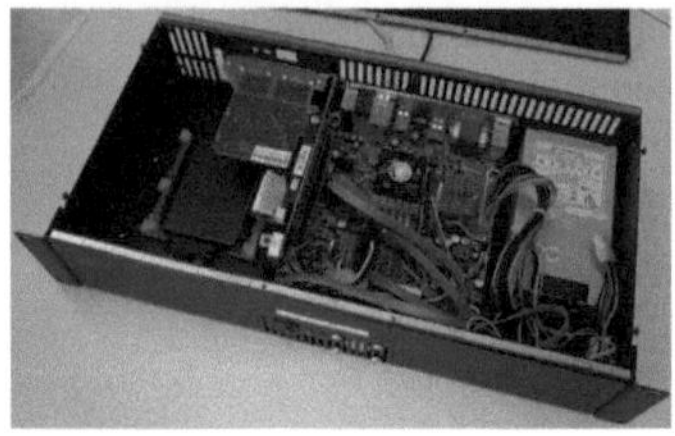

Fig. 6 Powerful linux PC running the complex software system

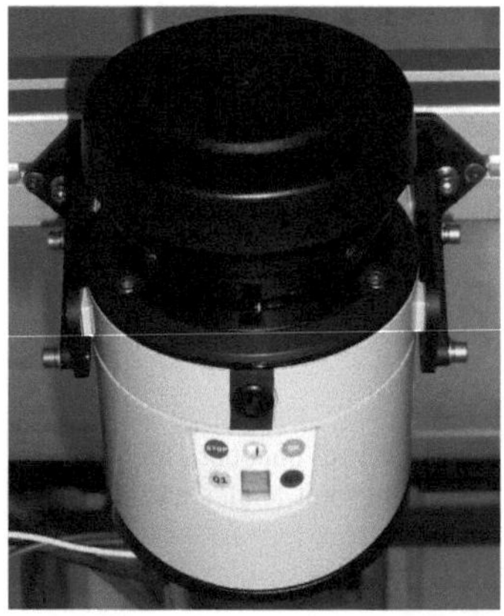

Fig. 7 Laser scanner for gathering exact distance information for the machine

terrain (Armbrust et al. 2011). After a brief description of the used behavior framework and the existing behavior network, Sect. 5 presents the integrated obstacle avoidance layer to guarantee safety during trajectory generation.

3 Low-Level and High-Level Safety Layers

In this work two different systems for safety are presented, which shall be clarified in this section. The low-level safety is a very basic system which is meant to prevent harm in the case of catastrophic control failure. It is designed as a standalone system which can bring the machine to an emergency stop if an imminent collision is detected. In this work, only the arm of the excavator is considered, but the system can be extended to also provide safety e.g. for the rear side.

The high-level safety is a concept which is embedded into the control architecture of the excavator. It provides implicit safety against collision with detected, known obstacles and also against self-collisions of the machine (the construction of the arm allows configurations which can damage the driver's cabin). In theory, the high-level safety should always be able to avoid any collisions so that the low-level system will never need to become active. Also, the high-level system is designed to work around a collision while the low-level system's only ability is the emergency halt.

4 Safety Fields for Collision Avoidance

To ensure a safe emergency stop of the bucket excavator during panning even in the event of non-responding control software or a disrupted messaging system, a "last line of defense", realized in hardware, has to be present. This solution is thought to react only if all other safety measures have failed, i.e. because of software or hardware malfunction. To this end, a specialized secondary safety system has to be used. The function of this approach is to switch on a collision-preventing subsystem before panning the excavator's superstructure.

Industrial grade laser scanners like the SICK S3xxx[1] family of sensors contain a feature called Protective Fields to switch a special output whenever a predefined safety field is violated. In this work we use a SICK LMS 151 which is not as rigorously certified as the S series but contains a Field Evaluation functionality which can be used as demonstrator of the safety system.

The working principle of these laser scanners is to emit laser pulses through a rotating mirror and to measure the phase shift of the returned signal. The measurements of each revolution are combined into a vector of distances. A safety field (or safety envelope) is a vector containing the minimum distances for each of distance vector's elements. If any of the measurements falls below its respective minimum a field violation is triggered.

The most problematic part of hardware-supported safety fields is the limited amount of available safety field definitions. The top-of-the-range models can store up to 42 fields, which must be defined offline and can be switched during operation. The LMS 151 offers 10 evaluation fields.

The approach presented here consists of three steps: (1) generating a representative set of potential arm poses, (2) clustering of similar arm poses to minimize the number of required safety envelopes, and (3) the computation of safety envelopes which both fit tightly around the associated arm poses and do not leave any portion of the arm uncovered.

4.1 Preparing a Set of Arm Poses

The generation of safety field descriptions begins with a set of arm poses which are likely to occur during normal operation. These poses are calculated in a nested loop and with distinct ranges and step sizes for each arm joint angle α_i. The step

[1] www.mysick.com

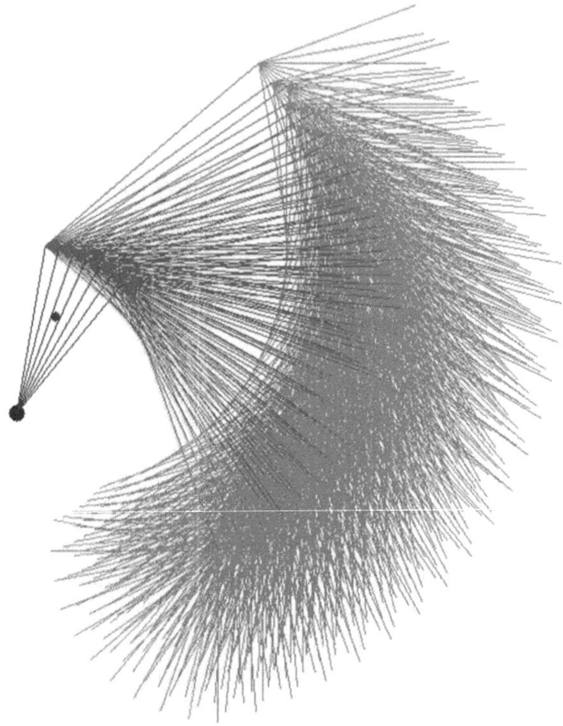

Fig. 8 Example of possible arm poses for a 3-joint-arm (*side view*). The *black dot* represents the first arm joint (the origin), the *red dot* is the position of a laser scanner

size of joints closer to the base needs to be chosen smaller, because of the bigger impact caused by a longer lever arm. The position J_i of each joint can be calculated using forward kinematics:

$$J_i := J_{i-1} + l_i \begin{pmatrix} \cos \sum_{k=0}^{i} \alpha_k \\ \sin \sum_{k=0}^{i} \alpha_k \end{pmatrix}, \quad J_0 := \begin{pmatrix} 0 \\ 0 \end{pmatrix} \tag{1}$$

where l_i is the length of the ith arm segment, and α_k are the joint angles. Figure 8 shows an example of several thousand arm poses.

4.2 Clustering of Arm Poses

The most important and interesting part is the grouping of the arm poses into a predefined number of clusters. As already mentioned, a safety scanner is only able to store a very small amount of safety field descriptions, in our case 10. To group the generated poses into a given number of groups a clustering technique needs to be employed. Since the number of clusters is known beforehand, the well-known k-means clustering has been chosen. This clustering method needs a distance function which is used as measure for intra-group similarity and inter-group dissimilarity.

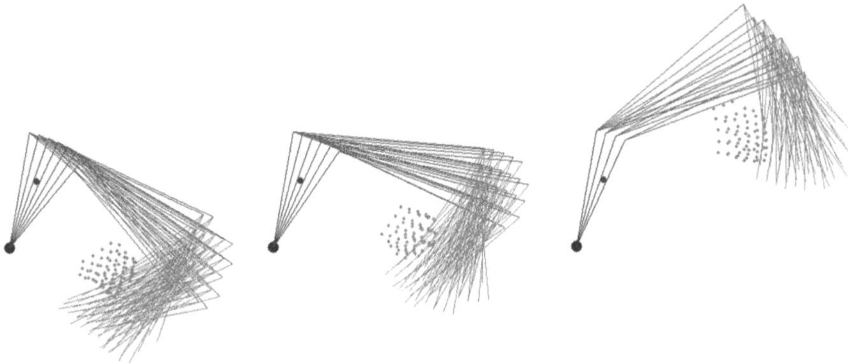

Fig. 9 Example of clustered arm poses using the center of mass (*green dots*)

Finding the right distance metric is the most crucial part of the clustering. The function should yield smoothly varying results when the arm pose is changed by small amounts, it should describe the arm pose in a coherent way, and it should have a small number of parameters (low dimensionality).

One such metric, which has also been found to give very good clustering results, is the Euclidean distance of the geometrical average of each arm pose. The geometrical average (or "center of mass") is easily calculated as

$$M = \frac{1}{N+1} \sum_{i=0}^{N} J_i \tag{2}$$

where $J_0 \ldots J_{N-1}$ are joint positions and J_N is the position of the tool center point. The Euclidean distance of average joint positions (and TCP) fulfills all the requirements listed above for a good metric for arm pose clustering. Figure 9 shows an example of three arm pose groups.

4.3 Calculation of Safety Fields

After having grouped similar arm poses into clusters a safety field has to be defined for each group. The definition of safety fields is done using a simple geometrical calculation. The sensor position P is defined relative to the first arm joint, which is positioned at the origin of the coordinate system. The safety envelopes are generated using ray intersection. From the position of the scanner rays are cast at a predefined angular resolution.

$$R_i := P + \begin{pmatrix} \cos \beta_i \\ \sin \beta_i \end{pmatrix}. \tag{3}$$

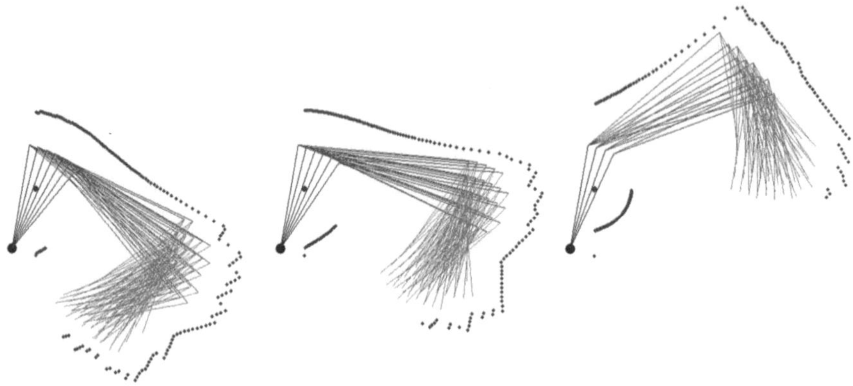

Fig. 10 Example of clustered arm poses with associated safety fields

The rays are then intersected with the segments of each arm pose. The longest distance (plus an additional safety margin) between an intersection point and the ray is stored as minimum needed distance for coverage. Figure 10 shows a few examples of arm pose groups and their respective safety fields.

5 Behavior-Based Obstacle Avoidance

As the previously presented safety layer guarantees that the machine does not hit obstacles, even in case of wrong high-level software decisions the behavior-based obstacle avoidance tries to guarantee the generation of collision-free trajectories which prevent from activation of low-level safety.

To make this possible, the control structure of the excavator has to be briefly explained first. The classic approach for control systems for autonomous mobile robots uses global knowledge to solve the task like in the sense-plan-paradigm (Brooks 1991). It uses all sensor information from the bottom layer to calculate the solution on the highest layer. This top-level solver gets very complex and difficult to implement. In behavior-based control systems like *iB2C*[2] the task is split into relatively simple behaviors following the behavior-based paradigm (Arkin 1998).

There is a set of decentralized behaviors, which get the information they need to perform their task. These behaviors have defined ports to connect them to a network and organize them in groups. One single behavior is usually easy to implement and can only solve relatively simple problems in most cases. More detailed information can be found in (Albiez et al. 2003) or (Proetzsch et al. 2007).

The behavior module is the result of the developments in (Albiez 2007) and (Proetzsch et al. 2005). Each behavior is wrapped into a uniform module (as shown

[2] Integrated behavior-based control.

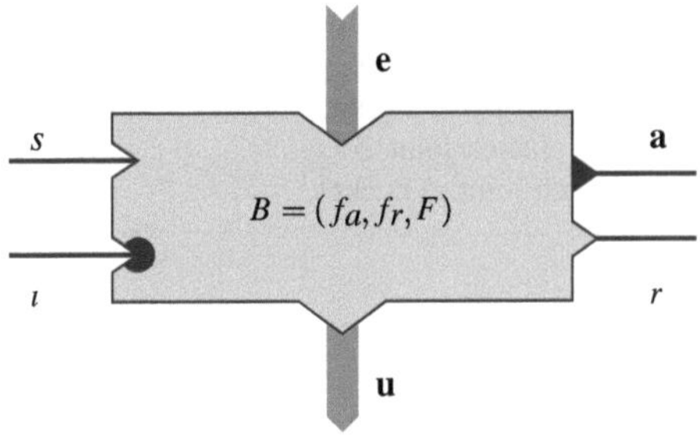

Fig. 11 Standard *iB2C* behavior module: the input ports are on the *left* (stimulation *s* and inhibition *i*) and output ports on the *right* (activity **a** and target rating *r*). With input **e** and output **u** arbitrary ports are provided

in Fig. 11). Standardized ports allow the reuse of behavior modules in a different context (Kiekbusch and Proetzsch 2011). The stimulation *s* stands for the relevance of the behavior ($s = 0$ means no stimulation, $s = 1$ full stimulation, values between 0 and 1 mean a partial stimulation). Inhibition *i* is used to suppress the behavior action from the outside and is the important port used for the obstacle avoidance. The activity *a* represents the current amount of influence of the behavior ($a = 1$ all output values have the highest impact and $a = 0$ means the behavior is inactive). The target rating signalizes how content the behavior is ($r = 1$ means maximum dissatisfaction and $r = 0$ total contentment).

One of the most difficult parts in behavior based controls is the fusion of the single behaviors. If there are different behaviors, with different goals that want to dictate the same output control value, a clever decision must be made. Derived from the context of the behaviors, different strategies are necessary. The *iB2C* offers three types of fusion behaviors (*maximum fusion*, *weighted average*, *weighted sum*), see (Proetzsch et al. 2010) for further details.

5.1 Behavior-Based Inverse Kinematics Solver

As it is an important issue of this document how the excavator arm can be inhibited, a short overview of the arm control is given here. It is realized with a behavior-based inverse kinematic solver, which works within the *iB2C* Framework (Pluzhnikov et al. 2012). The solver gets the desired position and orientation of the tool center point as input and generates six values for the different joint angles (shown in Fig. 12) as result.

In this control the distributed principle as mentioned above has been applied. There is no global control that evaluates a centralized solution for the task. Instead each joint has an own control to decide in which direction it rotates to solve the task. If a new desired pose is given to the system, every joint control requests its current angle and calculates only a small step (about 1°–4°) towards the given pose. The movement of all joints is then internally simulated and used as the origin for the next step. If the calculated pose is close enough to the desired pose the movement process is stopped by a supervisor module. This design has been

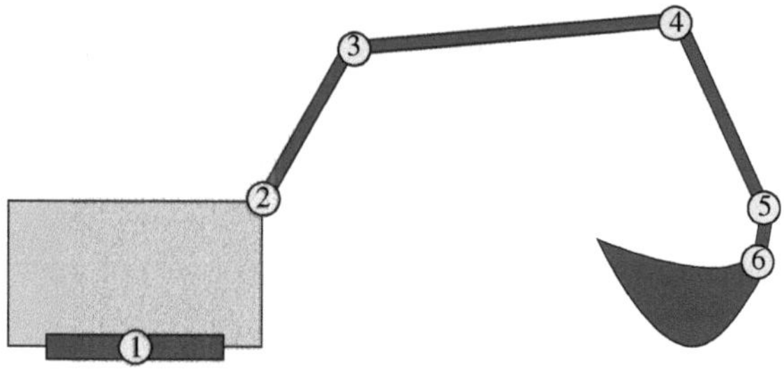

Fig. 12 Schematic view of the excavator arm. *1* Torso joint, *2* boom joint, *3* dipper arm joint, *4* stick joint, *5* bucket pitch joint, *6* bucket roll joint

realized with *iB2C* behavior modules. Each joints has two control parts, one to reach the desired position and one to adjust the orientation which are combined with a *weighted sum* fusion behavior. Each of these control parts consist of two behaviors to turn the joint in a positive or a negative direction, which then is combined by a *maximum fusion* behavior. These four behaviors per joint are also partially connected interconnected by inhibition ports, to avoid a too large steps of joints that lie in the same rotational plane.

5.2 Obstacle Avoidance

The newly developed behavior-based obstacle avoidance is then also connected to the inhibition ports for each joint. It uses the information gathered from internal models about the machine itself and objects in the environment to calculate the different workspace views for every component of the excavators digging arm. It has six parallel ports to request the nearest obstacles for every joint. Also the perpendicular foot for every component is calculated.

It is first checked if the obstacle distance is smaller than the component length. In this case a collision with the component is possible. The next check tests if the obstacle is lying inside of the inhibition range of the other dimensions. This has the following reasons: It is only necessary to consider an obstacle for the height limitation, if azimuth and length are lying inside a given range. Otherwise a obstacle that may be very near in height but with a totally different azimuth will cause an inhibition. But this would lead to unwanted effects, as it restricts the joint movements for no reason. And because we are interested in a collision with the component and not only with the joints, we use the perpendicular foot, that gives us the shortest distance to the component itself. Afterwards we differentiate between the case a minimum or a maximum has to be defined, based on the obstacles position. Only one of the limitations is set, because only one obstacle is considered, what prevents a inflation of limitations. The structure of the length and azimuth workspace calculations is equal, only with the difference that the azimuth limitations for all joints (except the last—bucket roll) are only calculated and then the maximum/minimum is published, because the azimuth can only be inhibited at

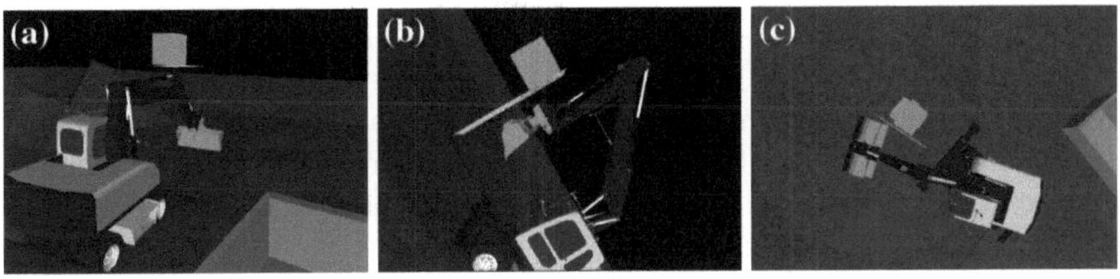

Fig. 13 Demonstration of the *WorkspaceLimiter*. **a** (*Left*) shows a height-limitation with a maximum, **b** (*center*) a length-limitation also maximum and **c** (*right*) shows a limitation for the azimuth

Table 1 The inhibition relation between joints and coordinate system axis

	Torso	Boom	Dipper arm	Stick	Bucket pitch	Bucket roll
Azimuth	•					•
Length		•	•	•	•	•
Height		•	•	•	•	•

the boom and bucket roll joint. For all vacant limitations a standard parameter is published, to reset a possible older value.

To validate the results and visualize the process a complex debug output has been implemented. If activated multiple planes are drawn directly in the simulation to represent the single limitations. Different colors symbolize minimums or maximums for all dimensions and joints. The series of images in Fig. 13 shows various settings.

There are three modules with similar functions to restrict the behaviors: One for height, length and for azimuth restrictions. They affect the joints as depicted in Table 1.

The modules calculate the restrictions for all joints they are responsible for in a parallel job. Therefore, the following tasks are performed:

- Fetch limitation values and current values for all elements
- Calculate the inhibition values for all joints
- Charge the values against each other and limit them to the boundings
- Publish the calculated values.

After all inhibition values have been calculated they are charged against each other. Because of the structure of the digging arm, for example an inhibition of the bucket means also an inhibition for the stick, dipper arm and the boom. Due to that fact it is necessary to add up all inhibitions along the element chain. But because the inhibition value has to lie between 0 and 1, it has to be limited afterwards.

6 Conclusion

In this document we have introduced the autonomous bucket excavator project and the demonstrator vehicle THOR. We presented a short overview of the Robotics Research Lab's behavior-based control system *iB2C* as well as its application for the calculation of inverse kinematics.

The novel parts of this document presented two separate research topics. First, a concept for a hardware-supported "last line of defense" collision prevention system during panning motions of our excavator. This system was designed to allow for automatic generation of a very limited amount of safety fields for any sensor position using only the kinematic description of the excavator.

Second, the utilization of *iB2C* for workspace limitation and (self-)collision avoidance. An existing behavior-based control structure was extended to generate smooth trajectories while avoiding known obstacles as well as configurations which could damage the vehicle itself.

References

Jan Albiez. *Verhaltensnetzwerke zur adaptiven Steuerung biologisch motivierter Laufmaschinen*. GCA Verlag, 2007.

Jan Albiez, Tobias Luksch, Karsten Berns, and Rüdiger Dillmann. An activation-based behavior control architecture for walking machines. *The International Journal on Robotics Research, Sage Publications*, 22:203–211, 2003.

R. Arkin. *Behaviour-Based Robotics*. MIT Press, 1998. ISBN-10: 0-262-01165-4; ISBN-13: 978-0-262-01165-5.

Christopher Armbrust, Martin Proetzsch, and Karsten Berns. Behaviour-based off-road robot navigation. *KI - Künstliche Intelligenz*, 25(2):155–160, May 2011. http://dx.doi.org/10.1007/s13218-011-0090-2.

R. A. Brooks. Intelligence without reason. A.i. memo no. 1293, Massachusetts Institute of Technology (MIT), Artificial Intelligence Laboratory, 1991.

Lisa Kiekbusch and Martin Proetzsch. Tutorial: Control system development using ib2c. Technical report, Robotics Research Lab, University of Kaiserslautern, 2011. unpublished.

Sergey Pluzhnikov, Daniel Schmidt, Jochen Hirth, and Karsten Berns. Behavior-based arm control for an autonomous bucket excavator. In *Commercial Vehicle Technology 2012 – Proceedings of the Commercial Vehicle Technology Symposium (CVT)*, pages 251–261, Kaiserslautern, Germany, March 14–15 2012.

M. Proetzsch, T. Luksch, and K. Berns. Fault-tolerant behavior-based motion control for offroad navigation. In *Proceedings of the 20th IEEE International Conference on Robotics and Automation (ICRA)*, pages 4697–4702, Barcelona, Spain, April 18-22 2005.

M. Proetzsch, T. Luksch, and K. Berns. The behaviour-based control architecture ib2c for complex robotic systems (extended version). unpublished, 2007.

Martin Proetzsch, Tobias Luksch, and Karsten Berns. Development of complex robotic systems using the behavior-based control architecture iB2C. *Robotics and Autonomous Systems*, 58(1):46–67, January 2010. doi:10.1016/j.robot.2009.07.027.

Testing Capacity for Space Technology Suppliers

A. Pisla and C. Vaida

Abstract Starting with industrial painting and entertainment devices, for a long time parallel kinematics is strongly associated with flight simulators. Outstanding studies of parallel kinematics were achieved, from the beginning of their existence, within different applications in aerospace industry. For over 20 years, remarkable results are also obtained at the Technical University in Cluj-Napoca in the field of parallel kinematics. After an extended overview, presented in the MeSRob 2012, regarding some results oriented on the Medical and Service robots (Pisla in New Trends in Medical and Service Robots—Theory and Integrated Applications. Springer, pp. 177–191, 2013) in the chapter a survey is performed regarding the requirements of space robotics for companies that are or will be prepared to become European suppliers in the next space era. Some of the major milestones in space exploration are illustrated in the first part of the chapter, followed by the expertise and capacity of our research center. The training aspects are becoming secondary elements as adapted training facility dictated by the company necessities. Therefore the applications are oriented on the service robots point of view, for testing technical devices, simulating biological experiments in extreme conditions, and as a facilitator of versatile and ergonomic "partner" in aerospace logistics.

Keywords Parallel kinematics · Stewart-Gough platform · Mechanical motion simulation · Aerospace applications and training

A. Pisla (✉) · C. Vaida
Technical University of Cluj-Napoca, Cluj-Napoca, Romania
e-mail: Adrian.Pisla@muri.utcluj.ro

C. Vaida
e-mail: Calin.Vaida@mep.utcluj.ro

A. Rodić et al. (eds.), *New Trends in Medical and Service Robots*,
Mechanisms and Machine Science 20, DOI: 10.1007/978-3-319-05431-5_25,

1 Trends and Necessities

The human evolution is based on cycles. Every activity is concerned, planned and achieved based on a group of different cycles. The space activity is not much different, people looks at the stars for different reasons. Astronomy is one of the oldest natural sciences, having the origins in the same time with the appearances of religions and astrology that connects the gods and spirits with stars.

The "western astronomy" originated between Tigris and Euphrates in Mesopotamia (3500 BC), in Babylon existing a stars catalogue at about 1200 BC and they used sexagesimal as base of numeration, transposed in our days in the 360° of a circle division by the Chalendas, naming the astronomers. Their tools are very precious until our days: the clock (time sharing) and the geometry (path definition) that leads us to the cycles in time and space (http://en.wikipedia.org/wiki/History_of_astronomy).

The modern space era could be considered to start around 1500 AD with Nicolaus Copernicus due to the heliocentric theory mathematically demonstrated (with geometrical instruments developed since the time of Ptolemy).

The next great discoveries are achieved around 1600 by great scientists like Galileo Galilei (that also developed an ×20 refractor telescope) and Johaness Keppler as mathematician in Graz, Austria and assistant of the Danish Tycho Brache. The works of Johannes Keppler is continued by Sir Isaac Newton, that together with the infinitesimal mathematics elevate the doubts about the Keppler heliocentric theory (1700 AD).

The 1750s focuses more on the conquest of the oceans but space benefits from Thomas Wright's theory that the Milky Way Galaxy is a disk-shape system. In the same time Leonhard Euler develops the Euler-Bernoulli beam-equation that leads to the plate theory and the finite elements analysis used nowadays.

1801 AD marks the discovery of the minor planets (the asteroids) that leads to a large observation network and researches in avoiding the collision with the planet Earth (in 2012 the Dawn unmanned orbiting spacecraft left the asteroid Vesta (http://en.wikipedia.org/wiki/4_Vesta), but will explore the Ceres from 2015. In 1850 3 astronomical objects are discovered (Fig. 1): Parthenope (a main belt asteroid), Victoria (a large main belt) and Egeria (a main-belt G-Type asteroid like Ceres) (Wiki 1800), marking the beginning of an era of exploration and discovery of astronomical objects.

The twentieth century is marked by smaller cycles within the aerospace activity and industry. In 1900, 12 new astronomical objects are discovered, 1903 Traian Vuia patented the first aeroplan-automobile, achieving the first self-propulsion flight with a machine heavier then the air, about which the Académie de Sciences de Paris mention: "*The problem of flight with a machine which weighs more than air cannot be solved and it is only a dream*" (http://www.ctie.monash.edu.au/hargrave/vuia.html). The 1957 marked several achievement within the Russian Space Programme, namely the successful launch of the first human made satellite Sputnik 1, followed by Sputnik 2 with the dog Laika on board.

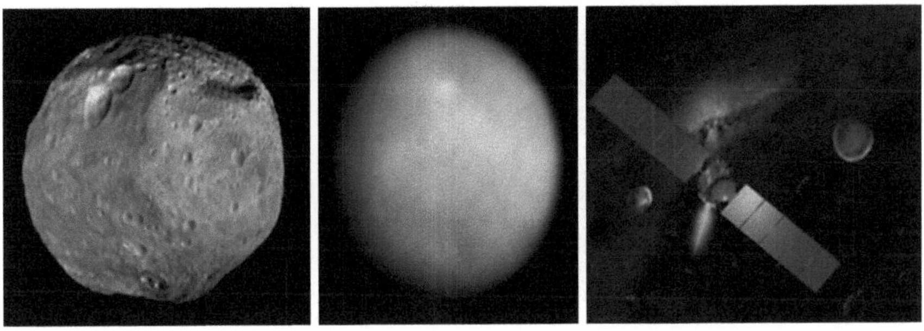

Fig. 1 From *left*, Ceres; Parthenope; Egeria and Victoria together with Dawn spacecraft

In 1958 the Americans launch their two first satellites Explorer 1 and Explorer 3 and took place the foundation of the National Aeronautics and Space Administration (NASA).

The next evolution was simply spectacular, marking many successful missions. 1961 is an important milestone in the space era marking the successful mission of the first man in outer space, the Russian Yuri Gagarin and the Vostok 1 mission followed by Alan Bartlet Shepard, the first American in outer space. Gus Grissom and Gherman Titov are the astronauts that follow their colleagues in the same very year.

Starting with 1970 we may talk about the successful space robotics, Luna 16 (Fig. 2) being the first robotic probe that landed on Moon and returned with soil probe on Earth.

Considering the cyclic activities, also in Robotics there are some milestones that mark the development cycles (http://heasarc.gsfc.nasa.gov/docs/heasarc/headates/1900.html):

- Osaka 1929, the first Japanese robot Gakutensoku ("Learning from the laws of nature"), an air actuated social robot that can change facial expression and move its hands and head;
- 1939 production of the remotely controlled teletank Shout-up TT26;
- 1954 the famous six-jack platform (parallel robot) was developed in UK by Gough and published in 1965 by D. Stewart.
- In 1968 Miomir Vukobratović introduced the Zero Moment Point for humanoid robots locomotion;
- 1970 the Lunokhod 1;
- 1973 Lunokhod 2;
- 1977 Voyager 1 and Voyager 2 space probes (Fig. 3);
- 1986 starts the humanoids series HONDA and the Navlab at Carnegie Mellon University, semi-autonomous vehicle, starting with top speed of 32 km/h, and a few years later ending with 110 km/h;
- 1993 starts the HONDA P series, humanoid robots;

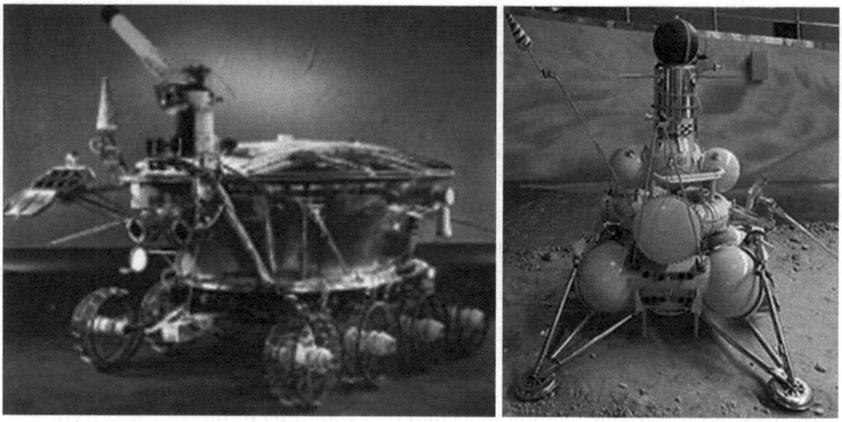

Fig. 2 The initial and the last version of the Russian moon space robot in the '70 (http://en.wikipedia.org/wiki/File:Lunokhod_1_(high_resolution).jpg)

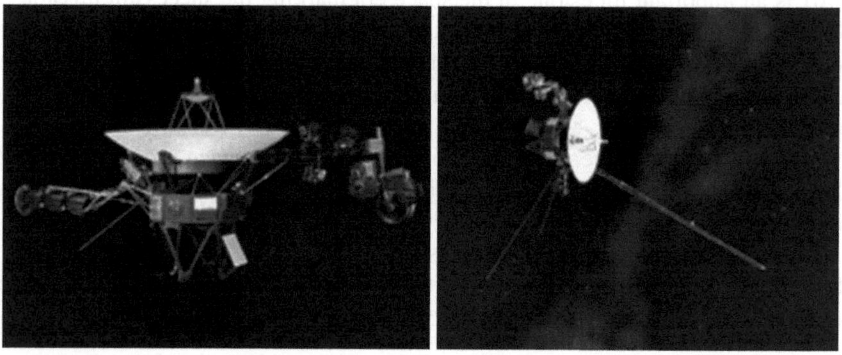

Fig. 3 Voyager 1 and Voyager 2 space probes (http://en.wikipedia.org/wiki/Voyager_1)

- 1996 the launch of the Mars Rover Pathfinder (Mars Pathfinder Mission: Rover Sojourner 2007);
- 1997 Carnegie Mellon University developed the Nomad Rover (Fig. 4);
- 2000 appears ASIMO by HONDA;
- 2001 MSS (Mobile Servicing System) Canadarm 2;
- 2002 at NASA Johnson Space Center (JSC) the Robonaut 2 (Fig. 5).

In 2004 a new series of Mars rover is launched: Opportunity and Spirit (Mars Pathfinder Mission: Rover Sojourner 2007; http://marsrovers.jpl.nasa.gov/home/index.html). Phoenix spacecraft. Dextre (2007) a two arms teleoperated robot part of the MSS Canadarm 2 (Fig. 6).

A new program for MARS started in 2011, with the Mars Rover Curiosity, leading to the design of the largest rover (http://marsrovers.jpl.nasa.gov/home/index.html;

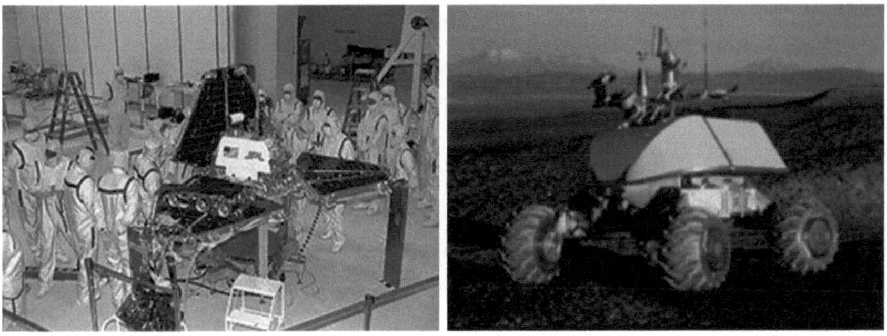

Fig. 4 The Mars Rover Pathfinder and the Nomad Rover (Chan et al. 2005)

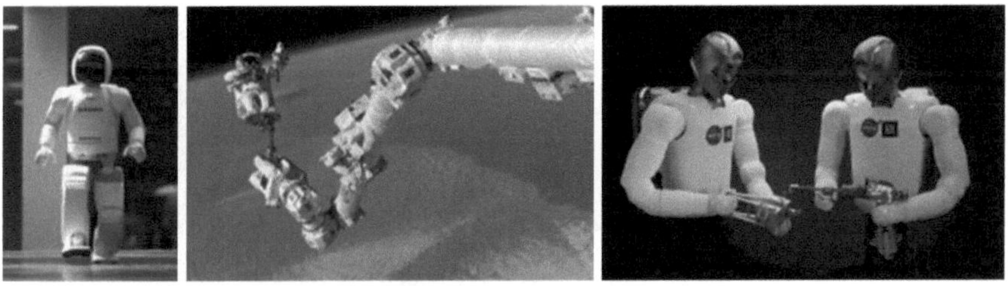

Fig. 5 The ASIMO; Canadarm 2; Robonaut 2

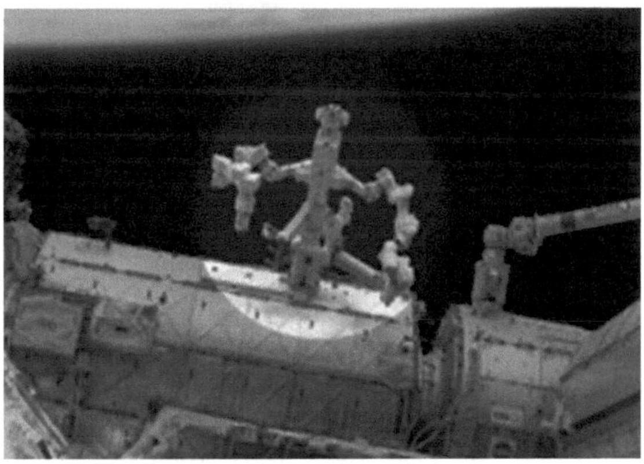

Fig. 6 The DEXTRE robot on the ISS

http://www.plm.automation.siemens.com/en_us/campaigns/mars-curiosity-rover/) (Fig. 7), intended to perform complex missions to investigate the Martian climate, geology, to assess the environmental conditions for microbial life and some preliminary studies for future human exploration (Figs. 8, 9).

We may conclude with the European Robot Arm (ERA) in 2011, the first robot arm able to be attached and work on to the Russian Segment of ISS to supplement the two Russian Strela cargo cranes, Fig. 10.

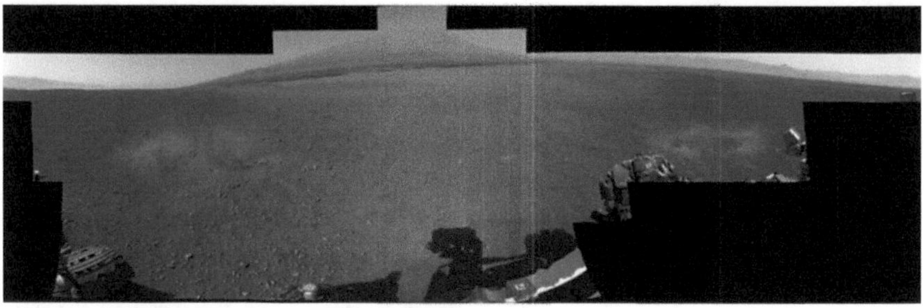

Fig. 7 The Curiosity first 360 degrees panorama image on Mars

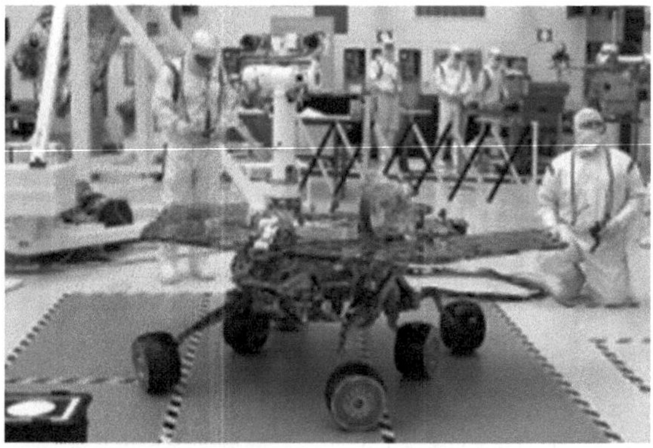

Fig. 8 The Opportunity Mars Rover

The ERA is designed and assembled by Dutch Space, EADS Company N.V, a global pan-European aerospace and defense corporation. The evolution of the Mars rovers is illustrated in Fig. 11 (http://marsrovers.jpl.nasa.gov/home/index.html).

The presented evolution has encouraged the setup of a Space Community, aspects totally confirmed within the discussions held with Mr. Claude Nicollier, at the Festival Robotique, in Lausanne, in April 2013 (https://festivalrobotique.epfl.ch/), spationaute by ESA (European Space Agency) and the first Swiss person in space with mission STS-46 in 1992. After he was selected by ESA in 1978, he joined the NASA group in 1980. It is very important to mention that Mr. Nicollier was 4 times in space 1992, 1993, 1996 and 1999, not only using space robots (namely Canadarm) but also participating at the elaboration of the HMI (Human Machine Interface), being a multiple licensed pilot, he also graduated in physical sciences within the Lausanne University.

At almost 60 years since the dawning of the space age, human behavior related to space exploration is still under construction. In (http://www.thespacereview.com/article/424/1) Jim Pass, Ph.D., lecturer in sociology at Long Beach City College, California and founder of Astrosociology.com, mentioned that "the overall approach from the "soft" scientists (social sciences) and the "hard"

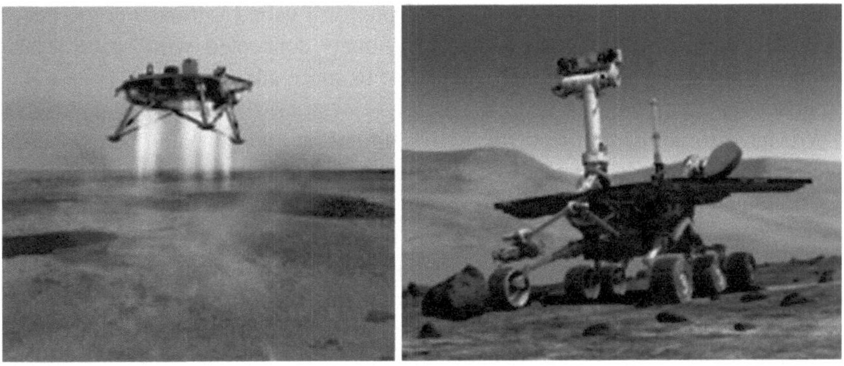

Fig. 9 The Opportunity Mars Rover, activity simulation

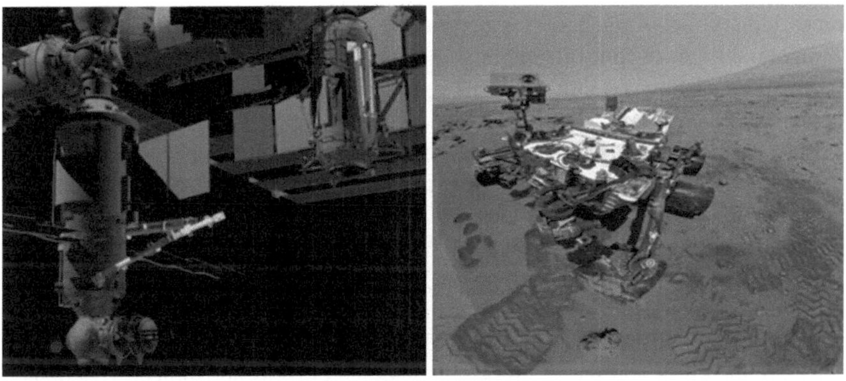

Fig. 10 The ERA Robot Arm and the Curiosity Mars Rover

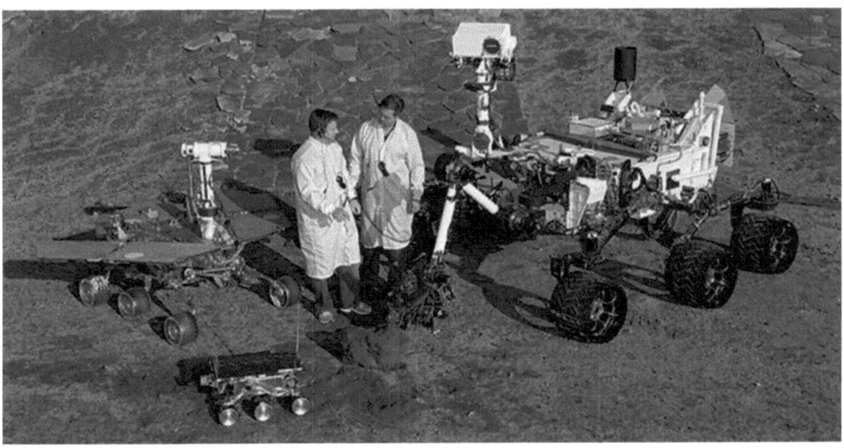

Fig. 11 Testing the three Mars Rovers

scientists (engineering) can be made on a platform called astrosociology, generating a structured space community, individuals connected with space related matters, from space scientists and engineers, to space advocates and space policy experts".

We have to admit the need for study cultural and social patterns and human interaction related to outer space ("an undiscovered asteroid will lead to no social reaction but an imminent collision with the Earth define a social chain reaction for taking measures").

Why should engineers or space scientist care about the social sciences as long as, in the space age, the most of the developments are made without them?

Jim Pass mentioned that the "behavioral patterns will interact to produce a particular quantity of social change once increasing the space exploration and becomes more essential to meeting social needs and solving social problems".

Currently the Outer space represents the low Earth orbit and we still mange a primitive, unreliable technology as the space tragedies demonstrate. But the social forces already acts, much of the aeronautics research are directly applicable to commercial flight or spin-offs applicable including medicine, materials processing, weather forecasting, communications applications that all together leads to different social behavior.

Like in medicine robotics, also in outer space applications is a vacuum of legislation, responsibility designation and implications control. The unknown qualities of space exploration demand maximum research and understanding, demanding collaboration not isolation (Wilcox et al. 2006).

Beyond Mars, human spaceflight will require more reliable spacecrafts. Engineers may design reliable habitats but they cannot design communities they need help for the establishment of space settlements in the future. The first people in space are the elites and the wealthy. The average citizens are subject to denials of the privilege of space travel.

As technology develops, societies must open space to the average person. In this context, space community refers to space settlements rather than the social network of space professionals.

Social/behavioral scientists are directly involved in planning space missions involving human and robotic spaceflight. The isolated space communities will need to be self-sustaining in all of their dimensions; social problems that will inevitably occur comprise a critical concern even while the physical environment continues to operate properly.

One of the first elements that demonstrate de social dimension of the space community is the new trends in development of the Airports area. Any development includes a technological and a social dimension creating a sort of Airport City (http://www.adp-i.com/index_en.html) (Fig. 12).

The Airport technology implies a wide range of facilities (Berbecar and Pisla 2009) from the one destined to light airplanes to the transcontinental ones. In the same time the new trends are including more robotics, taking into consideration he technology available to establish the safety, economical and environment friendly

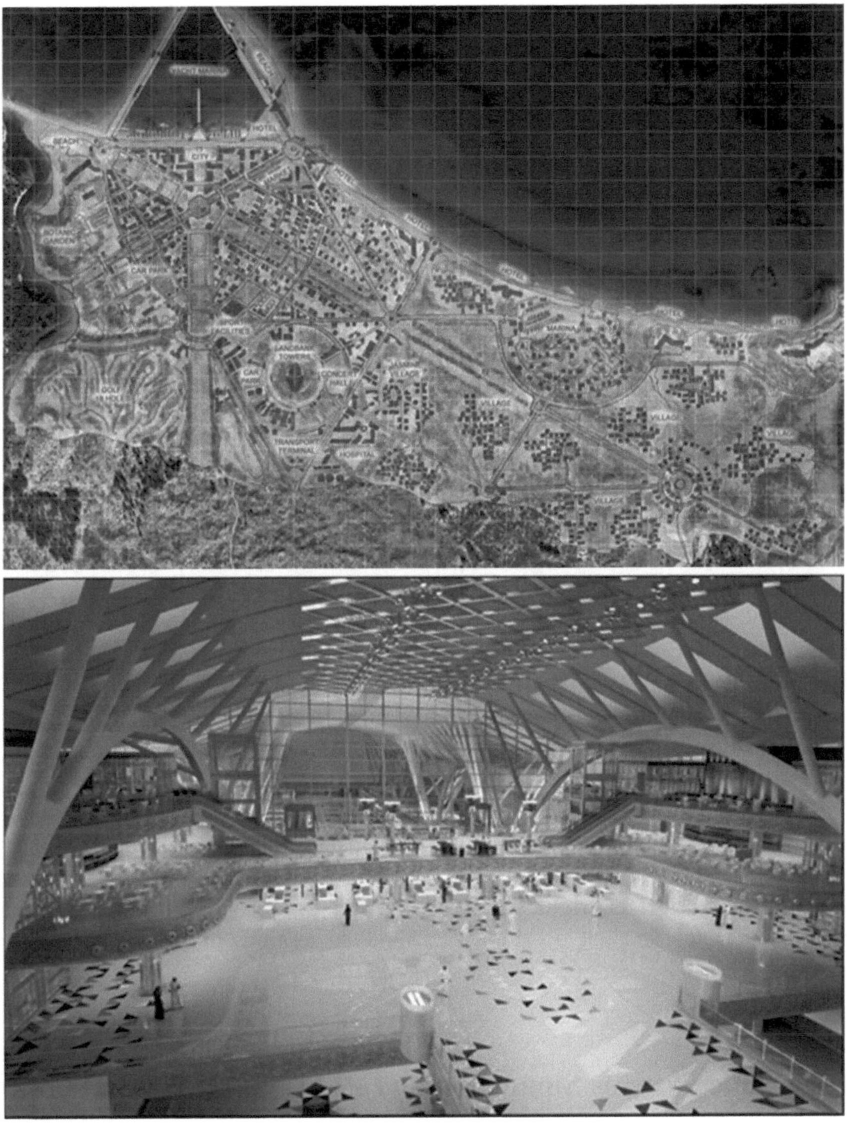

Fig. 12 Airport City perspectives

Personal Air Transportation System (PATS), that will increase the number of aircrafts and the number of pilots that must be trained and retrained.

The future is here considering that the *National Aeronautics and Space Administration* (NASA) has initiated already a project called “Small Aircraft Transportation System” (SATS), focused on the new aircraft design, airports development and economical foundation of the project.

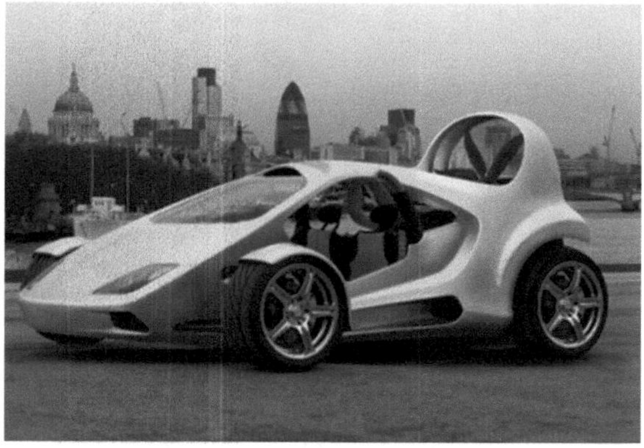

Fig. 13 Flying Car (http://news.kuwaittimes.net/2012/04/03/flying-car-gets-closer-to-reality-with-test-flight/)

With such desire the private industry is not far seeing a lot o opportunities in this area from building and service facilities to manufacturing and aircraft developments (PCSI) private commercial space industry.

The most spectacular example is SpaceX—Space Exploration technologies that "delivers outer space at bargain rates" (SpaceX 2012–2013; http://en.wikipedia.org/wiki/Voyager_1), providing infrastructure for low cost launch vehicles, due to the plans to reduce the launch cost by factor 10. But also lot of other applications like: GPS developments, tracking systems, car rentals, trains and combine communications, satellite surveillance, video monitoring, flight schools, wireless communication, airspace medicine, space travel, microgravity manufacturing and processing, space robotics and flying cars (Fig. 13).

Regardless the type of business each company requires a logistic system and a supply chain together with the supply chain management. Moreover to be successful in the space era it is to consider the PLM (Product Lifecycle Management) solutions that offer the right CAD/CAM/CAE/PDM tools doubled by a user friendly interface and the possibility to simulate motions and the dynamics of process.

2 Dynamic Systems Simulation and PLM

The engineering evolution can be extended to the management control by using specialized modules, repository for all documentation related to the design and the manufacture process specifications, with the ability to associate Word documents or a machine CNC programs with the corresponding parts, managing the lifecycle.

The service robots for the outer space are meant to work as standalone systems or assisting the astronauts. The next techno-economical demand is for "Space Technology Suppliers", capable to handle from prototypes to large series of manufacturing facilities, materials selection and processing, tooling, robots design

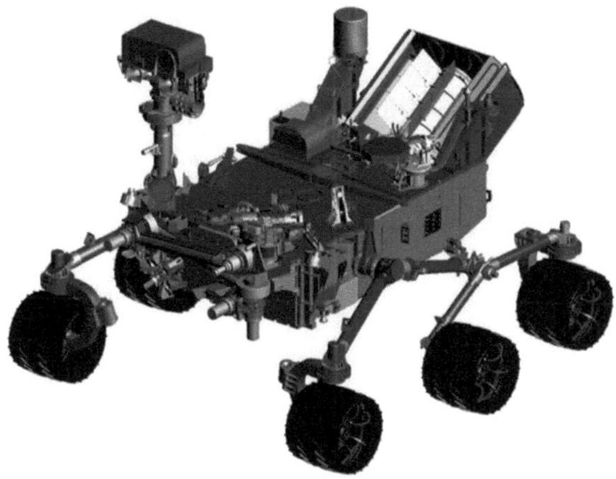

Fig. 14 Mars Rover designed with NX, courtesy of Siemens PLM

and control, development of the Man Machines Interfaces and the entire logistic chain much larger than the actual systems used in automotive or aviation industry.

In the same time the STS—space technology suppliers just appears but they will have to face the some problems Time and Money. The space age evolution demonstrates the cyclic evolution but also that the inner cycles are shorter and shorter, the time limits of a cycle being shortening by the amount of products and knowledge that must be delivered.

In this contest the adequate instruments make the difference, but without trained people are useless. Robots are replacing people but only by having highly skilled people behind. In this contest we combined to structures: one for training (the Authorized Training Center Siemens PLM); and the research and demonstration facility DSS (Dynamic Systems Simulation) laboratory. The first provide the instruments and the next researchers selection, the second testing facility.

CAD NX solutions, it is little to demonstrate as long as we may present a product designed with, namely the Curiosity rover (http://www.plm.automation.siemens.com/en_us/campaigns/mars-curiosity-rover/; http://www.maxonmotor.com/maxon/view/news/MEDIENMITTEILUNG-CURIOSITY), Fig. 14.

Siemens PLM CAD/CAM NX Team Center solutions are the most performant applications in aerospace industry.

NX-CAM, 5 CNC axes manufacturing management (Fig. 15).

FEA and NX Simulation solutions.

PDM NX MATLAB Simulation and Analysis (Fig. 16).

The Siemens PLM solution integrates a comprehensive set of tools that cover a large range of simulation tasks on different industrial area. Multi-body dynamics is compulsory for outer space robotics.

Flexible body dynamics can be implemented in assembly simulations allowing both rigid and flexible bodies to be combined in a single NX Motion simulation. A dynamic link can be created between NX Motion and MATLAB/Simulink, allowing to pass data in order to create a more accurate simulation.

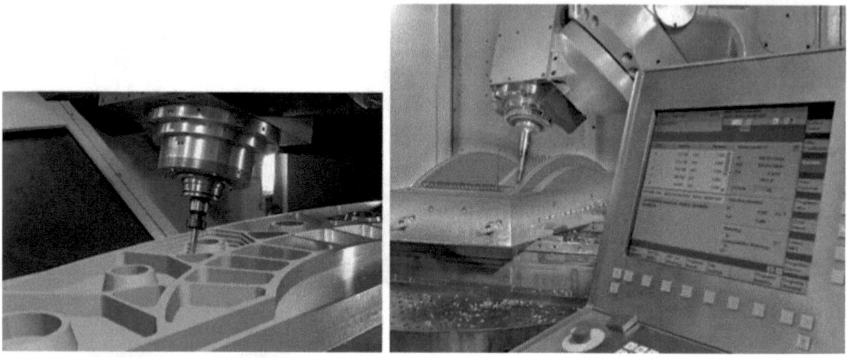

Fig. 15 Aluminum and special alloys manufacturing processes

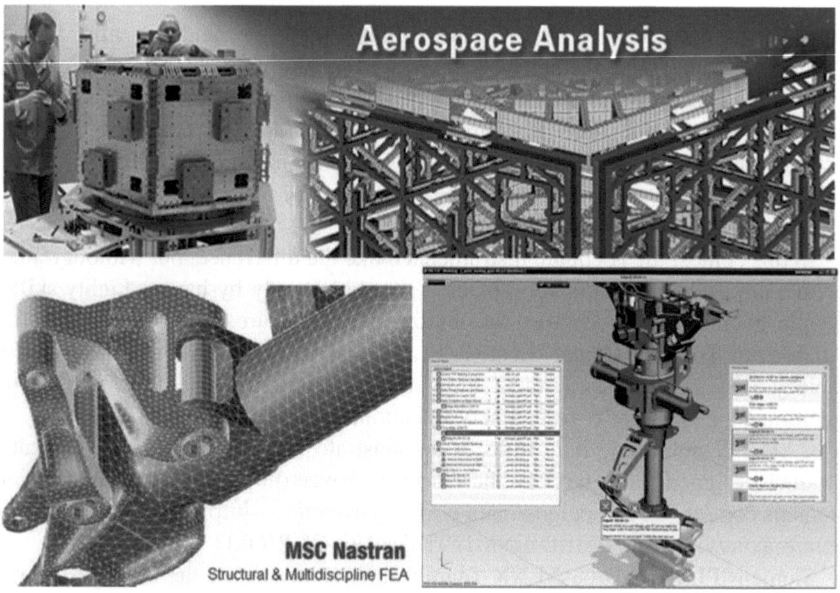

Fig. 16 Simulation and Analysis solutions from Siemens PLM

A forecasted activity is the combination between the digital environment analysis and the real tests. Starting with planning testing processes (measurement points, sensor settings, calibration process, testing scenario etc.) then using the physical test as feedback.

The digital-physical experimentation leads to better understanding of the process, more reliable results and reduce the number of physical tests, providing greater ability for tuning the simulation process.

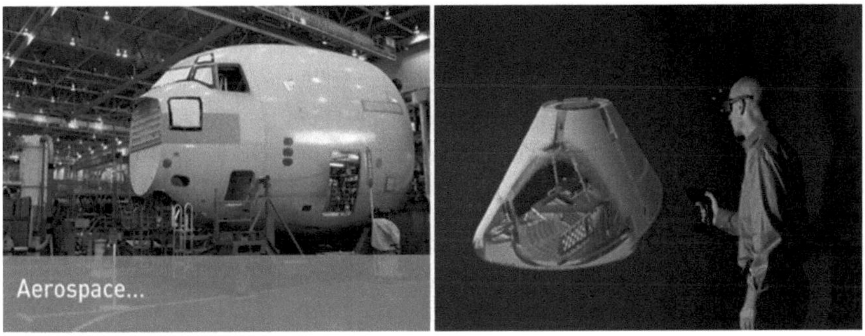

Fig. 17 An aerospace simulator

Within Siemens PLM the Synchronous Technology (ST) can pay huge dividends for the end user. Engineering and Management going hand in hand for the final product. Combined with the lightweight JT viewing techniques, NX allows the work with incredibly large datasets quickly and efficiently.

For the flows data management the Team Center module is doing what SAP can't manage at such a large number of simultaneous users.

It is not just a vision but NX actually fulfils to support an entire industry workflow, within a single system, while Siemens continues to increase the depth of functionality and HD3D bring clarity and richness to the often overwhelmingly complex and cryptic data in the data management system (Fig. 17).

The DSS (Dynamic Systems Simulation) laboratory is built up around a customized Stewart-Gough platform, starting from the idea to extend the parallel kinematics applications structural kinematical and dynamical research for open flying simulation system tailored to special demands.

3 STS Service Robots

Considering that the new set of activities will be oriented on outer space service robots, within (DSS), the actual Helicopter Mechanical Simulator (HMS) will be redesigned and oriented versus outer space to induce simulated shocks and controlled acceleration. The 3D and 6DOF may simulate non gravitational conditions in different environments and in contact with different other type of objects.

These facilities can be used for the robots control, devices behavior research and human operator training by generating the required simulated environment from the point of view of images, shocks, and vibration, temperature, communication and control panels, simulated in parallel as long as the outer service robots are defined, how we like to cote Mr. Kazuya YOSHIDA, from the Department of Aerospace Engineering, Tohoku University, Japan:

> Outer space service robotics is considered the ultimate field for the application of robotics technology due to the harsh environment, extreme temperatures, different gravity, vacuum conditions, high radiations and remote distance from Earth.

This may give unlimited opportunities to see HMS as a reference module for carrier service, device testing, MMI development, or as tool development facilitator, not mentioning the placement on rover systems. The approach starts from the already defined space robotics chapters. Therefore is to be reiterating this chapters and their content:

Orbital Robotics

Kinematics and Dynamics modeling of the in-floating robots
Coupling and contact dynamics
Remote control and teleoperated systems
TP (Tasks and Path) Lifecycle Management.

Intelligent Man Machine Interface IMMI

Command Ergonomics
Simulation and Training for transmission delay coordination
Haptic systems
Shared-Delegation and Hierarchy control (CDC—Compliant Dynamic Control).

Planetary robotics

Rover, service systems
Parallel kinematics in planetary exploration
Robotized manufacturing capacities
Robotized energetic and biological facilities.

A direction of studies that is continuing some previous activities and falls with success in all three chapters is considered to be the one oriented on applications of the parallel robots within low forces development systems.

This direction of activity is split in three branches of research, the evolution and the allocated resources depending on the number of researchers that can be involved.

The mentioned sub branches are:

- Coupling and contact dynamics
- Remote control and teleoperated systems, from the Orbital Robotics chapter and
- Shared-Delegation and Hierarchy control (CDC—Compliant Dynamic Control), from the Intelligent Man Machine Interface.

Within the outer space applications, the different gravity conditions define practically the implied processes as "Low forces processes"-LFP, characterized mainly by three elements: the considered process forces, resulting only from the manipulation; the process technology that implies a lot of wires, tubes and cables, that must be carried allover; the tool orientation and critical constant distance to the processed surface.

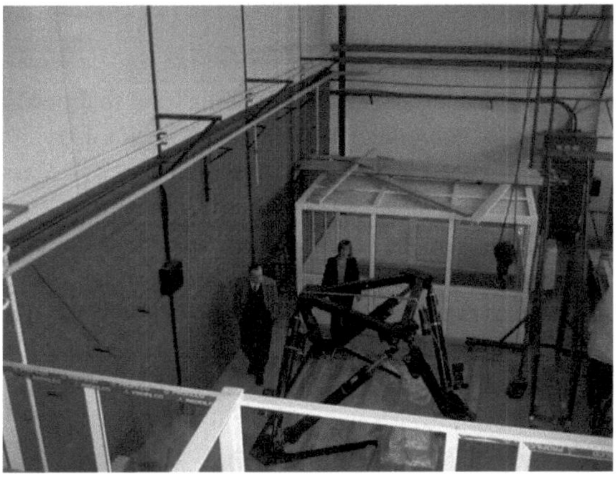

Fig. 18 The DSS laboratory development, TU Cluj-Napoca

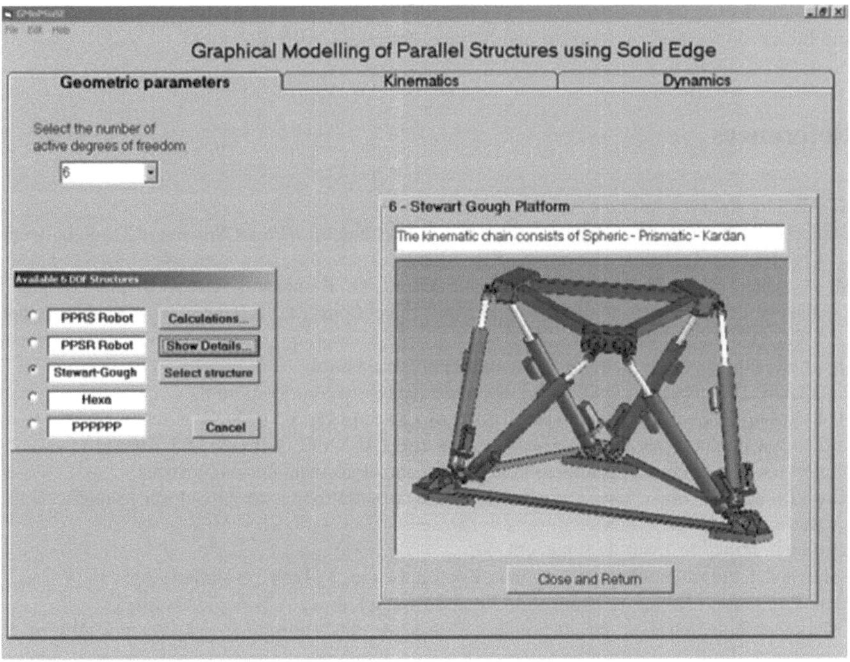

Fig. 19 The simulation control interface for the HMS applications

The mentioned elements are very important for the control, in managing the tasks together with the dynamic model but also from the singularities point of view (a delicate matter within parallel robots). Therefore a parallel system one for the SG-platform (Fig. 18) and another for the application (Fig. 19) are developed.

4 Conclusions

The chapter represents a survey intended to demonstrate that new space age starts with new requirements for manufactures (the space technology suppliers—STS). The DSS Laboratory evolution and trends have the capacity to assist them.

The human resources formation, expertise and consulting, availability of the right tools and know-how must be used within this type of activity.

Creating an independent research platform could be an advantage in combining the theory with practice in the same time the possibility to reveal the large number of opportunities for those that would like to enter into the space robotics area.

The existing software and hardware facilities, pertinent analysis, simulation and development tools will lead towards new, efficient and reliable solutions to comply with the ever new challenges in the exploration of space.

Acknowledgments This work was supported by a grant of the Romanian National Authority for Scientific Research, Programme for research—Space Technology and Advanced Research—STAR, project number 95 entitled "Instructor Operation Station designed for space applications" and by the Scopes International Grant IZ74Z0_137361/1 entitled "Creative Alliance in Research and Education focused on Medical and Service Robotics CARE-Robotics".

References

ADAP, http://www.adp-i.com/index_en.html;

Berbecar, F., Pisla, A.: Constructive Elements in Building up a Flight Simulator, Diploma work, Cluj-Napoca Technical University, 81p. (2009);

M. A. Chan, B. B. Bowen, W.T. Parry, J. Ormo, G. Komatsu, "Red rock and red planet diagenesis: Comparisons of Earth and Mars concretions", GSA Today, Vol. 15, No. 8, doi: 10.1130/1052-5173(2005)015, 2005.

Hargrave, http://www.ctie.monash.edu.au/hargrave/vuia.html;

HEASARC, http://heasarc.gsfc.nasa.gov/docs/heasarc/headates/1900.html;

History, http://en.wikipedia.org/wiki/History_of_astronomy;

http://www.maxonmotor.com/maxon/view/news/MEDIENMITTEILUNG-CURIOSITY;

http://www.plm.automation.siemens.com/en_us/campaigns/mars-curiosity-rover/;

Kuwait times net, http://news.kuwaittimes.net/2012/04/03/flying-car-gets-closer-to-reality-with-test-flight/;

Lausanne, https://festivalrobotique.epfl.ch/;

Lunokhod 1, http://en.wikipedia.org/wiki/File:Lunokhod_1_(high_resolution).jpg;

Mars Exploration Rover Missions, http://marsrovers.jpl.nasa.gov/home/index.html;

"Mars Pathfinder Mission: Rover Sojourner", NASA, 2007, http://mars.jpl.nasa.gov/MPF/rover/sojourner.html;

Pisla, A.: On Medical and Service Robots with Compliant Dynamic Control, New Trends in Medical and Service Robots – Theory and Integrated Applications, pp. 177-191, Springer, (2013);

Space Review, http://www.thespacereview.com/article/424/1;

SpaceX, Case study 2012–2013;

Voyager, http://en.wikipedia.org/wiki/Voyager_1;

Wiki 1800, http://en.wikipedia.org/wiki/Category:Astronomical_objects_discovered_in_1880;

Wiki Vesta, http://en.wikipedia.org/wiki/4_Vesta;

B. Wilcox, R. Ambrose, V. Kumar, "Assessment of International Research and Development in Robotics - SPACE ROBOTICS", 2006, http://www.wtec.org/robotics/;

MIX
Papier aus verantwortungsvollen Quellen
Paper from responsible sources
FSC® C105338
FSC
www.fsc.org

If you have any concerns about our products,
you can contact us on
ProductSafety@springernature.com

In case Publisher is established outside the EU,
the EU authorized representative is:
Springer Nature Customer Service Center GmbH
Europaplatz 3, 69115 Heidelberg, Germany

Printed by Libri Plureos GmbH
in Hamburg, Germany